NEUROSCIENCE FOR THE MENTAL HEALTH CLINICIAN

NEUROSCIENCE
FOR THE
MENTAL HEALTH
CLINICIAN

STEVEN R. PLISZKA

THE GUILFORD PRESS
New York   London

© 2003 The Guilford Press
A Division of Guilford Publications, Inc.
72 Spring Street, New York, NY 10012
www.guilford.com

Printed in the United States of America

This book is printed on acid-free paper.

Last digit is print number: 9 8 7 6 5 4 3 2 1

Library of Congress Cataloging-in-Publication Data

Pliszka, Steven R.
    Neuroscience for the mental health clinician / Steven R. Pliszka.
        p. cm.
Includes bibliographical references and index.
    ISBN 1-57230-811-7
    1. Neurosciences. I. Title.
RC341.P58 2002
616.89—dc21

2002012525

To my wife, Alice, and my son, Andrew, in gratitude for their patience and love. This book is also dedicated to the residents of the Division of Child and Adolescent Psychiatry at the University of Texas Health Science Center at San Antonio, whose hard work and eagerness to learn have been a major inspiration for this book.

About the Author

Steven R. Pliszka, MD, is Associate Professor and Chief of the Division of Child and Adolescent Psychiatry at the University of Texas Health Science Center at San Antonio. He was the recipient of a Career Development Award from the National Institute of Mental Health (NIMH) and currently has an NIMH grant to study attention-deficit/hyperactivity disorder using neuroimaging techniques. He has a very active clinical practice and teaches neurobiology to the Child and Adolescent Psychiatry residents. He lives in San Antonio with his wife, Alice, and son, Andrew.

Contents

1

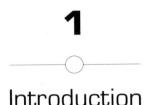

Introduction

WHY ANOTHER BOOK ON NEUROSCIENCE?

There are literally hundreds of books on the brain, so why should a mental health clinician read this one? Current books in the field of neuroscience fall into a number of areas, usually directed at specific audiences. There are textbooks of neuroanatomy that describe the physical structure of the brain. Neurochemistry or pharmacology texts give the chemical structures of the many neurotransmitters in the brain and describe the multitude of drugs that affect these transmitters. Psychopharmacology books give physicians "nuts-and-bolts" information about marketed pharmaceuticals in terms of their indications, dosages, and side effects. Physiological psychology textbooks aimed at graduate students focus on laboratory techniques and animal research. What appears to be missing is a book that can integrate the recent research on neurobiology for the practicing mental health clinician. This is true even for psychiatrists, despite their exposure to neuroscience and neuroanatomy in medical school. By the time psychiatrists finish residency, they often find that what they learned in neurology does not transfer well to the treatment of mental disorders. Clinical neurology focuses on strokes, epilepsy, and degenerative diseases of the brain that can have psychiatric sequelae, but even most psychiatrists do not encounter these disorders in their daily practice. What is of more interest to psychiatrists, and, I suggest, to the broader group of mental health practitioners is a book outlining the neurobiology of the disorders we see every day: depression, mania, anxiety, personality disorder, and attention-deficit/hyperactivity disorder (ADHD).

1

Take, for example, the fact that medications such as fluoxetine (Prozac) or sertraline (Zoloft) are effective in the treatment of major depressive disorder (MDD). These drugs are selective serotonin reuptake inhibitors (SSRIs), meaning that, at least acutely, they increase the amount of serotonin available to the neurons. But in this sentence are embedded a whole series of questions. Where exactly in the brain does serotonin reside? What role does it play in normal mood and behavior? What role, if any, does it play in the development of affective disorder? How does perturbing serotonin with medication improve depression? Finally, if serotonin is a critical link in treatment of depression, why are other agents that have no effect on serotonin also effective treatments for affective disorder? These are the sorts of questions this book seeks to answer about the many brain systems involved in mental disorders.

WHO SHOULD READ THIS BOOK?

This book is aimed primarily at practicing mental health clinicians (psychiatrists, psychologists, social workers, counselors, neurologists, developmental pediatricians) who are interested in how advances in neurobiology will ultimately lead to new treatments and social policies. This audience would include residents and interns in all these professions, as well as medical students in clinical psychiatry courses or rotations. It also should be highly useful as an introductory textbook for graduate students or upper-division undergraduates who seek a more clinically focused treatment of neurobiology. Many advanced neuroscience textbooks can be quite daunting in terms of their size and complexity. I think many students will find that this book can help them get their bearings before they move on to more advanced material. I assume knowledge of the *Diagnostic and Statistical Manual of Mental Disorders* (DSM-IV) classification of mental disorders, as well as college-level biology.

NEUROSCIENCE ISSUES
FOR MENTAL HEALTH CLINICIANS

The role of neuroscience in mental health goes well beyond the prescription of medication for specific mental disorders. The development of new techniques in genetics and brain imaging have the potential to significantly change our views of mental illnesses and, indeed, our view of the human condition itself. For some, this is a worrisome prospect: They are concerned that emphasizing the role of biology in mental illness will lead to a "reductionistic" view of mental illness, that complex mental disorders will be attributed to a single cause with medication as the only treatment. As this book shows, this reductionism is not the goal of clinical neuroscience. To place these issues in perspective, I give an overview of the history of the study of mental disorders germane to this issue.

EARLY DEVELOPMENTS

For hundreds of years, the severely mentally ill were cared for in asylums, where many were brutally treated. At the St. Mary of Bethlehem Hospital in London, patients were often displayed for the entertainment of the public. It is from this institution that the word "bedlam" acquired its popular meaning as a "place of uproar." Most modern people would profess to be horrified by the thought of going to see mental patients for entertainment, but let us not be too smug. Recently in a major city I noticed a man on the street, wearing a billboard that said, "America awake, Vice President Gore's body has been taken over by aliens." The man carried a bullhorn, with which he broadcast his warnings to all who passed by. The man probably suffered from bipolar disorder, but as people walked past they laughed and pointed. Admittedly, the man's behavior was funny—until you reflected that he was someone's son or spouse. That day, the people on the street of 21st century America were little different from the crowds at "Bedlam" in the 1400s.

Throughout the 17th and 18th centuries, however, there were movements to provide more humane care for persons in hospitals. The most notable of these was the "moral therapy" movement began by Philippe Pinel, who in 1795 ordered mentally ill inmates at the Paris hospital Salpêtrière released from chains. "Moral treatment" dominated psychiatry in the early part of the 19th century. In 1830 the British physician John Conolly started a movement to abolish mechanical restraints of patients; in 1841 limiting the use of restraint became the official policy of the Association of Medical Officers of Hospitals for the Insane (now the Royal College of Psychiatrists). Debates about how to deal with violent behavior in mental patients remain intense in our own time. During the 1800s the first debates began as to whether the causes of mental illness were primarily biological or psychological. In Germany, Johann Reil published *Rhapsodies about the Application of Psychotherapy to Mental Disturbances* (1803), which emphasized psychological factors, whereas in 1845 Wilhelm Griesinger wrote that mental diseases were brain diseases. As professor of psychiatry and neurology in Berlin, he had wide influence on European psychiatry. The discovery by Paul Broca and Carl Wernicke of specific brain lesions that caused speech and language deficits reinforced the view that disturbed behavior could be related to brain dysfunction. At this point, biological psychiatry entered a phase that led to great advancements on the one hand and tragedy on the other.

At the turn of the 20th century, Emil Kraepelin divided "insanity" into manic–depressive illness and "dementia praecox" (schizophrenia). In 1906 Alois Alzheimer discovered the relationship between early-onset dementia and a pathological lesion in the brain; this disorder now bears his name. At the turn of the 20th century, Ladislas von Meduna noted that convulsions reduced symptoms in schizophrenia; two Italian psychiatrists, Ugo Cerletti and Lucio Bini, developed a means of inducing convulsions by electroshock. Electroconvulsive therapy (ECT) proved highly effective for psychosis, particularly for affective disorder. Before antidepressants and antipsychotics were developed, ECT was the mainstay for treating these disorders. It remains a highly effective option for some patients today, despite the negative views that some lay people hold of it. At the turn of the 20th century, there was great optimism that the brain mechanisms underlying mental disorders would soon be unraveled.

THE PROBLEM OF EUGENICS

There were, however, other trends in biological psychiatry that were not so positive. In the late 19th century the French psychiatrists Bénédict-Augustin Morel and Valentin Magnan proposed the "theory of degeneration." This theory held that all mental illnesses were genetic and that mental illness often worsened from one generation to the next. The same was felt to be true for many neurological illnesses, such as epilepsy. The theory took on an ominous note, as degeneration was thought to cluster among the "lower classes" who often belonged to racial or ethnic minorities. This theory was the justification for the widespread sterilization of mentally ill and retarded patients in the late 19th and early 20th centuries. The Italian psychiatrist Cesare Lombroso proposed that criminal behavior was also the result of "degeneracy" and could be predicted by the physical features of an individual. Lombroso is viewed as the father of criminology, but his views led to much pessimism about the possibility of rehabilitating criminals. Again, this debate is with us today. The theory of degeneration spawned the "eugenics" movement in the early 20th century. Kraepelin had noted that many cases of manic–depressive illness ran in families, and in 1917 he established a Genealogical and Demographic Department at the Kaiser Wilhelm Institute of Psychiatry in Munich to study how mental illnesses were transmitted in families. The head of this department, Ernst Rüdin, took over the Institute on

Kraepelin's death in 1926. Rüdin became infamous as the author of the "Law to Prevent Hereditarily Sick Offspring," enacted by the Nazis in 1933. Hundreds of thousands of people with physical handicaps or mental illnesses were forcibly sterilized and later murdered in the Holocaust. In the United States, eugenics gained some ground, with forced sterilization often being practiced in facilities for the mentally ill or retarded. After World War II, particularly when the crimes of the Nazis were exposed, the eugenics movement was rightly abandoned. Today, some critics of modern psychiatry point to these horrors as reasons that the study of genetic or brain-based mechanisms of mental illness should not go forward. The implication is that any study of the brain with regard to human behavior will inevitably place society on a "slippery slope" that leads to genocide. It is important to bear in mind, however, that the Holocaust was not the result of the Nazis "slipping" into mass murder. Hitler's intent to eradicate the Jews and others he deemed inferior was a deliberate policy for which the pseudoscience of eugenics was not a necessary prerequisite. Moreover, "eugenics" and the "theory of degeneration" were not supportable even by the science of the time—it was the departure from the scientific method that allowed the eugenics movement to spread. There is no parallel between the modern study of neurobiological factors in mental illness and the pseudoscientific views of Morel, Lombroso, and Rüdin; this becomes clear as the reader progresses through the chapters on specific mental disorders. It is critical for the sophisticated clinician to be able to articulate how our modern studies differ fundamentally from the pseudoscience of the past.

PSYCHOANALYSIS AND THE DECLINE OF BIOLOGICAL PSYCHIATRY

As pointed out by Samuel Barondes in his book *Mood Genes*, it was not just the excesses of the eugenics movement that led to the decline of the study of biological factors in mental illnesses. Biological factors became viewed as irrelevant to mental illness when psychoanalysis began to grow. At the end of the 19th century, neurologists used their expanding knowledge of the nervous system to associate specific neurological symptoms (e.g., paralysis) to lesions in the brain. Certain disturbances in behavior, however, could not be explained by neuroanatomy. Many people of the time suffered from what was called "neurasthenia"—a syndrome of tiredness, weakness, and somatic complaints (i.e., nonspecific aches and pains). The description of the disorder was quite similar to the modern disorders of chronic fatigue syndrome or fibromyalgia—conditions that today also defy medical understanding. Other patients, particularly women, suffered from hysteria—for instance, paralysis of a limb not related to a neurological lesion. The neurologist Jean-Martin Charcot found that these symptoms could be relieved by hypnosis. At this same time, Sigmund Freud was also using hypnosis to treat hysteria, but he developed a different technique, free association, that seemed just as effective in removing the symptoms. As patients talked in open-ended manner, they often reported dreams and memories of a sexual nature. Freud developed the theory that unconscious thoughts, particularly sexual ones about which the patient felt guilty, caused the hysteria. There is controversy among historians as to how Freud arrived at this conclusion. Freud had first developed a "theory of seduction," which stated that hysteria arose as a sequelae of sexual abuse during childhood. He presented this hypothesis to the Society for Psychiatry and Neurology in 1896. He presented 18 cases, but the audience rejected his reasoning; his lecture, Freud said, "had an icy reception from the donkeys." Critics of Freud suggested that he abandoned this seduction theory because it was poorly received by the medical community of the time. Allegedly, he then revised his theory to state that, between the ages of 3 and 5, all children had sexual feelings toward the parent of the opposite sex and that fixation in this "oedipal" stage led to neurosis. An alternative view has it that he encountered sexual fantasies of this sort in so many of his patients that he came to view actual sexual abuse as an improbable mechanism of neurosis. Thus he revised his theory, and neuroses were viewed as stemming from unconscious conflicts. Psychoanalysis was born.

The impact of Freud on 20th-century culture was profound. In the repressive atmosphere of the Victorian time, people were not expected to have any sexual feelings—this was especially true of women. Children were regularly beaten for masturbation or even wetting the bed. (See George Orwell's "Such, Such Were the Joys" for a chilling look at a childhood in the early 1900s). Hysteria was more common among women. It is reasonable to speculate that the highly restricted lifestyle women led—corsets, hours of domestic labor, lack of access to careers, complete domination by husbands or fathers—led to the high rates of hysteria noted at the time. Indeed, both men and women of the time were more likely to be more anxious ("neurotic") than we are today. Imagine the relief for so many of these individuals when they had the opportunity to talk to a doctor who did not condemn them for revealing thoughts of a forbidden nature.

Psychiatrists of the era viewed psychoanalysis as a major advance. Most of the treatment techniques of the time (ECT, lobotomy) were relevant only for severely ill patients in mental hospitals. These methods were of little use for the neurotic patient who came to the office (and could afford to pay for treatment). In 1909, Freud gave a series of lectures at Clark University in Worcester, Massachusetts, and took American psychiatry by storm. Indeed, psychoanalysis was embraced much more strongly in the United States than in Europe. The only other competing theory that addressed the development of personality was John Watson's behaviorism. Watson postulated that all behavior arose from the effects of conditioning; he speculated that any child could be conditioned to produce any sort of behavior. Yet Watson had little to say regarding mental illness; only Freud appeared to offer a treatment that was viewed as thoughtful and humane. Indeed, after World War II, psychoanalysis gained even more adherents among American psychiatrists. By this time, B. F. Skinner had further developed behaviorism, elucidating the principles of operant conditioning (which play a fundamental role in many modern psychological treatments, including behavior modification and cognitive therapy). Yet behavior modification, in the postwar years, was viewed by mental health professionals as authoritarian. Skinner himself reinforced this view by publishing two books (*Beyond Freedom and Dignity* and *Walden Two*) in which he stated that free will did not exist and that human beings were best governed by conditioning them to produce prosocial behaviors. Psychoanalysis seemed free of any coercion at all. The patient came to the office, talked freely to the analyst, and developed a relationship ("transference") with the analyst that replicated an earlier (parental) relationship. The transference could then be interpreted; with insight the patient's symptoms would remit.

There is no doubt that psychoanalysis helped many neurotic patients. Freudian psychology led to many changes in attitudes about child rearing. Benjamin Spock, the famous pediatrician, was heavily influenced by Freudian ideas; his child-care books led to more benevolent treatment of children (feeding on demand, more humane toilet training, healthier attitudes about sex). Other "interpersonal" psychotherapy techniques evolved from psychoanalysis, including family therapy and group therapy. In the period 1940–1970, many American psychoanalysts began to claim that all mental illnesses, including schizophrenia and manic–depressive illness, were caused by psychological conflicts that could be ameliorated through psychoanalytic psychotherapy. Often parents, mainly mothers, were blamed for their offsprings' mental disorders. Particularly cruel was the concept of the "schizophrenogenic mother," which proposed that schizophrenia was caused by the mother appearing to love but unconsciously rejecting the child. In a series of widely read books, Bruno Bettelheim theorized that autism was caused by parental rejection and that only a "parentectomy" (i.e., removing the child from the home) could lead to a cure. Those who champion the concept that mental illnesses have only "environmental" or "psychological" causes often feel that they are occupying the high moral ground—defending the patient against a deterministic biological theory. They often fail to notice that their own theories of mental illness, in the absence of proof, blame parents and families for a child's problem and thus cause enormous pain and suffering. It would be analogous to denying the biological nature of cancer and telling the parents of a child with leukemia that their failure to have a loving relationship with the child led to the illness. A generation of psychiatrists was taught nonsense. They spent hours listening to schizophrenic patients describe hallucinations and attempted to interpret them. Behavioral treatments were shunted aside as pointless because they treated only "symptoms" and did not get at "deeper conflicts." Psychiatry became divorced from medicine, and the medical knowledge of psychiatrists declined.

It is not, however, the intent of this book to bury Freud. In fact, I show that some of his ideas (albeit formulated in more precise language) may in fact be validated by neuroscience. It is clear that the brain does process information at an unconscious level, as shown in the action of the amygdala, a part of the brain critical to emotional response. Freud conceptualized the id, a part of the psyche that operated on the pleasure principle—that is, it drove the individual to seek gratification and was restrained by the ego and superego. In examining substance abuse, I examine a particular circuit in the brain that responds very strongly to cues in the environment associated with reward.

In the public mind, psychoanalysis is considered the prototypical psychotherapy. The "couch" and a therapist using a nondirective approach are what most people envision when they think of a psychiatrist, psychologist, or therapist. In this book, however, I draw from the rich body of research in clinical psychology, particularly neuropsychology. Within psychology many psychosocial factors, such as parent–child interactions, school environments, neighborhood factors, abuse, and neglect, have been extensively studied and shown to have a large role in the etiology of mental illness. Not everyone who is exposed to such stressors develops a mental illness, however, and two people exposed to the same trauma may develop very different illnesses. One of my goals is to examine how factors intrinsic to the brain (genetic or prenatal insults) interact with environmental factors. Another, equally important goal is to study how environmental factors change the brain—for instance, an enriched, stimulating environment may facilitate the development of dendritic branching in neurons. Already data exist, which I examine in Chapter 11, on the ways in which cognitive-behavior therapy may alter brain metabolism in patients with obsessive–compulsive disorder. Years before the development of neuroimaging techniques, neuropsychology developed methods of carefully measuring attention, memory, visual–spatial, language, and executive functioning (planning) skills. Use of such tests in patients who suffered damage to specific areas of the brain led to theories about the localization of such cognitive functions. Today, these tests can be used in healthy persons undergoing neuroimaging to see what areas of the brain are activated by different types of cognitive tasks. We can then see how patients with learning disabilities are different from controls in these brain regions. Clearly, the field of psychology is a critical partner in clinical neuroscience.

THE DEVELOPMENT OF PHARMACOLOGICAL APPROACHES TO PSYCHOPATHOLOGY

Biological psychiatry did not completely decline during the post-World War II years. Almost by accident, a revolution in the treatment of serious mental illness came about in the 1950s. Medications were discovered for the treatment of depression and psychosis. In the late 1940s the French surgeon Henri Laborit was seeking a drug that would be a more effective sedating agent for patients undergoing medical procedures. Paul Charpentier had synthesized chlorpromazine, which Laborit administered to patients, noticing its sedating properties. Thinking it would be a safer alternative than restraint for violent mentally ill patients, Laborit persuaded psychiatrists in Paris to administer it to severely psychotic patients. In 1952 Delay, Deniker, and Hart reported that not only did the drug sedate agitated patients but it also improved the patients' underlying psychosis. Reminiscent of Pinel two centuries earlier, restraints were removed from patients throughout the mental hospitals of Paris. Thorazine was discovered.

Tuberculosis was the scourge of the late 19th and early 20th centuries. Two drugs, iproniazid and isoniazid, were developed to combat them. While these drugs were undergoing trials, R. G. Bloch and colleagues reported in 1954 that about 20% of the patients developed symptoms very similar to mania. Intrigued, in 1958 Nathan Kline tried these drugs in severely depressed patients and found them to be highly effective in improving mood. It was soon noted that these drugs inhibited monoamine oxidase, an enzyme that breaks down norepinephrine, serotonin, and dopamine, three brain neurotransmitters that play a critical role in modulating behavior. Also in 1958, the drug imipramine was noted to be very similar in structure to chlorpromazine and thus underwent trials for the treatment of psychosis. It did not work for psychosis, but depressed patients were found to benefit greatly. R. Kuhn showed imipramine to be effective for the treatment of depression, and a whole class of tricyclic antidepressants was later developed. Like the mono-amine oxidase inhibitors, these drugs were found to affect norepin-ephrine and serotonin, a fact that stimulated much research in the 1970s and 1980s into the role of these neurotransmitters in depression and ma-nia.

In the 1940s the psychiatrist John Cade was thinking about the pos-sible causes of mania. He speculated that an unknown hormonal sub-stance that could be detected in the urine of manic patients might cause the illness. He injected guinea pigs with urine from manic patients; to make the urate in the urine dissolve, he added lithium. The guinea pigs became sedated. In an intuitive leap, Cade realized that the lithium, rather than something in the urine, might be causing this sedative effect. He tried the same experiment with lithium carbonate and got the same results. Cade knew that lithium had been used in treatment of "gouty mania" in the mid-19th century, and after taking lithium carbonate him-self, he administered it to several seriously manic patients, with good re-sults. Although lithium treatment took longer to be accepted than antipsychotics, by the 1970s it was the primary treatment for mania. Since then, other "mood stabilizers," particularly anticonvulsant medi-cation, have been shown to be effective for bipolar disorder.

These advances in treatment led to research on the etiology of men-tal disorders by reasoning backward from the effect of the drug. Because antipsychotics blocked dopamine in the brain, researchers formulated a dopamine theory of schizophrenia. If antidepressants increased the amount of serotonin or norepinephrine (at least acutely), then this sug-gested that low levels of these neurotransmitters caused depression. Neu-roscience has moved beyond these simple models. The advent of new techniques in genetics and neuroimaging will allow us to ask which ar-eas of the brain are dysfunctional in mental disorders. We must also inte-grate data from the psychosocial sciences into our models.

The first section of this book reviews neuroanatomy and neuro-chemistry; the second section applies this knowledge to the study of spe-cific mental disorders. In the epilogue, I discuss the implications of these findings for the future of the mental health profession and social policies on mental disorders. In a book of this type, it is of course impossible to cover every study and every theory of the biology of mental disorders, particularly as quickly as the field is expanding. Thus I have sought to summarize and highlight. Each chapter must be read with the caveat that a new breakthrough in genetics or neuroimaging could change every-thing. Nonetheless, this book provides the fundamentals to allow the mental health professional to place these advances in their proper per-spective.

REFERENCES

Barondes, S. H. (1998). *Mood genes: Hunting for origins of mania and depression*. New York: Freeman.

Bloch, R. G., Dooneif, A. S., & Buchberg, A. S. (1954). The clinical effect of isoniazid and iproniazid in the treatment of pulmonary tuberculosis. *Archives of Internal Medicine, 40,* 900.

Cade, J. F. J. (1949). Lithium salts in the treatment of psychotic excitement. *Medical Journal of Australia, 36,* 349–352.

Colp, R. (2000). History of psychiatry. In B.J.Sadock & V. A. Sadock (Eds.), *Comprehensive textbook of psychiatry* (7th ed., pp. 3301–3332). Philadelphia: Lippincott Williams & Wilkins.

Delay, J., Deniker, P., & Hart, J. M. (1952). Utilisation en thérapeutique psychiatrique d'une phénothiazine d'action centrale élective (4560 RP). *Annales Médico-Psychologiques, 110,* 112–120.

Gay, P. (1998). *Freud: A life for our time.* New York: Norton.

Kline, N. S. (1958). Clinical experience with iproniazid (Marsilid). *Journal of Clinical and Experimental Neuropsychology, 19*(Suppl. 1), 72–78.

Kraepelin, E. (1915). *Manic-depressive insanity and paranoia,* translated (1921) by R. M. Barclary & G. M. Robertson. Edinburgh: E and S Livingstone.

Kuhn, R. (1958). The treatment of depressive states with G22355 (imipramine hydrochloride). *American Journal of Psychiatry, 115,* 459–464.

Orwell, G. (1961). Such, such were the joys. *The Orwell Reader* Edited by R. H. Rovere. London: Harvest Books.

Reil, J. C. (1968). *Rhapsodieen über die Anwendung der psychischen Curmethode auf Geis teszerüttungen* Halle, 1803; reprint. Amsterdam: Bonset.

Shorter, E. (1997). *A history of psychiatry.* New York: Wiley.

Skinner, B. F. (1971). *Beyond freedom and dignity.* New York: Knopf.

Skinner, B. F. (1976). *Walden two.* Englewood Cliffs, NJ: Prentice-Hall.

I

BASIC PRINCIPLES OF NEUROSCIENCE

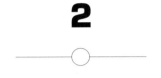

Draw the Brain

INTRODUCTION TO CLINICAL NEUROANATOMY

Of the all the topics presented in this book, it is neuroanatomy that the mental health clinician is most likely to find anxiety provoking. Clinicians other than psychiatrists may not have had any neuroscience courses, either at the undergraduate or graduate level. Pick up a neuroanatomy textbook, and it is easy to get lost after the first chapter. Even if one had had the time to learn the difference between the substantia nigra compacta and the substantia nigra reticulata, what relevance does it have to clinical work? Even psychiatrists find that they lose their grip on the neuroanatomy they learned in medical school, as little of it seems to matter in the day-to-day care of patients. Yet, as the neuroscience of mental disorders advances, a basic understanding of neuroanatomy will be critical to being a good consumer of the clinical neuroscience literature; more important, it is impossible to make any sense of information regarding neurotransmitters or brain imaging without this anatomical foundation.

Mental health clinicians without a strong science background need not shrink from the task—neuroanatomy can be made simple without being simplistic. This chapter has two major goals: to give the reader a grasp of the major structures involved in cognitive, motor, and emotional behaviors and to provide a three-dimensional grasp of how these structures relate to each other. This is most easily done by drawing the structures as you read. Indeed, it would be wise to draw them several times, so that you can reproduce them from memory. Once you have a grasp of the anatomy, it will be easier to understand where the neurotransmitters (dopamine, norepinephrine, etc.) work in the brain (Chapters 3 and 4). You will then be prepared to take the step of understanding how the brain produces behaviors and feelings (Chapter 5). These drawings are not intended to be exact anatomical replicas of the brain. They have been designed so that those without great artistic ability (like myself) can reproduce them.

STEP 1: THE BRAIN'S EXTERIOR

Get a stack of typing paper and some number 2 pencils. Draw the cortex, and then draw two vertical lines below the cortex to represent the brain stem (Figure 2.1). A quarter circle drawn between the brain stem and the back of the cortex illustrates the cerebellum. Draw a vertical line in the middle of the cortex; this shows the central sulcus (Latin for "a furrow or ditch"). It divides the frontal from the parietal lobe. The frontal lobes are involved in *action*. The very tips of the frontal lobes are involved in planning a motor movement; as you move toward the central sulcus, the areas of the frontal lobe become more involved in specific motor acts. Right in front of the central sulcus is the precentral gyrus (Greek for "circle," not to be confused with "gyro," the popular Greek food). The precentral gyrus contains neurons that send axons all the way to the spinal cord; each part of the precentral gyrus influences a particular group of muscles. Behind the central sulcus is the postcentral gyrus. This area receives information from the skin (after several relays); thus it is termed the primary somatosensory cortex. The area behind the postcentral gyrus to the rear of the cortex is the parietal lobe. The posterior part of the cortex is the occipital lobe. The lateral sulcus (or Sylvian fissure) separates the parietal from the temporal cortex. If the frontal lobes are involved in *doing*, then the parietal, occipital, and temporal lobes are involved in *perceiving* and *processing*. As noted, the postcentral gyrus receives somatosensory (touch) information. The occipital area receives visual information, and the superior temporal gyrus receives auditory information. Throughout the parietal and temporal lobes, information from these modalities is integrated, and perception occurs. I discuss this in more detail in Chapter 7, but for now let's understand some differences in the way the parietal and temporal lobes process information. The parietal areas are concerned with "where" the objects we perceive are located in space, whereas the temporal lobe seems concerned with "what" they are (object identification). The parietal lobe also appears to be important in constructing our internal map of our own bodies, as well as our map of the external world. This is particularly true of the right parietal lobe, which also seems critical to maintaining alertness to what goes on around us.

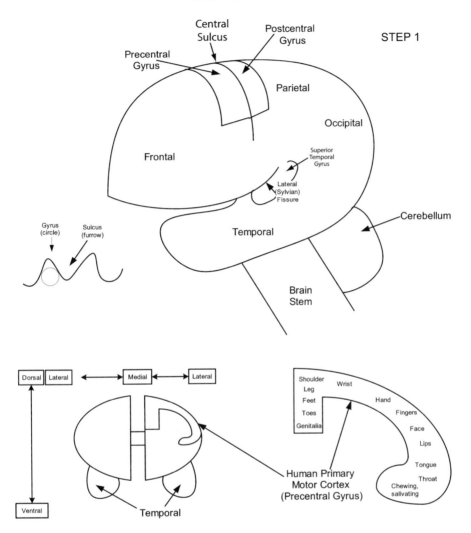

FIGURE 2.1. Basic structure of the brain

This is a good time to be certain that you understand the terminology used to navigate around the brain. When looking from the side, we are taking a lateral view—the front is the anterior and the rear is the posterior. In the bottom part of Figure 2.1, we are taking a front (anterior) view. Thus we see the far right and left sides of the brain (lateral), and the area toward the midline of the brain is referred to as "medial." Finally, the top of the brain is referred to as "dorsal"(from the Latin meaning "back") and the bottom of the brain as "ventral" (from the

Latin meaning "belly"). Many structures of the brain are named using these terms to define their position. Also presented in the bottom half of Figure 2.1 is an enlargement of the precentral gyrus, showing which parts of it influence which motor group.

STEP 2: LOOKING INSIDE THE BRAIN

In Step 2 (Figure 2.2), we have removed the left side of the cortex. On the medial side of the right cortex, draw the corpus callosum. This is a mass of white matter (axons) that connects the two hemispheres and allows them to communicate with each other.

STEP 3: ADDING THE HIPPOCAMPUS AND AMYGDALA

Below the cortex, draw a cylinder to represent the brain stem (Figure 2.3). On the back (dorsal side) of the brain stem, draw two "bumps"; these are the superior colliculi (plural of *colliculus*, Latin for "mound"). Below the left superior colliculi, draw another bump, the left inferior colliculus. You cannot see the right inferior colliculus because it is behind the brain stem. The four colliculi together are referred to as the "tegmentum" or "tegmental plate" (*tegmen* is Latin for "roof or covering"). It forms the roof of the cerebral aqueduct of Sylvius, which you can also draw in. (This carries the cerebrospinal fluid, or CSF, from the third ventricle to the fourth.) The superior colliculi help govern eye movements, and the inferior colliculi help orient us in response to auditory stimuli. In Step 2 (Figure 2.2) we took off the right half of the cortex; now we are going put back a small piece of the right temporal lobe (ventral temporal lobe). Attached to it, draw the hippocampus, which looks like a horn.

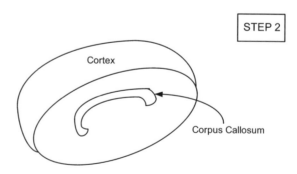

FIGURE 2.2. Medial view of the cortex

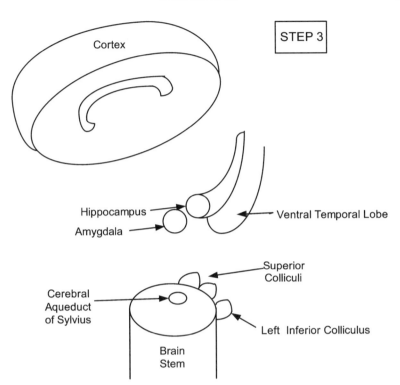

STEP 3

Cortex

Hippocampus

Amygdala

Ventral Temporal Lobe

Superior Colliculi

Cerebral Aqueduct of Sylvius

Left Inferior Colliculus

Brain Stem

FIGURE 2.3. Relationship of hippocampus and temporal lobe

Normally, you can't see the hippocampus from the outside of the brain. The hippocampus is discussed in more detail in future chapters, as it plays a role in both memory and anxiety. Its importance is best illustrated by the case of H. M., a man who had both of his hippocampi (there is one on each side) removed in the 1950s. This was necessary because he had severe epileptic seizures that seemed to emanate from around his medial temporal lobes, where the hippocampus is located. After his surgery he appeared to recover completely. There was no neurological abnormality that would be apparent to the layman. However, H. M. lost all ability to access or form new long-term memories. If he met a new person, he would forget the person five minutes after he or she left the room. He would read the newspaper over and over again, with no memory of what he had read previously. The aide at the nursing home who cared for him had to introduce himself every morning even after many years; when the aide died and H. M. was told of it, he asked, "Who's he?" Thus the hippocampus is critical in shifting experience from short-term memory stores into long-term memory. Recent studies (which are reviewed in Chapter 10) suggest that the hippocampus may play a role in posttraumatic stress disorder. Early physical or emotional abuse may cause changes in the hippocampus.

Just anterior to the hippocampus sits the amygdala—it also plays a role in memory. The amygdala is key in the formation (as opposed to the maintenance) of fear; it is also critical to our abilities to recognize the biological significance of stimuli, such as identifying edible substances or interpreting sexual signals. It is strongly activated by perceptions of faces with emotional content (particularly angry affect). In primates, the amygdala plays a greater role in the management of affect and memory relative to the hippocampus than it does in lower mammals such as rats. The amygdala's role in processing affectively laden stimuli is discussed at length in Chapter 5.

STEP 4: THE FORNIX AND MAMMILLARY BODY

The next step is simple, but does require some three-dimensional thinking (Figure 2.4). Information is coming into the hippocampus through the ventral part of the temporal lobe. After processing, the information (discussed in Chapter 5) passes out of the hippocampus through the fornix. This structure starts as broad band of axons (white matter) that move up and toward the middle of the brain (i.e., dorsally and medially). *Fornix* is Latin for "arch," and these axons do form an arch. As they approach the midline, the axons compress together, then turn vertically (ventrally) and form a column. This column terminates in the mammillary body. There is a mammillary body on each side of the midline of the brain, and these are visible on the underside of the brain. They looked like breasts to the medieval (male) anatomists, hence their name. At this point you may become distraught, wondering, What do these structures do? Let me ask your forbearance; once you understand the anatomy, the discussion of function will be much easier.

STEP 5: TAKING ANOTHER VIEW:
ADDING THE THALAMUS

In Figure 2.5, we are looking directly at the front (anterior view) of the brain. You can see the anterior (front end) of the hippocampus. Again, the fornix rises from the hippocampus and forms an arch, then funnels into a column and dives ventrally to reach the mammillary body (MB). In this anterior view, the arch-like nature of the fornix can be seen more clearly. Beneath the arch, we now draw an egg-like structure, the

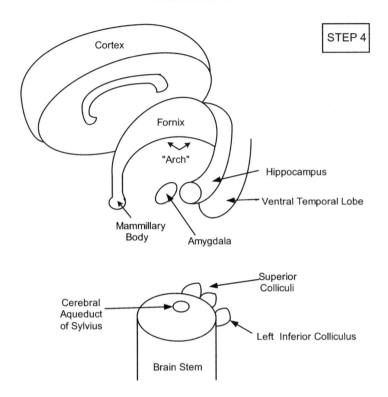

FIGURE 2.4. Fornix and mammillary body

thalamus. The thalamus is a relay station. Information from the sensory organs stops off here before being sent on to the cortex. Also here are "motor nuclei," in which motor commands from the frontal cortex and the basal ganglia (discussed in Chapter 5) are processed. Draw a much smaller egg-like structure below the thalamus; this is the "subthalamic nucleus," appropriately named as it is below the thalamus. It is also involved in motor behavior.

STEP 6: THE CAUDATE AND PUTAMEN

In this step, we first draw the structure (Figure 2.6), and in the next step we see where it fits in the brain. The important thing to bear in mind is that the caudate and putamen are one structure. Together, they are called the "neostriatum" (*neo*, or new, because they are a later evolutionary development in higher animals). The caudate and putamen resembles a

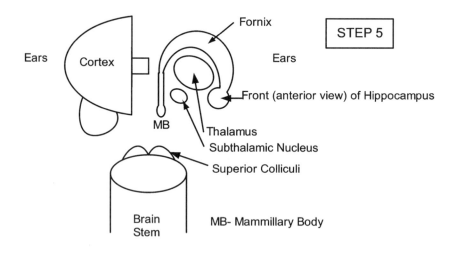

FIGURE 2.5. Looking at the brain from the front (anterior view)

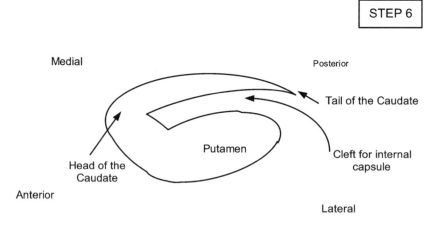

FIGURE 2.6. The caudate and putamen (neostriatum)

tadpole, with the putamen appearing as a large head. At the anterior part of the putamen, the structure bends around 180 degrees and bulges out slightly. This forms the head of the caudate. The caudate runs backward (posteriorly) and tapers into the body, and then bends downward (ventrally) to form the tail of the caudate. (Actually, *caudate* is Latin for "tail," so we are really saying, the "tail of the tail"; but if it doesn't bother neuroanatomists, why should it bother us?) There is a space between the putamen and the caudate; through this cleft runs the "internal capsule." These are the axons from the frontal lobe neurons that are making their way to the caudate and putamen, the brain stem, and ultimately to the spinal cord, where they help direct the motor neurons that directly control the muscles. The caudate and putamen form part of the basal ganglia, which also include the globus pallidus. The globus pallidus are medial to (just inside) the putamen. You cannot see the globus pallidus in Figure 2.6 because we are looking at the lateral side of the putamen.

STEP 7: VISUALIZING THE GLOBUS PALLIDUS

In Step 7A (Figure 2.7a), we are looking at the caudate and putamen from a lateral view. To see the globus pallidus, first cut off the tail of the caudate, then imagine that you are turning the putamen and the head of the caudate around so that you are now looking at it from behind (a posterior view; Figure 2.7b). Now you can see the globus pallidus clinging to the medial side of the putamen. *Pallidus* is Latin for "pale"—it is named for the color of the tissue in the fresh brain. The globus pallidus is divided into two parts: the interna, which is closer to the midline of the brain, and the externa, which lies next to the putamen. Notice also two "globular" structures on the bottom (ventral) of the neostriatum and globus pallidus. These structures are the ventral striatum and ventral pallidal area, respectively. The ventral striatum is a more primitive structure. Whereas the neostriatum is involved in initiating more complex motor acts and plays a role in linking cognition to motor behavior, the ventral striatum is more concerned with those behaviors related to survival, particularly aggression, sexuality, and eating. The neostriatum converses with the frontal lobes; the ventral striatum converses with the limbic parts of the cortex, that is, those related to emotion. The nucleus accumbens lies within the ventral striatum. Animals will self-stimulate this area via an implanted electrode; the animals also will press a button to inject drugs of abuse directly into this area. It is thought that the circuitry of the ventral striatum is critical to the experience of reward. This is more fully explored in discussing substance abuse disorders in Chapter 10.

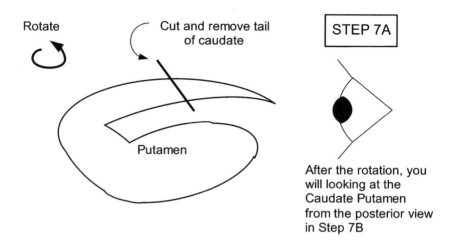

FIGURE 2.7a. Different views of the neostriatum

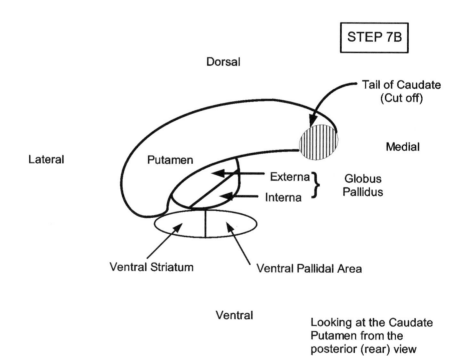

FIGURE 2.7b. Visualizing the globus pallidus

STEP 8: WHERE DOES THE STRIATUM FIT?

Step 8 (Figure 2.8) recreates Step 4 (Figure 2.4). Insert the thalamus under the "arch" of the fornix. Insert the smaller subthalamic nucleus beneath it. Insert the neostriatum (i.e., the caudate and putamen) just anterior to the fornix. Note that I have used dotted lines on the column of the fornix to indicate that the caudate is passing anterior to (in front of) this structure. Below (ventral to) the neostriatum, you should now draw an oval to represent the ventral striatum. We are now also in a position to see the purpose of the cleft between the putamen and the caudate. As shown in Figure 2.8, axons from the frontal cortex (those concerned with motor behavior) come together to pass ventrally through this cleft. Some neurons branch off to reach the caudate and putamen, others proceed to the thalamus, and others continue ventrally to the spinal cord. These axons form the ventral corticospinal tracts. One neuron in the precentral gyrus can send an axon through the "internal capsule" down

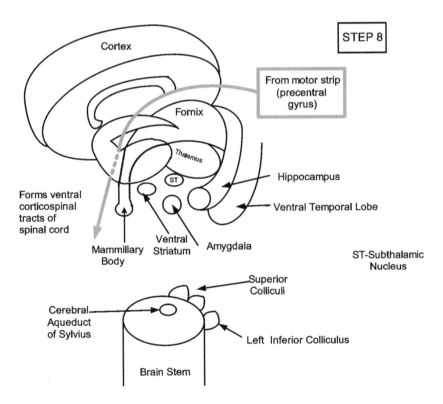

FIGURE 2.8. Putting it together

to the spinal cord. All the axons from the precentral gyrus are bunched together as they exit the internal capsule and appear on the ventral side of the brain stem; this area is called the "pyramid." Why the pyramid? Because many of the neurons in the precentral gyrus that contribute their axons to this bulge are triangular in shape (i.e., "pyramidal"), the bulge is given that name. Before proceeding to the spinal cord, the neurons decussate; that is, they cross to the other side of the spinal cord. For this reason, strokes that occur on one side of the brain impair movements on the opposite side of the body.

STEP 9: A FIRST ATTEMPT
AT FUNCTIONAL NEUROANATOMY;
UNDERSTANDING THE PAPEZ CIRCUIT

The Papez circuit is part of the limbic system and is very much involved in emotion and memory. In Step 9 (Figure 2.9), you should redraw Step 4 (Figure 2.4), then again add the egg-shaped thalamus. Leave out the neostriatum for the time being. Label the corpus callosum (the white matter, i.e., axons, connecting the two hemispheres). Around the corpus callosum runs the cingulate gyrus, which is a critical part of the limbic system. Below the thalamus, sketch in the hypothalamus (*hypo* is Greek for "below"). The hypothalamus is involved in many bodily functions, but for now let's note that it is the head ganglion of the sympathetic nervous system; that is, it influences the "fight or flight" reaction. Information about the *current* state of the world enters the temporal lobe (1) and is then transferred to the hippocampus (2). After processing in the hippocampus (covered in more detail in Chapter 5), the information is transferred via the fornix to the mammillary body (3) and then from the mammillary body to the anterior thalamus (4). The anterior thalamus sends the information to the cingulate gyrus, where it interacts with older information in long-term memory stores (5), and then it returns to the hippocampus (6). Thus the hippocampus is in a position to compare information about the current state of the world with information from the past and to make a determination as to whether what we are currently experiencing is familiar or not. Furthermore, the hippocampus can project to the hypothalamus (7) to activate the sympathetic nervous system. If our adrenaline begins flowing (as it does if the hippocampus matches the current state of the world to a painful memory), we experience anxiety. Thus you can see how damage to the hippocampus might lead to inappropriate levels of anxiety when there is no danger around (as in panic attacks or posttraumatic stress disorder). The physiology of anxiety is surely more complicated than this (involving the amygdala as well); this example illustrates how neuroanatomy is relevant to behavior.

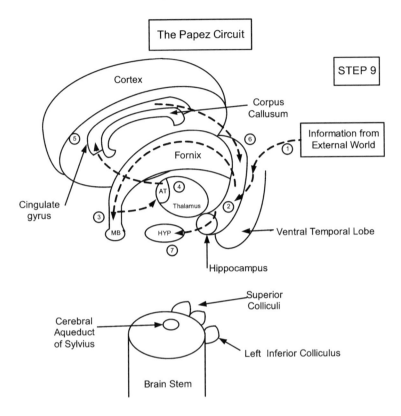

FIGURE 2.9. Functional neuroanatomy

STEP 10: THE BASAL GANGLIA
AND THEIR CONNECTIONS

There is no need to draw Step 10 (Figure 2.10); it is included to allow you to understand the connections of the striatum and globus pallidus that you drew in Steps 7 and 8. Two circuits are illustrated: the limbic striatum circuit on the left side of the figure and the sensory–motor striatum circuit on the right. The sensory–motor circuit involves higher level, more complex motor acts, whereas the limbic circuit involves motor behaviors related to the pursuit of rewarding ("appetitive") stimuli. You will note that the limbic striatal circuits include the nucleus accumbens that I described previously as being involved in processing stimuli related to reward. Let us examine this circuit first. For now, we do not take up the functional aspects of the circuit but focus on how the circuit is put together. Notice that information flows back and forth between the cingulate gyrus (limbic cortex) and the dorsomedial nucleus of

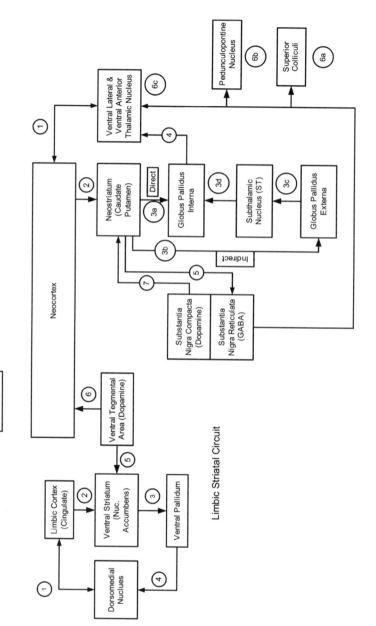

FIGURE 2.10. The basal ganglia and their connections

STEP 10

Neostriatal (Sensory-Motor) Circuits

Limbic Striatal Circuit

28

the thalamus (1). The limbic cortex sends information in a one-way direction to the ventral striatum (2). From the ventral striatum the information flows to the ventral pallidum (3) and then back to the dorsomedial thalamus (4). Note the box labeled "ventral tegmental area." Anatomically, this area lies ventral to the tegmentum, the structure formed by the superior and inferior colliculi (see Step 4). The cell bodies of these neurons produce the neurotransmitter dopamine that is released at synapses in the prefrontal cortex and ventral striatum (nucleus accumbens). The pathway from the ventral tegmental area (VTA) to the nucleus accumbens (5) is quite interesting. If an electrode is inserted into this pathway in a mouse, the animal will press a button to stimulate the pathway with electricity, causing the neuron to release dopamine into the accumbens. If a very small tube is surgically placed in the accumbens, an animal will inject cocaine into the area, which causes a very sudden release of dopamine. Later chapters explore how this mechanism is relevant to substance abuse disorders. A final part of this circuit involves the projection of dopamine neurons from the VTA to the neocortex (6). This pathway, the "mesocortical" dopamine pathway, may play a critical role in the pathophysiology of attention-deficit/hyperactivity disorder and psychotic disorders. It may also play an important role in "working memory"—the ability of the brain to hold information "online" while plans for an appropriate response to the current environment are made.

The sensory–motor striatum, shown on the right side of Figure 2.10, is more complicated, but it follows a circuit parallel to that of the limbic striatum. Again, there is an interchange of information between the frontal lobes and the thalamic nuclei, this time with the ventral anterior and ventral lateral nuclei (1). The frontal lobes also send information to the neostriatum (2). There are three pathways out of the neostriatum. Two of these pathways project to different parts of the globus pallidus. The direct pathway goes immediately to the globus pallidus interna (3a). The indirect pathway projects to the globus pallidus externa (3b). Information is then transferred to the subthalamic nucleus (3c), and from there it is passed on to the globus pallidus interna (3d). From the interna, the information flows back to the ventral lateral and ventral anterior thalamic nuclei (4). The third pathway from the neostriatum also flows to a part of the substantia nigra (see the following discussion), the reticulata (5). The reticulata differs from the substantia nigra compacta in that it uses γ (gamma)-aminobutyric acid (GABA) as a neurotransmitter, whereas the compacta, like the VTA, uses dopamine. GABA is an inhibitory transmitter; it turns off neuronal impulses. The reticulata then projects to and releases GABA into three structures, as shown in Figure 2.10: the superior colliculi (6a), which play a role in eye movements; the pedunculopontine nucleus (which is found in the brain stem and governs major muscles of the trunk involved in balance, standing, and walking) (6b); and the ventral lateral and ventral anterior thalamic nuclei (6c).

I explore motor behavior in depth in Chapter 5, but, for now, I summarize the role of the two parts of the substantia nigra. The reticulata uses the inhibitory neurotransmitter GABA; when GABA is released into these three areas, there are no eye movements, truncal, or walking movements, and when the thalamic motor nuclei are inhibited, further higher level motor movements are also inhibited. Furthermore, the substantia nigra reticulata is tonically active, that is, the neurons are nearly always firing. Thus motor movement is prevented; for the person to move, this inhibitory influence must be withdrawn. The substantia nigra compacta, through the influence of dopamine on the neostriatum (7), plays a major role in removing this inhibitory influence and allowing the initiation of new behaviors. This is why persons with Parkinson's disease (in which dopamine is depleted in the compacta) lose the ability to initiate new motor action; the movements they can produce are slow and jerky.

The focus of this chapter was to present the brain in three dimensions (3-D) and to familiarize you as to how these structures fit together. In the following chapters, I focus on specific neurotransmitters. There are specific pathways in the brain for each neurotransmitter, and we draw in these pathways in the next chapters. It would be cumbersome to draw a 3-D picture each time we wish to consider a different neurotransmitter. Therefore, once you have mastered the 3-D structure of the brain in Steps 1–9, you should draw the general brain figure shown in Figure 2.11. You are looking at a lateral view (from the side of the brain), but one half of the brain has been removed to allow you to visualize the hippocampus, the fornix, and the caudate putamen (neostriatum). At this point, the globus pallidus cannot be seen, but remember that it is medial to the striatum. The fornix is represented as a simple tube. I have added one more structure to those we have already discussed—the stria terminalis. Like the fornix, it carries the axons of neurons, it connects the amygdala to the hypothalamus, and it is also a means by which neurotransmitters reach the amygdala from the brain stem. See Plate 1 (opposite p. 120) for a detailed color illustration of the entire cerebral hemispheres.

The first step, understanding the neuroanatomy of the brain, is complete. The next step is to understand how neurons communicate internally and with each other. We can then look at how the different parts of the brain work together to generate behaviors, cognition, and emotions.

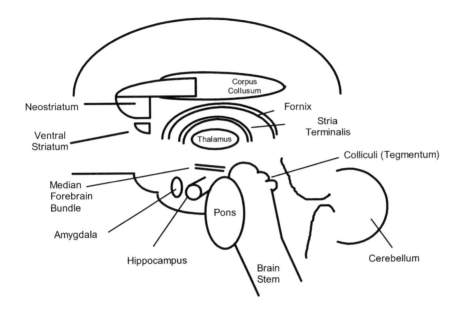

FIGURE 2.11. A simplified view of the brain

REFERENCES

Alexander, G. E., DeLong, M. R., & Strick, P. L. (1986). Parallel organization of functionally segregated cricuits linking basal ganglia and cortex. *Annual Review of Neuroscience, 9,* 357–381.

Brodal, P. (1992). *The central nervous system: Structure and function.* New York: Oxford University Press.

Chevalier, G., & Deniau, J. M. (1990). Disinhibition as a basic process in the expression of striatal functions. *Trends in Neuroscience, 13,* 277–280.

Koob, G. F., & Nestler, E. J. (1997). The neurobiology of drug addiction. In S. Salloway, P. Malloy, & J. L. Cummings (Eds.), *The neuropsychiatry of limbic and subcortical disorders* (pp. 179–194). Washington, DC: American Psychiatric Press.

Mega, M. S., Cummings, J. L., Salloway, S., & Malloy, P. (2000). The limbic system: An anatomic, phylogenetic, and clinical perspective. In S. Salloway, P. Cummings, & P. Malloy (Eds.), *The neuropsychiatry of limbic and subcortical disorders* (pp. 3–18). Washington, DC: American Psychiatric Press.

Purves, D., Augustine, G. J., Fitzpatrick, D., Katz, L. C., LaMantia, A. S., & McNamara, J. O. (1997). *Neuroscience.* Durham, NC: Sinauer Associates.

Wilson, C. J. (1998). Basal ganglia. In G. M. Shepherd (Ed.), *The synaptic organization of the brain* (pp. 329–375). New York: Oxford University Press.

Wise, R. A., & Bozarth, M. A. (1987). Brain mechanisms of drug reward and euphoria. *Psychiatric Medicine, 3,* 445–460.

3

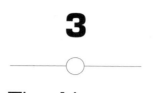

The Neuron

The neuron is the microprocessor of the brain. The basic unit of the brain's circuitry is shown in Figure 3.1. Hundreds of dendrites project from the cell body; these dendrites in turn are covered with thousands of receptors. Axons from other neurons form synapses on these dendrites. The axons release neurotransmitters onto these receptors. A particular neuron may receive input from 1 to 100,000 different axons. Thus the neuron is not a simple relay; this complex input is integrated so that the neuron may formulate a response. A single axon may signal one neuron, or the axon may branch to send signals to thousands of neurons. Because there are 100 billion neurons in the brain, with each having hundreds of connections to each other, the complexity of the brain circuitry is self-evident. The receptors produce many different types of signals within the neuron. The most significant signals the neuron produces are electrical transmissions called action potentials. These electrical signals travel down the axon, and when they reach the synaptic buton (at the end of the axon), the neuron releases its own neurotransmitter onto the neighboring dendrites.

When a neurotransmitter binds to a receptor, the neuron is affected in a variety of ways as shown in the bottom of Figure 3.1. Three types of receptors in neurons concern us in this chapter. The first is the *ligand-gated ionotropic* receptor, numbered 1 in the figure. When a neurotransmitter binds to this receptor, it causes a channel to open in the neuronal membrane, and through this channel ions may flow. *Ions* are positively or electrically charged atoms—the ions involved in neuronal functioning

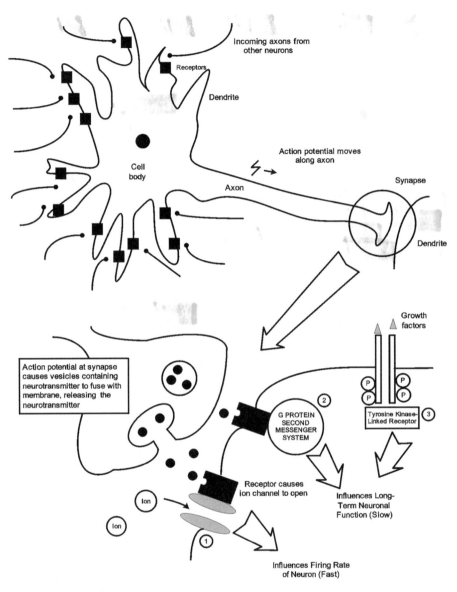

FIGURE 3.1. Fundamentals of neurotransmission

are sodium (Na⁺), potassium (K⁺), chloride (Cl⁻), and calcium (Ca²⁺). The flow of these ions in or out of the neuron is the critical factor in stimulating or inhibiting the neuron's firing (action potential). The two other receptor systems have more subtle effects on the neuron that may be relevant to the mechanisms of mental illness and the effects of psychotropic drugs. The receptor labeled 2 stimulates the "G protein second messenger system." The neurotransmitter is the first message. When the G protein is activated, it turns an enzyme in the cytoplasm on or off; this action has long-term effects on neuronal function. Although the effects of the ionotropic receptor turn on and off within milliseconds, the processes set in motion by the G protein may last anywhere from milliseconds to weeks. Receptors linked to G protein are often referred to as "metabotropic" receptors because they affect long-term cellular processes. The final type of receptor I examine is the tyrosine kinase-linked receptor (TKR). This receptor actually protrudes through the cell membrane. When a neurotransmitter (referred to as a "growth factor") binds to the part of TKR outside the membrane, phosphate groups bind to inner portions of TKR. TKR, through a complex series of steps that are examined later, activates an enzyme called Ras. Ras, in turn, can affect the transcription of DNA and the process of cell proliferation. Mutant forms of Ras have been linked to various cancers. In the brain, growth factors (small chains of amino acids, or peptides) bind to TKR receptors and play a major role in preventing neuronal death. In animals, high levels of stress reduce the amount of growth factors released, and that, in turn, causes neuronal atrophy. Thus the processes governed by the TKR receptors may be highly relevant to stress-induced psychiatric disorders.

HOW DO NEURONS FIRE?

Neurons maintain an electrical charge, like tiny batteries. I first show how this voltage is produced; then it will be clear how the neuron generates the action potential that ultimately causes the release of the neurotransmitter. Figure 3.2 illustrates how the "membrane potential" is produced.

Figure 3.2a shows a neuron with K⁺, Cl⁻ and Na⁺ ion channels. Each channel can admit only one type of ion, and Na⁺ channels are much less permeable than K⁺ and Cl⁻; that is, Na⁺ has more difficulty flowing in or out of the neuron than the other two ions. In Figure 3.2a, we first add potassium chloride (KCl) to the solution. The K⁺ and Cl⁻ distribute themselves on each side of the membrane. (mM, millimolar, is a measure of the concentration of the ions.)

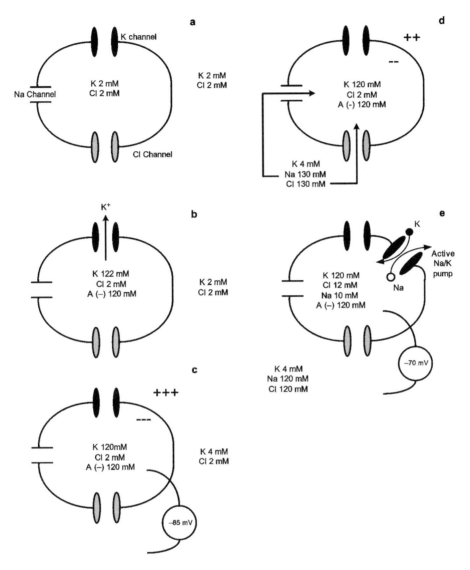

FIGURE 3.2. Understanding the neuron membrane potential

In Figure 3.2b, 122 mM of K⁺ ions are injected inside the neuron, but these K+ ions are associated with 120 mM of negatively charged proteins (A⁻). These large proteins *cannot* pass through the ion channels or the membrane. Because there is now an excess of K⁺ inside the neuron, K⁺ begins to flow out of the neuron, down its *concentration* gradient. Because the proteins cannot follow the K⁺ ions, a separation of charge is created. The positively charged K⁺ ions move out, leaving the negatively charged proteins behind. With more K⁺ on the outside than inside, the inside is negatively charged. After only a small amount of K⁺ has flowed out, enough of a charge separation has built up that K⁺ can no longer flow out against the *electrical* gradient. Figure 2c shows the neuron after the K⁺ has reached equilibrium—the electrical and concentration gradients are balanced. Because there is an unequal distribution of charge, a potential (i.e., a voltage difference) is set up. The inside and outside of the neuron are analogous to the positive and negative terminals of a battery. This potential is calculated by the Nernst equation:

$$V_m = \frac{RT}{zF} \ln \frac{[K_{out}]}{[K_{in}]}$$

For the mathematically inclined, V_m is the membrane potential, R is the universal gas constant (8.31 joules/mole K⁺), T is the temperature in degrees Kelvin (297°), z is the valence (1 for K⁺) and F is the Faraday (96,500 coulombs/mole). The natural log, ln, can converted to log (base 10) by multiplying by 2.3. The ratio on the K⁺ ion concentration is 4 mM/120 mM, or .0333. Thus the membrane potential, if it were based only on K⁺, would be about −85 mV.

The cell is no longer at osmotic equilibrium because of the large concentration of negative proteins inside the cell. Water would flow into the cell and cause it to burst. This does not happen, however, because of the large concentration of NaCl in the extracellular fluid. As shown in Figure 3.2d, when NaCl is added, Na⁺ begins to flow down its concentration gradient, as well as down its electrical gradient. Cl⁻ follows Na⁺ as the negative ion. However, Na⁺ and Cl⁻ channels are significantly less permeable relative to K⁺ channels. Subsequently, equilibrium is established as the flow of K⁺ *out* of the cell balances the flow of Na⁺ and Cl⁻ *into* the cell. The membrane potential is again given by the Nernst equation, taking into account the fact that the permeability (p) of the membrane to Na⁺ and Cl⁻ is considerably less than that for K⁺.

$$V_m = \frac{RT}{zF} \ln \frac{[K_{out}] + p[Na_{out}] + p[Cl_{in}]}{[K_{in}] + p[Na_{in}] + p[Cl_{out}]}$$

$$V_m = \frac{8.31 \cdot 297}{96,500} 2.4 \log \frac{4 \text{ mM} + 0.3 \cdot 120 \text{ mM} + .1 \cdot 10 \text{ mM}}{120 \text{ mM} + 0.3 \cdot 10 \text{ mM} + .1 \cdot 130 \text{ mM}}$$

$$V_m \approx -70 \text{ mV}$$

This is shown in Figure 3.2e. Like any battery, the neuron would "run down" and lose its charge if there were not an active process that maintains the membrane potential. Left to itself, Na^+ ions would leak into the neuron and K^+ ions would leak out to the point that no charge was left. Thus the neuron must actively pump K^+ and Na^+ ions in and out of the cell, respectively. This pump is shown in Figure 3.2e. This requires considerable energy, and thus neurons require a steady supply of oxygen and glucose. Hence neurons are highly sensitive to damage when deprived of their blood supply, as in a stroke.

THE ACTION POTENTIAL

Figures 3.3 and 3.4 take us through the mechanism that leads to the generation of an action potential. Figure 3.3a shows the neuron at rest. There are two ligand-gated channels that are closed and two passive open channels, one for Na^+ and one for K^+. These are the channels involved in the production of the membrane potential that I just discussed. On either side of them are the "voltage-gated" ion channels, which remain closed at rest. These are the channels that will ultimately trigger the action potential. In Figure 3.3b, a neurotransmitter binds to the receptor and causes the ion channels to open. Na^+ flows into the cell, and K^+ flows out. *This localized flow of ions, by itself, does not trigger the action potential.* Rather, it produces voltage changes around the area of the receptors. The membrane in that particular area becomes more positive relative to areas around it. The key to triggering the action potential is whether enough neurotransmitter has been released to open sufficient ligand-gated channels, which in turn produces the electrical change needed to open the voltage-gated Na^+ channels.

This process is shown in Figure 3.4a. When the voltage-gated channels open, Na^+ rushes into the cell, down its concentration gradient. This action causes the inside of the cell to become more positive relative to the outside; this is shown in the graph at the bottom of the figure. The neuron has become "depolarized." In Figure 3.4b, the neurotransmitter has disengaged from the receptor, closing the ligand-gated channel. The depolarization has now caused the voltage-gated K^+ channels to open,

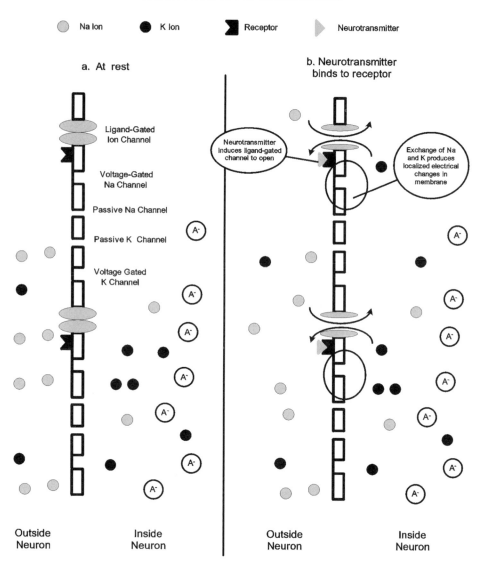

FIGURE 3.3. Understanding the action potential (a). The neuron at rest (b) A neurotransmitter binds to the ionotrophic receptor

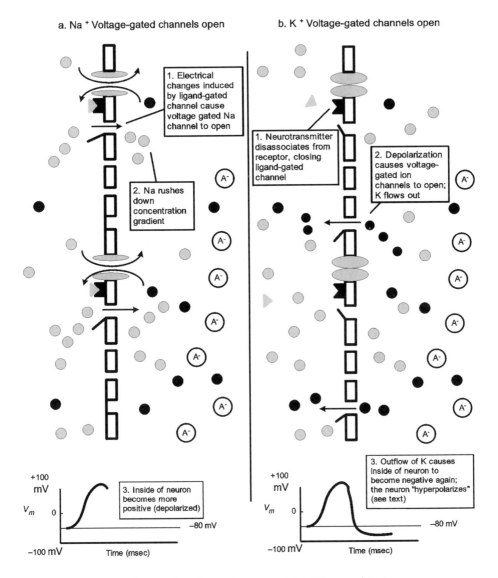

FIGURE 3.4. Understanding the action potential (a) Entry of Na⁺ causes membrane potential to become positive (b) Outflow of K⁺ restores negative membrane potential and induces hyperpolarization

and K^+ rushes out of the cell down its concentration gradient. As shown in the graph in the lower part of 3.4b, the membrane potential returns to being negatively charged (inside compared to outside). Notice that the neuron "overshoots"; that is, the membrane is more negatively charged than it was before the action potential was triggered. This happens because so much K^+ has flowed out of the neuron through its voltage-gated channels. This process is referred to as "hyperpolarization." The neuron enters a refractory period in which it is more difficult for it to generate another action potential. Because the membrane is so negative on the inside relative to the outside, much more neurotransmitter will be required to induce the opening of enough voltage-gated Na^+ channels to fire another action potential. After several minutes, the membrane will drift back up to –70 mV, and the neuron may fire again. *The neuron can regulate its firing rate by adjusting the size of the post-action-potential hyperpolarization.* If the neuron leaves the voltage-gated K^+ channel open for a longer time, the membrane is more hyperpolarized, and the refractory period is longer. If the neuron shuts off the K^+ voltage-gated channel earlier, then the membrane is not so hyperpolarized (because less K^+ flowed out), and the neuron can fire again sooner. Later in the chapter, I show how the second messenger systems accomplish this task.

Figure 3.5a shows how the action potential propagates down the axon. When the ligand-gated channel is opened by a neurotransmitter, Na^+ flows in (1). As I have discussed, the voltage changes caused by this inflow of Na+ cause the voltage-gated channels to open (2), further increasing the flow of Na^+ into the neuron (3). Now, the voltage changes induced in Step 3 flow further down the axon, inducing the next group of voltage-gated channels to open (4). Once again, more Na^+ flows in (5), and these voltage changes will be transmitted to the next of set of voltage-gated channels. The process continues until the action potential reaches the end of the axon.

Figure 3.5b shows how the action potential leads to the release of the neurotransmitter. Previously, an organelle within the neuron, the endosome, pinched off a small sphere called a vesicle (1). The vesicle fills with the neurotransmitter (2) and then moves to the edge of the membrane, a process referred to as "docking" (3).When the action potential reaches the end of the axon (4), it causes the opening of voltage-gated calcium channels (5). Now, when the calcium enters the end of the neuron, enzymes are activated that fuse the vesicle to the membrane, disgorging the neurotransmitter into the synaptic cleft (6).

a. Propagating the action potential down the axon

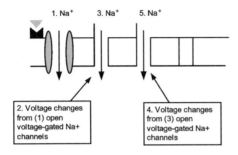

1. Na⁺   3. Na⁺   5. Na⁺

2. Voltage changes from (1) open voltage-gated Na+ channels

4. Voltage changes from (3) open voltage-gated Na+ channels

b. Release of neurotransmitter

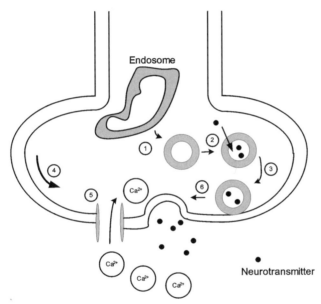

Endosome

Neurotransmitter

FIGURE 3.5. Propagation of the action potential and release of neurotransmitter

THE G PROTEIN SYSTEM

Figure 3.6 shows this important second messenger system. At rest, the G protein is attached to the inside of the neuron membrane, facing the cytoplasm of the cell. It is only very loosely associated with its receptor. When the neurotransmitter stimulates the receptor, it changes shape such that the G protein can bind to it. A G protein consists of three parts: α, β, and γ. There are over 35 types of G protein. Most of the amino acid structure of the α subunit is what varies from one type of G protein to another. These differences in the α subunit convey different functions to the G protein, and usually the β-γ units are very similar from one G protein to the next. The α subunit, during the resting state, is bound to a molecule of guanosine diphosphate (GDP). When the G protein associates with the receptor, another shape change occurs such that guanosine

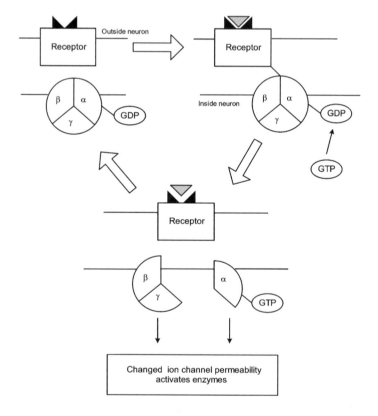

FIGURE 3.6. The action of G proteins associated with the metabotropic receptor

triphosphate (GTP) replaces the GDP. When this occurs, the G protein splits into an α-GTP and β-γ subunit. These pieces of the G protein become active and change ion channel permeability and activate enzymes in the neuronal cytoplasm. Two critical enzymes so activated are adenylyl cyclase and phospholipase C. I explore their actions next.

ADENYLYL CYCLASE

Adenosine triphosphate (ATP) is a molecule of adenosine (one of the bases in DNA) with a chain of three phosphate groups attached to it. The enzyme adenylyl cyclase transforms ATP into cyclic adenosine monophosphate (cAMP). The enzyme cleaves off two phosphates and makes a circular bond out the final phosphate left on the adenosine molecule. Figure 3.7 shows how G proteins are involved in this process.

Two different receptors are shown at the top of the figure. The receptor on the left is linked to a G protein with an α_s subunit; this indicates that this G protein stimulates adenylyl cyclase. In contrast, the receptor on the right is linked to a different G protein, one with an α_i subunit; its effect is to inhibit the activity of adenylyl cyclase. If the adenylyl cyclase is stimulated via G-α_s, the enzyme becomes active, transforming ATP into cAMP. Cyclic AMP can then activate a number of cytoplasmic enzymes. For now I focus on protein kinase A (PKA). A kinase is an enzyme that puts two molecules together. A principal function of kinases in the neuron is to attach phosphate groups to proteins and thus regulate their function. The PKA is composed of four parts: two catalytic units, which actually add the phosphates, and two regulatory subunits, which bind cAMP. When two cAMP molecules bind to PKA, it breaks apart; the catalytic units can then enter the nucleus of the neuron. Here they place a phosphate group on a protein called CRE-binding protein (CREB). CRE stands for "cAMP-response element"; as shown in the figure, CRE is a segment of the DNA that CREB can bind to. When CREB does bind to CRE, it facilitates the transcription of the nearby gene. New proteins can be synthesized, which will be critical in the long-term life of the neuron.

THE PHOSPHOINOSITIDE SYSTEM

The phosphoinositol (PI) system helps regulate the level of calcium in the neuron. In discussing the action potential, I observed that the neuron had a low level of Na^+ inside, whereas the Na^+ level in the bloodstream (i.e., the extracellular fluid) was high, much like seawater. Thus, when

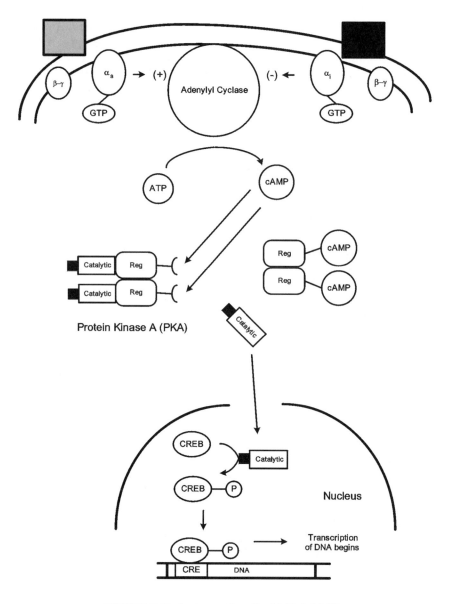

FIGURE 3.7. Actions of cyclic AMP (cAMP)

cells first evolved, they developed mechanisms to pump Na⁺ out of them, so that the chemical milieu inside of the cell is very different from the sea around them. When animals emerged on land, they had to develop mechanisms to bring the ocean with them. The plasma of blood has a similar concentration of ions as seawater; our kidneys and hormones work to maintain this balance of salts. Calcium is present in high concentrations in seawater and in our bloodstream, yet it is maintained at low levels inside cells. The concentration of Ca inside neurons is 1/10,000th of that found outside the cell. In the neuron, like other cells, there is an organelle termed the "endoplasmic reticulum." This structure contains high levels of calcium similar to those found outside the cells. Why all this trouble to regulate calcium? In discussing adenylyl cyclase, I pointed out how cAMP activates protein kinase A by binding to it. Nature found phosphorylation an efficient way to regulate cell activities, but high levels of calcium make the chemical reaction needed to add or cleave off the phosphate group very difficult. Hence, cells evolved ways to keep their intracellular calcium low. A bonus of this system is that by subtly adjusting calcium levels, neurons can regulate the activity of a wide variety of proteins within themselves.

The top half of Figure 3.8 shows a molecule called phosphatidy-linositol 4,5-biphosphate (PIP_2). This complex molecule has three parts. Inositol is a six-carbon ring with hydroxyl (oxygen–hydrogen, –OH) attached to each carbon. Because oxygen carries an electrical charge (i.e., it is polar), it likes being in water (hydrophilic). This part of the molecule sits in the cytoplasm of the neuron. The inositol molecule is linked to a molecule of glycerol, which is a three-carbon chain with a hydroxyl group on each carbon. Inositol binds to one of the carbons, but long fatty acids bind to the other two carbons. These fatty acids are "oily," and water and oil don't mix. They are hydrophobic and remain inserted into the membrane. At rest, the PIP_2 molecule is all in one piece.

When a neurotransmitter attaches to a receptor linked to the PI system, the α-GTP subunit activates the enzyme phospholipase C. This enzyme, which is attached to the membrane, splits the PIP_2 molecule into two parts (bottom half of figure). The inositol part of the molecule is set free in the cytoplasm as inositol triphosphate (IP_3). IP_3 attaches to a receptor on the endoplasmic reticulum—this opens a calcium channel, and calcium flows out of the reticulum into the cytoplasm. This rise in calcium activates another enzyme, calmodulin. Back at the membrane, the piece of the PIP_2 molecule left behind is called diacylglycerol (DAG). DAG, in turn, activates protein kinase C (PKC), which also phosphorylates cytoplasmic enzymes. IP_3 is then recycled to produce more PIP_2. The enzymes activated by the PI system play critical roles in the neuron's life. Excessive activation of PKC can lead to tumors. Calmodulin can activate

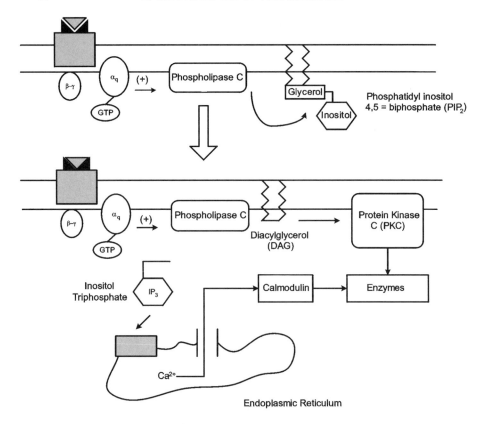

FIGURE 3.8. The phosphatidylinositol 4,5-biphosphate (PIP_2) second messenger system

the enzyme nitric oxide synthase, which produces minute amounts of nitric oxide (NO) gas that can diffuse to other neurons. This may be a critical step in memory formation (see Chapter 6). Calcium-activated enzymes are crucial in the formation of synaptic vesicles and efficient neurotransmitter release.

HOW SECOND MESSENGER SYSTEMS WORK TOGETHER

Figure 3.9 shows how the second messenger systems regulate one major facet of neuron function: how frequently the neuron can fire an action potential. In the top left graph of the figure, a neuron is stimulated with the neurotransmitter glutamate; the glutamate stimulates sufficient ligand-gated ion channels to trigger action potentials. In the top right graph, the neuron is again stimulated with glutamate, but this time the neurotransmitters norepinephrine (NE) and acetylcholine (Ach) are stimulating the neuron as well. Notice that even though the same amount of glutamate is used, the neuron responds more vigorously in the presence of NE or Ach. The bottom half of the figure illustrates how this occurs. Remember that the ability of the neuron to fire again is governed by the degree of hyperpolarization—the more K^+ that leaves the cell, the more negative the membrane becomes, and the more difficult it is to fire another action potential. By decreasing the K^+ outflow, the hyperpolarization is decreased, and the neuron can fire sooner. When NE binds to its receptor, adenylyl cyclase in activated by the G protein system. Cyclic AMP is formed, which activates PKA. PKA phosphorylates the K^+ channel, making it less permeable to K^+

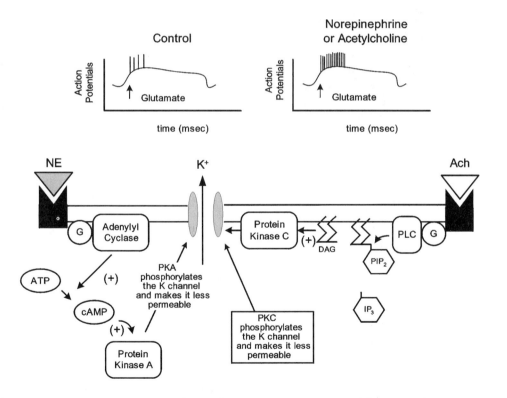

FIGURE 3.9. Interaction of second messenger systems to modify neuronal excitability. Abstracted with permission from Nicoll, R. A. (1988)

and reducing the outflow of K^+. Ach, by binding to one of its receptors, activates a G protein that turns on phospholipase C (PLC), achieving the same result. PIP_2 is cleaved, and DAG activates PKC. PKC, like PKA, phosphorylates the K^+ channel, reducing the hyperpolarization.

GROWTH FACTORS AND THE TYROSINE KINASE RECEPTOR (TKR) SYSTEM

Growth factors play a crucial role in neuron proliferation and survival. Specific growth factors that are possibly relevant to mental disorders are discussed in later chapters. Traditional neurotransmitters are small molecules, whereas growth factors are small chains of amino acids (peptides). Most neurotransmitters are unidirectional in that they are released by the presynaptic neuron and bind to a receptor on the postsynaptic neuron. Growth factors, on other hand, can reach a target neuron by three different ways. Other cells in the brain besides neurons can produce growth factors and release them onto a neuron. The postsynaptic neuron can release a growth factor that travels back to the presynaptic neuron to bind to a receptor there, thus becoming a retrograde messenger. Figure 3.10 shows how growth factors transmit their signal to the cell nucleus, so as to activate the transcription of DNA. The receptors for these growth factors are *monomeric* proteins that span the neuron's membrane (1). When growth factors bind to them, their shape alters such that they associate in pairs, becoming *dimers* (2). Once *dimerized,* the receptor binds four phosphate molecules, converting them into an active enzyme. A special protein called Ras is bound nearby to the inside of the neuronal membrane. Like the G protein, it binds a molecule of GDP in the inactive state. When the receptor has its four phosphates, activation occurs (3). An adapter protein binds to the receptor. This adapter has two parts, or domains (SH2 and SH3; I give details about them in a later chapter). The adapter protein recruits another protein, SOS, and together they build a bridge to Ras. Now, GTP can replace GDP, and Ras is active. Active Ras converts another protein, Raf. Raf links with yet another protein, MEK (the "M" in "MEK" stands for "MAP," or mitogen-activated protein kinase, and the "E" stands for extracellularly regulated kinase). So MEK phosphoralytes MAP, which in turn phosphorylates other proteins and enzymes involved in the life of the neuron. Neurons often require regular stimulation by a variety of growth factors to avoid cell death; the absence of these factors may result in the deleterious effects of stress on the brain.

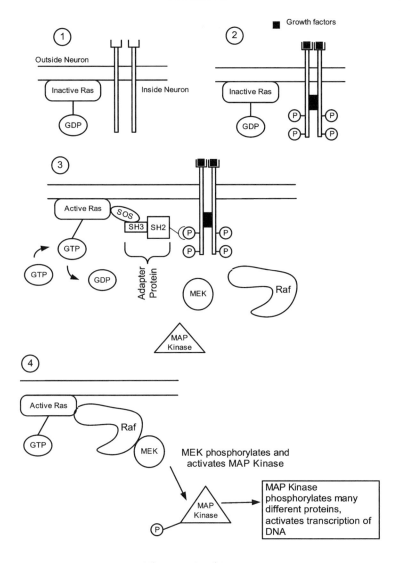

FIGURE 3.10. The tyrosine kinase receptor system

SUMMARY

I have examined the mechanisms by which neurotransmitters invoke responses in neurons. They may open ion channels and trigger the firing of the neuron. They may also open ion channels that further hyperpolarize and thus inhibit firing. Through G proteins, they activate enzymes that control calcium levels or initiate the transcription of DNA. Finally, growth factors set in motion a series of complex events critical to neuronal survival. It is important to note that is not the neurotransmitter but the structure of the receptor that conveys which of these mechanisms is used. Some neurotransmitters only open ion channels; others only act through G proteins; still others bind to arrays of receptors, each of which uses a different mechanism. In the next chapter, I examine the anatomy and function of each of the major neurotransmitters thought to be involved in mental disorders.

REFERENCES

Fisher, S. K., & Agranoff, B. W. (1999). Phosphoinositides. In G. J. Siegel, B. W. Agranoff, R. W. Albers, S. K. Fisher, & M. D. Uhler (Eds.), *Basic neurochemistry: Molecular, cellular and medical aspects* (6th ed., pp. 415–432). Philadelphia: Lippincott Williams & Wilkins.

Hille, B., & Catterall, W. A. (1999). Electrical excitability and ion channels. In G. J. Siegel, B. W. Agranoff, R. W. Albers, S. K. Fisher, & M. D. Uhler (Eds.), *Basic neurochemistry: Molecular, cellular and medical aspects* (6th ed., pp. 119–138). Philadelphia: Lippincott Williams & Wilkins.

Landreth, G. E. (1999). Growth factors. In G. J. Siegel, B. W. Agranoff, R. W. Albers, S. K. Fisher, & M. D. Uhler (Eds.), *Basic neurochemistry: Molecular, cellular and medical aspects* (6th ed., pp. 383–400). Philadelphia: Lippincott Williams & Wilkins.

Lodish, H., Berk, A., Zipursky, S. L., Matsudaira, P., Baltimore, D., & Darnell, J. (2000). *Molecular cell biology* (4th ed.). New York: Freeman.

Nestler, E. J., & Duman, R. S. (1999). G proteins. In G. J. Siegel, B. W. Agranoff, R. W. Albers, S. K. Fisher, & M. D. Uhler (Eds.), *Basic neurochemistry: Molecular, cellular and medical aspects* (6th ed., pp. 401–414). Philadelphia: Lippincott Williams & Wilkins.

Nicoll, R. A. (1988). The coupling of neurotransmitter receptors to ion channels in the brain. *Science, 241,* 545–551.

Putney, J. W. Jr. (1999). Calcium. In G. J. Siegel, B. W. Agranoff, R. W. Albers, S. K. Fisher, & M. D. Uhler (Eds.), *Basic neurochemistry: Molecular, cellular and medical aspects* (6th ed., pp. 453–470). Philadelphia: Lippincott Williams & Wilkins.

Shepherd, G. M. (1994). *Neurobiology* (3rd ed.). New York: Oxford University Press.

4

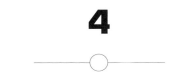

Neurotransmitters

I have examined the neuroanatomy of the brain and the mechanisms by which chemical neurotransmitters convey their messages to the interior of the neuron. The next step is to examine some of the major neurotransmitter systems believed to be involved in the genesis of mental disorders. For each of these neurotransmitter systems, several questions need to be answered:

1. Where in the brain is the neurotransmitter system located? What is its origin (where the cell bodies of the neurons are found) and to where do these axons project? The place in the brain where the neurotransmitter is released is the *terminal field*.
2. How many different types of receptors does the neurotransmitter bind to? Are these receptors ionotropic (directly influencing ion flow and affecting the probability of an action potential) or metabotropic (using second messengers to influence the long-term function of the neuron)?
3. What are the behavioral effects of neurotransmitter system activity in the brain? This last question is the most complex to answer, and in this chapter I lay the groundwork for understanding how dysfunction in neurotransmitter systems might lead to mental disorders.

GLUTAMATE

Glutamate is an amino acid that does not cross into the brain from the bloodstream. The brain synthesizes it from glucose and other nutrients. Glutamate is the principal excitatory neurotransmitter in the brain; even minute amounts of glutamate can trigger action potentials. Figure 4.1 shows the glutamate pathways in the brain.

Pathway (1) in the figure is one of the longest in the brain. The cell bodies originate in the cortex, and the axons descend through the internal capsule (the cleft between the putamen and caudate). The axons continue their descent and then branch off to the pons and to the red nucleus in the brain stem. Here they excite motor neurons that govern a wide variety of muscles. In the brain stem, these axons cross to the other side of the body (decussation) then proceed down the spinal cord. At each level of the spinal cord, they excite motor neurons that actually cause muscles to contract. Due to the decussation, a stroke on one side of the cortex will cause weakness on the opposite side of the body. Pathway (2) is equally important in governing motor behavior. These cell bodies also originate in the cortex and project to the neostriatum (caudate and putamen). Pathway (3) projects from the prefrontal cortex to the ventral striatum; this pathway is

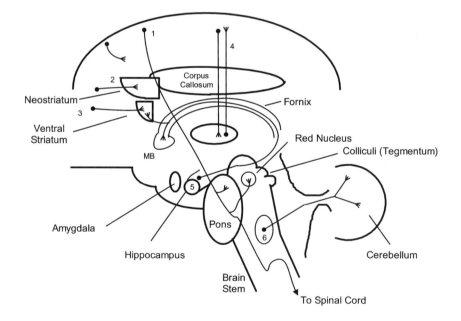

FIGURE 4.1. The glutamate pathways

key in our later study of the limbic system and behaviors related to reward-ing stimuli. Pathway (4) shows an excitatory "motor loop" between the cortex and the thalamus. These neurons excite each other, and this circuit is active while an ongoing motor activity is being executed. This "loop" must be interrupted for the ongoing motor activity to stop and a new ac-tion to be initiated. Information from the hippocampus uses a glutamate pathway; these axons project though the fornix to reach the mammillary body (5). This pathway is part of the Papez circuit examined in Chapter 2. A large number of glutamate neurons have cell bodies in the inferior olive of the brain stem (6), which project to the cerebellum. These neurons are involved in motor coordination. Finally, although they are not shown on the figure, neurons with long axons exchange information between hemi-spheres (transversing the corpus callosum) and between the various lobes within a hemisphere.

Figure 4.2 shows the wide variety of receptors that glutamate can bind to. Receptors are often named for the chemical that binds to the

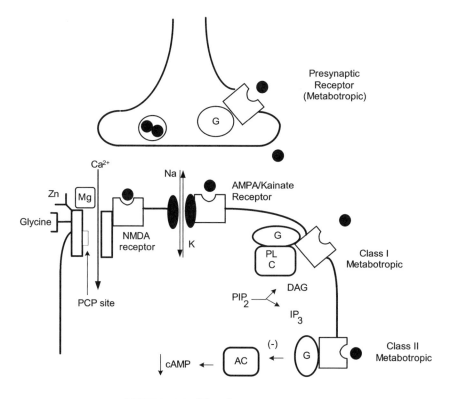

FIGURE 4.2. The glutamate receptors

receptor in the laboratory, even when these substances are not found in the brain. There are three types of ionotrophic glutamate receptors: α-amino-3-hydroxy-5-methylisoxazole-4-proprionic acid (AMPA), kainate, and N-methyl-D-aspartate (NMDA). The first two are very similar, and I discuss them as one. As shown in the figure, when glutamate binds to the AMPA/kainate receptor, it opens a ligand-gated ion channel, and Na^+ and K^+ are exchanged; this leads to the opening of voltage-gated Na^+ channels, and an action potential is triggered. The NMDA receptor is a most interesting ionotropic receptor. Calcium flows through the channel, where it will activate a series of neuronal enzymes. Several things must happen, however, before the channel will open and admit calcium. First, glutamate and the amino acid glycine must both bind to receptor sites, as shown in the figure. The metal zinc (Zn) can enhance the opening of the channel but is not required. Once glutamate and glycine open the channel, the calcium still cannot enter, because when the neuron is at rest, a magnesium (Mg) ion blocks the channel. It is only when the neuron has been depolarized by the action of sufficient AMPA/kainate receptors that the Mg ion "moves out of the way" and the calcium enters. This process turns out to be critical in learning and memory, as we shall see in Chapter 6. Also of interest to the study of schizophrenia and drug abuse, the drug phencyclidine (PCP) blocks the calcium from entering the neuron. PCP is a powerful hallucinogen; thus the NMDA receptor may play a role in the pathophysiology of psychosis.

Glutamate also binds to receptors that are metabotropic in nature. Class I glutamate metabotropic receptors use a G protein which activates PLC, cleaving PIP_2 into DAG and IP_3. Class II metabotropic receptors ultimately inhibit adenylyl cyclase (AC), which leads to a decrease in the amount of cAMP. The metabotropic receptors activate enzymes that phosphorylate the voltage-gated calcium channels in the neuron, deactivating them. Remember that the voltage-gated calcium channels cause the release of neurotransmitter, so the metabotropic receptors achieve the opposite of the AMPA/kainate receptors, that is, less excitability. Why should this be so? Perhaps this is a mechanism by which the neuron keeps itself from being overstimulated. Metabotropic receptors are also found presynaptically, where they also decrease the release of glutamate and thus regulate excitability.

GAMMA (γ)-AMINOBUTYRIC ACID

Gamma (γ)-aminobutyric acid (GABA) is synthesized from glutamate in the brain. It is the principal inhibitory neurotransmitter in the central nervous system. Its pathways are shown in Figure 4.3. Notice the large number of small neurons spread throughout the cortex (1). These small interneurons inhibit their target neurons from firing, thus maintaining the overall level of neuronal excitability at a manageable level. The "long" GABA pathways are complex. One pathway (2) originates in the neostriatum and terminates in the globus pallidus interna (GPi). These axons synapse on other GABA cell bodies in the GPi, which in turn project to the thalamus (3). Another set of GABA neurons leaves the neostriatum (4) and projects to the globus pallidus externa (GPe). Again, they synapse on GABA neurons in the GPe; these neurons (5) project to the subthalamic nucleus (STN). A GABA pathway (6) starts in the neostriatum and ends in the substantia nigra reticulata (SNr). From the SNr, GABA pathways (7) spread out to three locations: the thalamus, the superior colliculi, and the pedunculopontine nuclei (PPN). Parts of the thalamus, as we saw with the glutamate pathways, make up the motor circuitry. The superior colliculi are important for eye movements. The PPN helps govern the muscles of the trunk. The SNr is "tonically active," releasing GABA onto these structures, inhibiting their neurons. If the motor circuits of the thalamus, the colliculi, and the PPN are turned off, there is no movement. When a new movement is desired, the cortex and neostriatum work together to shut off the SNr, thus making the movement possible.

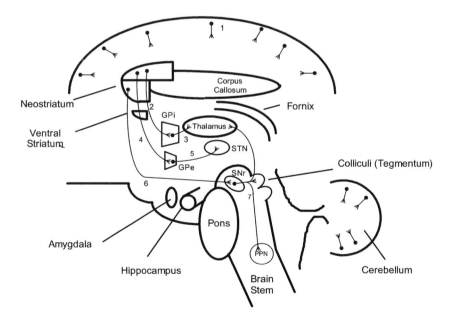

FIGURE 4.3. The GABA pathways

GABA has two receptors, $GABA_A$ and $GABA_B$. The $GABA_A$ receptor is ionotropic; the $GABA_B$ is metabotropic. As shown in the left side of Figure 4.4, the $GABA_A$ receptor is linked to a chloride channel. When GABA binds to the receptor, the channel is opened, and chloride can flow into the neuron. This increases the negative charge inside the neuron, hyperpolarizing it and making the neuron less likely to fire. The right side of Figure 4.4 shows the $GABA_A$ receptor in more detail. It is composed of five proteins. The site to which $GABA_A$ binds is found between the α and β subunits. Also part of the α subunit is the benzodiazepine site, where drugs such as diazepam (Valium) bind. When an antianxiety drug such as a benzodiazepine binds to this site, the GABA is more potent at opening the channel. Benzodiazepines are also potent anticonvulsants. If neurons are firing inappropriately during a seizure, benzodiazepines will enhance GABA's inhibitory effect, terminating the seizure. Inside the channel there is a site at which barbiturate drugs such as phenobarbital bind, also increasing the flow of chloride into the neuron. These drugs also have an anticonvulsant effect. There are multiple subtypes of these units. The α unit has six subtypes, the β four subtypes, and the γ three. $GABA_A$ receptors in different parts of the brain have varying α, β, and γ subunits; these subunits convey differing sensitivities to benzodiazepines.

$GABA_B$ receptors are metabotropic and inhibit adenylyl cyclase. As shown in Figure 3.9 in the Chapter 3, this would lead to reductions in cAMP, and with less phosphorylation of the potassium channels (due to less activity of PKA), there would be greater outflow of K^+. This, too, would hyperpolarize the neuron and decrease the firing rate, though on a longer time scale. $GABA_B$ receptors are found both pre- and post-synaptically.

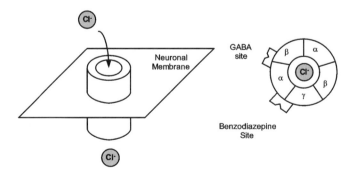

FIGURE 4.4. The $GABA_A$ receptor

ACETYLCHOLINE

Acetylcholine (Ach) is the neurotransmitter used by neurons that innervate the muscles. Stimulation of Ach receptors on muscles results in their contraction. Ach and norepinephrine are the principal neurotransmitters of the autonomic nervous system, which is examined at the end of this chapter. Within the brain, the role of Ach is less clear, though it quite likely plays critical roles in learning and alertness. Drugs that block Ach can produce deficits in cognition; in toxic doses they produce psychotic symptoms. These effects can be found with some psychotropics, such as the tricyclic antidepressants, as well as with a number of nonpsychiatric drugs. Ach central neurons deteriorate in Alzheimer's disease, although treating dementia with Ach agonists has met with mixed results. The diverse Ach pathways are shown in Figure 4.5. The first major pathway (1) originates in the dorsal tegmental area and projects to the thalamus. This pathway is part of the "reticular activating system," the array of inputs from the brain stem to the thalamus and cortex the

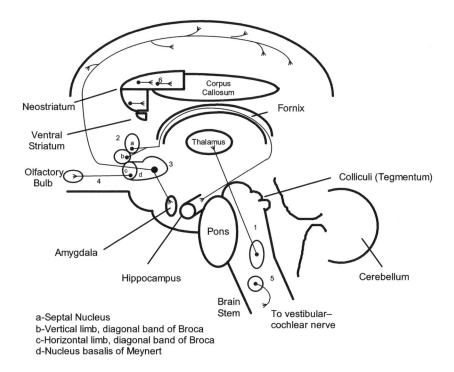

a-Septal Nucleus
b-Vertical limb, diagonal band of Broca
c-Horizontal limb, diagonal band of Broca
d-Nucleus basalis of Meynert

FIGURE 4.5. The acetylcholine pathways

govern the level of arousal and alertness. The second Ach pathway begins in the septal nucleus (2) and sends its axons through the fornix to reach the hippocampus (a). In Chapter 2 I discussed the role of the hippocampus in memory, and I return to this issue in depth in Chapter 6. These Ach inputs from the septal nucleus are critical in regulating the firing rhythm of the hippocampus. This may be part of the reason that deterioration of Ach cell bodies impairs memory in patients with Alzheimer's. Just ventral to the septal nucleus is a group of Ach neurons that together are called the Ach forebrain complex (3). These are the vertical limb of the diagonal band of Broca (b), the horizontal limb of the diagonal band of Broca (c), and, the largest of the three, the nucleus basalis of Meynert (d). These neurons send their axons through the cortex and also to the amygdala. Ach neurons project to the olfactory bulb (4), and brain stem Ach neurons project to the vestibular–cochlear nerve, which is important in balance (5). This is the reason anticholinergic drugs such as Dramamine are helpful in motion sickness. Finally, there are small Ach interneurons throughout the neostriatum; these are important in attenuating the Parkinsonian effects of the older antipsychotic medications.

When Ach is released from its neurons, it can bind to one of two major types of receptors—nicotinic and muscarinic. Nicotinic receptors are ionotropic. As with the AMPA/kainate glutamate receptors, when Ach binds to them, an ion channel is opened that ultimately leads to the firing of an action potential. Nicotinic receptors are found on the muscles and can activate action potentials within the brain, as well. In the brain and the autonomic nervous system, Ach also binds to muscarinic receptors that are metabotropic. G proteins that lead to a variety of actions are activated. Within the brain Ach can regulate the refractory period of the neuron through the activation of adenylyl cyclase and the phosphorylation of K channels. The neurons become more responsive to stimuli; perhaps this accounts for the greater arousal noted in an animal when the Ach system is active. To understand the action of Ach in the body, it is necessary to review the functions of the autonomic nervous system, as shown in Figure 4.6.

The autonomic nervous system governs many of the body's basic functions: heart rate, respiratory rate and volume, digestion, and sexual function, among others. It is subdivided into the parasympathetic and sympathetic systems. The parasympathetic system slows heart rate, enhances digestion and defecation, and, with sexual arousal, causes erection of the penis. It helps meet the body's physical needs. In contrast, the sympathetic nervous system increases heart rate, shifts blood flow away from the periphery and into the muscles, and inhibits digestion. Part of the sympathetic response involves the release of epinephrine (adrenaline) into the bloodstream. This is the "fight or flight" reaction. Sympathetic activa-

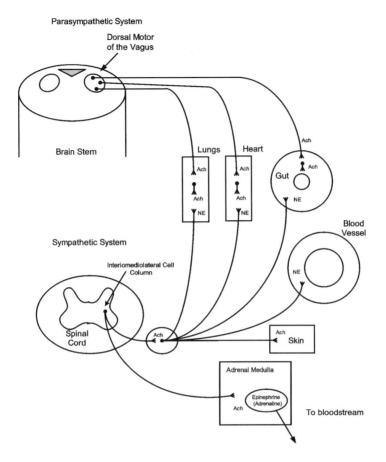

FIGURE 4.6. Overview of the sympathetic and parasympathetic nervous systems

tion leads to high arousal and the experience of agitation, anger, and/or anxiety. The top part of Figure 4.6 shows the parasympathetic nervous system. It is a two-neuron chain. Neurons in the dorsal motor nucleus of the brain stem send axons out into the vagus nerve, which travels, in different branches, to the heart, lungs, and gut. These are termed the "preganglionic" neurons, and they release Ach onto smaller "postganglionic" parasympathetic neurons. Ach binds to muscarinic receptors on these neurons, causing them in turn to release Ach onto muscarinic receptors on the heart, lungs, and gut. When this happens, heart rate is slowed, gut motility increases, and the bronchi are restricted. There are also preganglionic parasympathetic neurons in the sacral (lowest) area of the spinal cord; these project to the bladder, rectum, and sexual organs. These connections are not shown on the diagram.

The bottom part of Figure 4.6 shows the sympathetic nervous system (SNS). The preganglionic nerves have their origins in the middle part of the spinal cord, in a column of cells that run from just below the neck to above the sacrum. This is the intermediolateral (IML) cell column; from here the axons project to a line of ganglia along the outside of the spinal column, where they release Ach onto the second neuron in the sympathetic connection. The postganglionic neurons release the neurotransmitter norepinephrine (NE) onto muscles in the heart and blood vessels. This release causes heart rate to rise and blood vessels to constrict, and blood flows more readily to muscles. NE is released onto the bronchi of the lungs, causing them to open up so the person can breathe more deeply and get more oxygen to the blood. (Asthma inhalers mimic the effect of NE in the lungs.) The IML also sends Ach neurons to the adrenal medulla (the adrenal glands sits atop the kidney), and here Ach causes the release of epinephrine (EPI; adrenaline) into the blood stream. EPI, too, increases heart rate and causes constriction of blood vessels.

NOREPINEPHRINE

The first thing to bear in mind regarding NE is that it is found peripherally in both the SNS and within the brain. Figure 4.7 (top) shows the complex projections of the central NE system. The cell bodies of most NE neurons in the brain are found in the locus coeruleus (LC) in the brain stem. From here the axons of NE neurons project to many different areas of the brain. Some travel down to the spinal cord, where they synapse on neurons that are receiving sensory information from the skin and internal organs. LC neurons do not communicate directly with the IML. NE neurons project to the pons and cerebellum, but their most important projections are to the cortex, and these projections are very widespread. In Figure 4.7, the size and darkness of the circles represent the densities of the cortical NE projections. NE neurons are most dense in the primary somatosensory cortex, but LC neurons strongly innervate the frontal lobes. LC neurons also project to the temporal cortex, although this is not shown in the figure. LC neurons branch off to enter the fornix and stria terminalis that lead to the hippocampus and amygdala, respectively. These structures also receive NE input via smaller, direct branches, as shown in the figure. Finally, NE neurons from the LC project to the dorsal raphe, where serotonin cell bodies are found. Thus NE plays a role in governing the output of the serotonin system.

The LC is not the only source of NE within the brain. A second set of NE-containing neurons is found just below (caudally to) the LC.

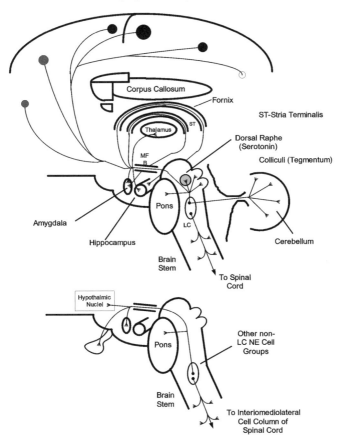

FIGURE 4.7. The norepinephrine pathways

These NE neurons project to the spinal cord, where they synapse on the IML, influencing the SNS directly. These neurons also project to the hypothalamus, where they help regulate "releasing factors," molecules that travel to the pituitary and regulate a wide variety of hormones. This structure is shown in the bottom part of Figure 4.7.

NE has a variety of receptors that it can bind to; divided broadly into α and β categories, they are further divided into subtypes, as shown in Table 4.1. The table shows their different second messenger systems. None of the NE receptors are ionotropic; all are metabotropic. α_1 and β receptors are found only on the postsynaptic neuron, whereas α_2 receptors are found both pre- and postsynatically. Presynaptically, α_2 recep-

TABLE 4.1. Norepinephrine Receptors and Their Actions

	Alpha receptors						Beta receptors		
	α_{1A}	α_{1B}	α_{1D}	α_{2A}	α_{2B}	α_{2C}	β_1	β_2	β_3
Second messenger system	?	↑IP$_3$	Open Ca channels	Inhibit adenylyl cyclase			Activate adenylyl cyclase		
Location in brain				Frontal cortex	Brain stem		Varies from one area of brain to another		
Location in body (PNS)	Blood vessels; leads to contraction			Platelets; enhances clotting	?	?	Heart[a]	Liver[b] Lungs[c]	Fat tissue[d]
Pre-/postsynaptic	Postsynaptic			Both pre- and postsynaptic; presynaptic receptors decrease NE release					
Human chromosome	2	5	8	10	2	4	10	5	8

[a]NE in bloodstream increases heart rate.
[b]NE leads to increase in blood sugar (glucose).
[c]NE opens bronchi in lungs, increases oxygenation of blood.
[d]Breakdown of fat.

tors, when stimulated by NE, reduce NE release and LC firing. Figure 4.8 shows NE receptors in both the brain and the periphery.

What is the role of such a wide distribution of NE neurons? Barry Jacobs has summarized studies of the functioning of LC in cats. In these experiments, an electrode is inserted (under anesthesia) into the brain stem of a cat in order to record the firing of the LC neurons. The cat awakes and behaves normally. (Because the tissue of the brain itself feels no pain, the procedure bothers the cat very little.) During sleep, the LC is essentially turned off. When an animal is awake, the LC fires at a very slow rate; but if a novel stimulus appears in the environment, it fires a volley of action potentials. If the stimuli are repeated and have no significance for the animal, the LC stops firing after several repetitions of the stimulus. When the animal is grooming or eating, the LC also decreases its firing rate. If a predator appears, the LC fires vigorously, and plasma NE rises. It may not be threat per se but rather any signal that is part of a learned scenario that triggers the LC—the stimuli signals that something is about to happen, based on past experience.

Marius Usher, Gary Aston-Jones, and colleagues have presented a model of LC function based on the activity of LC neurons in awake primates, applying a technology similar to that used in the cat studies just described. Monkeys learned to press a switch when a target appeared and were rewarded with a drink of juice. Nontargets also appeared on the screen, and the monkey had to learn not to press the switch. (This task is similar to the continuous performance test, a measure on which individuals with ADHD often do poorly.) They found that as the monkeys learned the task, the LC fired in response to the target, but that it ceased to fire when the distractors appeared. The LC also responded when the reward appeared. This quick bursting of the LC in response to stimuli is referred to as the "phasic activity." Usher and colleagues also measured the ongoing activity of the LC in between the appearance of the stimuli. They found the baseline activity of the LC varied. The monkey's best performance was obtained when the LC baseline activity was low and phasic bursts were associated with the targets. In contrast, if the LC baseline activity was high, the monkeys made many more false alarms. Usher and Aston-Jones suggested that LC activity showed a U-shaped relationship to attention. At very low levels of tonic LC activity,

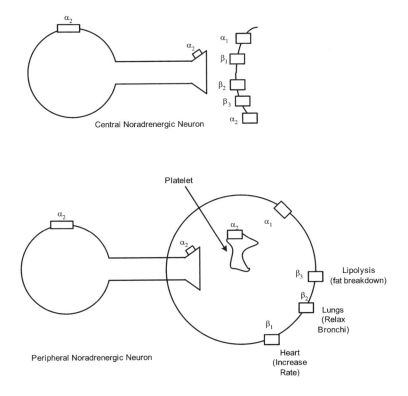

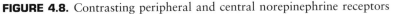

FIGURE 4.8. Contrasting peripheral and central norepinephrine receptors

the animal is sedated and inattentive and not responsive to the environment. At moderate levels of NE activity, the animal is alert, and the LC responds crisply to stimuli in the environment that are novel or have meaning. At high levels of LC activity, the animal becomes very aroused and responds to multiple (and perhaps irrelevant) events in the environment.

What does NE do to its target neurons? I showed in Chapter 3 that NE can enhance the "signal to noise" ratio for neurons. That is, the baseline activity of the targeted neuron declines, and it becomes more responsive to input. Thus part of NE activity may help "tune" the neurons to help them process and prioritize incoming information about the current state of the world. This is not the whole story, however. LC projections to the amygdala and hippocampus probably play a major role in fear and anxiety modulation and in memory (Chapters 5 and 6). NE input to the cortex plays a role in working memory and executive function (Chapter 7).

To fully comprehend how the NE system is involved in the brain's reaction to stimuli in the environment, we must understand how the central NE system and the SNS work together, even though there are no direct anatomical links between them. Figure 4.9 shows this relationship.

Information about external stimuli in the environment reaches the brain through vision, hearing and touch (somatosensory function). This information is integrated in the cortex to form our perception of the world. When stimuli are being sent to the cortex, the brain stem is alerted as well; neurons within the paragigantocellularis (PGi) are activated (1). The PGi has projections both to the LC (2) and to the spinal cord, where it activates the IML (3). The SNS is activated. The LC projects throughout the cortex, as we saw in Figure 4.7. As described previously, the stimuli might be associated with some experience. For instance, an animal might recognize a predator. The animal will be ready because the SNS has been activated already by the PGi. On the other, the stimulus might be meaningless, so the IML should be turned off. How would this happen?

Note the position of the hypothalamus in this circuit. It is receiving information from the prefrontal cortex and the cingulate gyrus (4). The prefrontal cortex may be responding to the stimuli in light of long-term plans, as opposed to immediate needs. The cingulate, along with the amygdala and hippocampus, accesses past memories about the stimulus, as well the relevance of the stimulus to current biological needs. The hypothalamus is also receiving information from the nucleus tractus solitarius (NTS). The NTS is in touch with the biological state of the body (fluid balance, glucose level, etc.). All of this information is weighted at the hypothalamus (5), which can send two major outputs

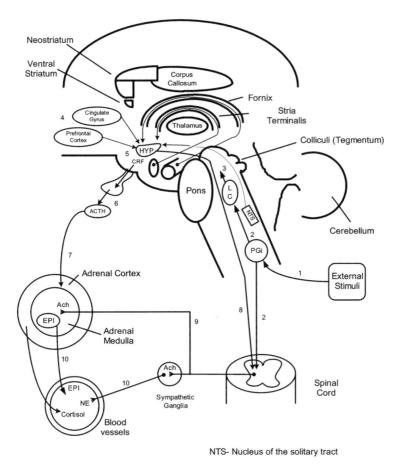

FIGURE 4.9. The norepinephrine system and the stress response

that govern the stress response. First, it releases corticotropin releasing factor (CRF) to the pituitary, and the pituitary responds by releasing adrenocorticotropic hormone (ACTH) (6). ACTH travels through the bloodstream to the adrenal medulla, where it causes the medulla to release cortisol. The hypothalamus also projects directly to the IML (7), where the SNS can be activated directly. EPI (adrenaline) is released into the bloodstream. The fight-or-flight reaction can begin.

In anxiety disorders, this circuitry may be too easily triggered. CRF, injected artificially, is a powerful anxiety-producing agent, and drugs that block the effects of CRF may be good antianxiety agents. Darlene Francis, Michael Meany and a group of investigators at McGill University have studied the NE system in mother rats in the postpartum period. During the first weeks of life, mother rats groom and lick their pups; if this does not occur (i.e., maternal neglect), the baby rats develop a hyperresponsive CRF–ACTH system. The "neglected" baby rats also produce greater activation of the SNS in response to stress. I return to this theme in Chapter 11.

DOPAMINE SYSTEM

Dopamine cell bodies are located primarily in two major groupings, shown in Figure 4.10. The first is the substantia nigra compacta (SNc). The axons of these neurons project to the striatum (1); this route is termed the "nigrostriatal pathway." Parkinson's disease is related to a deterioration of the SNc neurons. In Chapter 5 I show how a loss of dopamine input to the neostriatum can lead to the symptoms of Parkinson's: rigidity of muscles and slow movements (bradykinesia). The second major grouping is the ventral tegmental area (VTA). The axons of these neurons travel forward through the median forebrain bundle and then spread out to innervate two regions: the prefrontal cortex and the ventral striatum (2). These two routes are the mesocorticol and mesolimbic dopamine pathways, respectively. Many pharmacology textbooks display rat brains in which dopamine projects only to the prefrontal cortex. In primates (including humans), dopamine projections are much more widespread. As shown in Figure 4.10, the densest dopamine projections are to the primary motor cortex, although the other frontal areas are strongly innervated as well. Virtually no dopamine is found in the primary somatosensory cortex (where NE was at its densest), and very little is found in the occipital cortex. We do find substantial dopamine projections to the parietal and temporal lobes. DA and NE also innervate different levels of the cortex. NE neurons project to deeper layers of the cortex, DA to areas closer to the surface of the brain.

The projections from the VTA to the ventral striatum are of particular interest to the study of drug abuse and addiction. This pathway has some interesting properties in animals. As we saw in the studies of the LC, a very thin electrode can be inserted into a rat's brain such that its end is placed in the VTA. Once the animal recovers from the surgery, it roams its cage. The electrode is connected to a lever; when the animal presses the lever, the electrode stimulates the VTA-ventral striatum pathway. This causes action potentials to be fired in the axons, and dopamine is released into the nucleus accumbens (a subset of neurons within the ventral striatum). The rat finds this rewarding and will continue to press the bar to receive the stimulation.

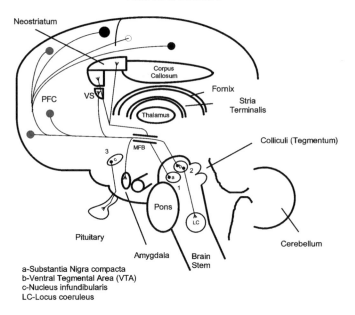

Neostriatum

Corpus
Callosum

Fornix

PFC VS

Stria
Terminalis

Thalamus

Colliculi (Tegmentum)

3 MFB

2

1

Pons

LC

Pituitary

Cerebellum

Amygdala   Brain
Stem

a-Substantia Nigra compacta
b-Ventral Tegmental Area (VTA)
c-Nucleus infundibularis
LC-Locus coeruleus

FIGURE 4.10. The dopamine pathways

Another type of experiment can be done with rats. A very thin glass tube can be inserted directly into the nucleus accumbens. These rats will then press levers that directly release cocaine into the accumbens. The cocaine blocks the reuptake of dopamine, increasing the amount of dopamine in the accumbens. Thus the VTA–accumbens pathway is a critical aspect of the brain's reward circuitry. Understanding its function may lead to clues as to why some individuals are more prone to drug abuse and addiction. The smallest of the dopamine pathways is the tuberoinfundibular (3). The axons of these neurons release dopamine into the pituitary, where the dopamine inhibits the release of the hormone prolactin. In females, prolactin promotes breast development; in males, its role is unclear. Older antipsychotic drugs block dopamine receptors in the pituitary, leading to an increase in prolactin. In females treated with this drug, this can sometimes lead to unwanted production of milk (galactorrhea) in a small number of patients. Finally there is a small dopamine pathway from the VTA to the cerebellar vermis. The vermis is a midline structure in the cerebellum that is important in regulating emotional arousal. I examine this structure, later as it is one of many suggested to be involved in ADHD.

There are five subtypes of dopamine receptors, as shown in Table 4.2. They are divided into two families. The "D_1 family" consists of the

TABLE 4.2. Dopamine Receptors

	D_1	D_2	D_3	D_4	D_5
Second messenger system	Activate adenylyl cyclase	Inhibit adenylyl cyclase			Activate adenylyl cyclase
Location in brain	Neo- and ventral striatum, cortex?	Neo- and ventral striatum	Ventral striatum, hypothalamus	Frontal cortex, medulla, midbrain	Hippocampus, hypothalamus
Pre-/postsynaptic	Postsynaptic	Both pre- and postsynaptic	Postsynaptic	Postsynaptic	Postsynaptic
Human chromosome	5	11	3	11	4
Affinity for dopamine[a]	2,000	2,000	30	450	250

[a]The smaller the number, the more tightly dopamine binds to the receptor.

D_1 and D_5 receptors. Both of these receptors are linked to G proteins that stimulate adenylyl cyclase. In contrast, the D_2, D_3, and D_4 receptors are linked to G proteins that inhibit adenylyl cyclase and that are referred to as the "D_2 family." The dopamine receptors have very different distributions in the brain. D_1 and D_2 are found almost predominantly in the neostriatum, whereas D3 receptors are found in the nucleus accumbens, where they may play a significant role in the pleasure circuit described previously. D_3 receptors are the most sensitive, requiring less dopamine to trigger them than the others. The D_1 and D_4 receptors are found in the cortex, and D_5 in the hypothalamus and the hippocampus.

Dopamine's role in the brain appears related to motor behavior and action. If dopamine is depleted from the SNc, we lose our ability to initiate movement. In monkeys, dopamine neurons in the SNc fire just before the neurons in the frontal lobe whenever a learned motor movement is about to be executed. If dopamine receptors in the frontal cortex of monkeys are blocked, the monkeys' ability to plan motor movements and keep the location of an object in mind is disrupted.

SEROTONIN

Figure 4.11 shows the diverse pathways of the serotonin (5-hydroxytryptamine, or 5-HT) system. Serotonin, as a neurotransmitter, appeared very early in evolution. It is found in the nervous system of the sea slug

(*Aplysia*), where it plays a role in the animal's memory: Serotonin facilitated the withdrawal of the creature's gill in response to an event that had been previously associated with a noxious stimuli. Serotonin neurons influence the leech's ability to swim through the water and latch onto a warm body. I provide these examples to illustrate the fact that serotonin must play some crucial role in the nervous system if it appeared so early in evolution and had been conserved in higher animals, including humans. Serotonin is widely distributed in the brain stem. I am concerned here with the three major nuclei termed "raphe." The dorsal (a) and median (b) raphe project to a wide variety of areas in the brain. The dorsal raphe (dotted line) proceeds through the median forebrain bundle, but before doing so it innervates the dopamine-containing neurons of the SNc and the VTA, thus influencing the output of the dopamine system. It projects to the striatum (both caudate–putamen and ventral striatum) and the entire cortex. The median raphe also sends its projections through the median forebrain bundle. Separate projections then proceed through the stria terminalis and the fornix to reach the amygdala and hippocampus, respectively. The median raphe also projects to

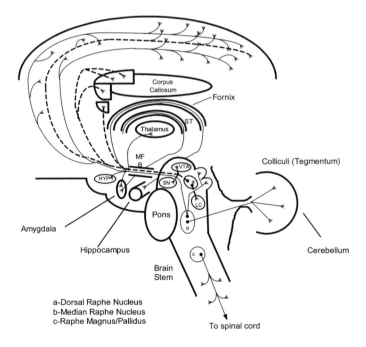

FIGURE 4.11. The serotonin pathways

the cortex, as well as the superior colliculi and cerebellum. There are serotonin inputs to the hypothalamus, particularly to a subset of this area,
the nucleus suprachiasmaticus. This nucleus is critical in regulating circadian rhythm, such as the sleep–wake cycle.

The raphe magnus/pallidus (c) projects downward (caudally) to the
spinal cord, where it modulates sensory input. It may play a role here in
"gating" pain stimuli, and thus drugs that affect serotonin often play a
role in pain management. These serotonin neurons also synapse on motor neurons, so serotonin clearly plays a role in movement, particularly
in setting the strength of reflexes. Finally, these serotonin neurons also
synapse on the IML, thus playing a role in the output of the SNS.

A dizzying array of serotonin receptor subtypes exists, as shown in
Table 4.3. A group of scientists, known informally as the "serotonin club,"
meet and discuss all the different ways the 14 known subtypes should be
labeled. 5-HT_1 receptors all inhibit adenylyl cyclase, whereas 5-HT_2 receptors all increase IP_3 and DAG through phospholipase C. The 5-HT_3
receptor is the only ionotropic receptor; all the others are metabotropic.
All of the receptor subtypes are widely distributed in the brain.

The function of the serotonin system is as complex as its distribution. In humans, it has been implicated in depression, anxiety, aggressive
behavior, obesity and other eating disorders, migraine, sexual dysfunction, and chronic pain. Drugs that affect serotonin are often helpful in
all these conditions. Obviously, this system influences a wide variety of
brain and bodily functions. One clue to serotonin's function is its relationship to, and its differences from, the NE and dopamine systems. LC
neurons play a role in modulating attention and working memory. The
dopamine system has as one of its key functions the modulation of motor behavior. The serotonin system sits in between these systems. NE
projects to the raphe, where it can activate the serotonin system through
α_1 postsynaptic receptors. Serotonin, in turn, projects to the VTA and
SN, where it strongly influences the release of dopamine into the brain.
NE enhances the effect of sensory input on the brain, but when serotonin is released onto the cortical neurons, they become less responsive to
input. Thus serotonin may play a role in deciding when sufficient time
has been spent processing information and a "hand-off" to the motor
systems is needed. Dopamine in turn can facilitate action. Serotonergic
neurons project not only to the cell bodies of the VTA and SN, but to the
ends of the dopamine axons. This makes the effect of serotonin on dopamine neurons complex. In some situations, serotonin may inhibit the release of dopamine neurons complex. In other situations, serotonin may
inhibit the release of dopamine, but at least in humans it appears to enhance serotonin release. There are very strong correlations between the

TABLE 4.3. Serotonin Receptors

Serotonin receptor	Receptor subtype	Second messenger system	Location in brain	Pre-/ postsynaptic	Human chromosome
5-HT$_1$	1A	Inhibit adenylyl cyclase	Hippocampus, amygdala, entorhinal cortex	Both pre- and postsynaptic	5
	1B		?		?
	1D		?		1
	1E		Cortex?		?
	1F		Cortex, striatum, hippocampus		3
5-HT$_2$	2A	Increase IP$_3$ and DAG	Cortex, neo- and ventral striatum	Postsynaptic	13
	2B		Throughout	?	2
	2C		Choroid plexus, cortex, globus pallidus, substantia nigra, spinal cord	?	X
5-HT$_3$	ionotropic	None	Hippocampus, entorhinal cortex, amygdala, ventral striatum, spinal cord, GI tract	Postsynaptic	?
5-HT$_4$		Activate adenylyl cyclase	?		?
5-HT$_5$	5A	Inhibit adenylyl cyclase	?		7
	5B	?			2
5-HT$_6$		?			?
5-HT$_7$			Cortex, thalamus, hypothalamus, amygdala, superior colliculus		10

levels of dopamine and serotonin metabolites in the cerebrospinal fluid. When humans are administered the drug fenfluramine, it causes a release of serotonin. Positron emission tomography (PET) studies in normal volunteers show that this increase in serotonin also causes a release in dopamine. Volunteers are given radioactive raclopride, which binds to dopamine receptors. The PET study shows how much raclopride is attached to the receptor. When the fenfluramine is given, the amount of raclopride bound to the receptor declines, because the higher amount of newly released dopamine competes with the raclopride for a place on the receptor. The differing effects of serotonin on dopamine release will be important to keep in mind when we study the actions of antipsychotic medications in Chapter 12. In the spinal cord, serotonin increases the excitability of motor neurons so they can react more quickly to a stimulus. Serotonin may facilitate action through activation of the dopamine system. Serotonin, through its influence on the hypothalamus, also governs feeding, sleeping, and many vegetative functions. Thus serotonin is likely to be involved not only in depressive disorders (in which sleep and appetite are disturbed) but also in impulse control disorders, sitting as it does between taking in information (the NE system) and taking action on that information (the dopamine system). Jeffery Gray and Neil McVaughton have suggested that the NE–serotonin system is part of a "behavioral inhibition system," that is, a brain mechanism tuned to responding to fear- or anxiety-producing stimuli. In contrast, dopamine pathways are suggested to be part of a "behavioral activation system" designed to seek out pleasurable stimuli (or engage in active escape from harmful stimuli). Adaptive behavior depends on a balance between fearful, inhibited behavior and active, pleasure-seeking activities. Serotonin may play a particular role in achieving this balance. This idea becomes clearer in later chapters that examine its role in depression, anxiety and aggression.

PEPTIDES

I now take up a very different set of neurotransmitters, the peptides. Rather than small molecules, peptides are chains of amino acids. The neurotransmitters studied so far are released and act only within the synaptic cleft of the neuron; they do not diffuse throughout the brain. They are rapidly broken down or taken back up into the neuron to quickly terminate their action. In contrast, peptides can diffuse and act at sites in the brain away from their release site, although, like classical neurotransmitters, they have receptors that are also highly localized. Sometimes, the peptide is released along with a conventional neurotransmitter. Whereas the small chemical neurotransmitter acts rapidly, as described previously, the effects of the peptide are more prolonged. There are scores of peptides. CRF, mentioned earlier, is one of these. Cholecystokinin, which was originally found in the gut and is involved in digestion, is also found in the brain. It may be involved in panic attacks. I return to it in Chapter 11. For now I focus on the endogenous opiates, substance P, and oxytocin. I introduce others in later chapters.

The pain-reducing and addictive potentials of morphine, heroin, and other opiate drugs are well known. The brain produces three natural, or endogenous opiates of its own: β-endorphin, enkephalin, and dynorphin. Small neurons that release these substances are found throughout the brain and spinal cord. In the spinal cord, they are concentrated in the pain-receiving area. Enkephalin and dynorphin neurons are found in the caudate putamen, from which they project to the globus pallidus; in these neurons the peptides are coreleased with GABA. The endogenous opiates bind to three types of receptors: δ (delta), κ (kappa), and μ (mu). β-endorphin and morphine bind most tightly to the μ receptor, whereas dynorphin binds strongly to the κ receptor. The enkephalins have greater affinity for the δ receptors. All of the endogenous opiate receptors inhibit adenylyl cyclase.

Recently, a chemical called [11^C]carfentanil has been developed. This positron-emitting substance can be injected safely into humans, and it binds to μ receptors in the brain so that they can be visualized on a PET scan. Jon-Kar Zubieta and colleagues performed PET scans on 20 human volunteers while they were exposed to painful stimuli; the participants also rated the amount of pain they were in. Opiate receptor activation during painful stimuli was found in many regions, including the anterior cingulate, prefrontal cortex, thalamus, and hypothalamus. Interestingly, the amount of opiate receptor activation correlated with how intensely the participants experienced pain. The greater the opiate receptor activation in the nucleus accumbens, amygdala, anterior cingulate, and thalamus, the less intense the participants rated the pain. This raises the interesting question of whether people with lower levels of opiate receptor activation would have a lower tolerance for pain. The opiate system will be discussed more fully in Chapter 10.

Substance P is a peptide that was discovered in the 1930s. It was extracted from gut tissues as a dry powder, so the discovers called it "P" in their notebooks. Although it was first discovered in intestines, it was later found in the nervous system, where it plays a major role in transmitting pain signals. Skin trauma triggers the firing of substance P neurons that terminate in the spinal cord. Chili peppers contain capsaicin, which stimulates the release of substance P. Within the brain substance P neurons project from the caudate putamen to the globus pallidus (similar to the enkephalins/dynorphins); they are also found throughout the brain as small interneurons. Substance P is involved not only in pain but also in the regulation of attachment behavior. Mark Kramer and colleagues injected agonists of substance P into guinea pigs, causing them to make vocalizations similar to those the animals make when under stress. When guinea pigs are separated from their mothers, they normally make distress calls. These calls are eliminated if the animals are infused with antagonists of substance P. In a clinical trial with depressed patients, a substance P antagonist drug was found to be an effective antidepressant.

Oxytocin neurons were first found in the hypothalamus, from which they project to the posterior pituitary. When oxytocin is released in pregnant females, it initiates uterine contractions, and it also triggers milk ejection in nursing mothers. The sound of a crying infant causes hypothalamic neurons to release oxytocin. Oxytocin is found in males, as well, and it has been show to play a role in bonding and sexual behavior. Carmichael and colleagues had human participants engage in sexual intercourse while blood oxytocin levels were assessed. There was a positive correlation between the number and intensity of orgasms and plasma oxytocin levels in both males and females. Prairie voles (a type of rodent), who are monogamous and who engage in high levels of maternal behavior with their offspring, have much higher oxytocin receptor density than species of voles who are polygamous. Again, it must be emphasized that there are many more brain peptides than can be covered in this book.

GROWTH FACTORS

The final group of neurotransmitters I consider are the growth factors. Growth factors are also peptides; they transmit their signals to the neuron via the tyrosine kinase receptor (TKR) system that was reviewed in Chapter 3. Growth factors can be produced by support cells (glia) of the nervous system, as well as by neurons themselves. As their name implies, they are critical early in development for neuronal division and growth, but they continue to be important throughout the life of the animal in preventing neuronal death. We are particularly interested in a subgroup of the growth factors, the neurotrophins, which support the differentiation and survival of specific subsets of neurons. These neurotrophins are nerve growth factor (NGF), brain-derived neurotrophic factor (BDNF), and neurotrophins 3 (NT3) and 4/5 (NT 4/5). Neurotrophins may be released from anywhere in the brain. Often the postsynaptic neuron will release a neurotrophin back onto its presynaptic neuron. NGF is needed for sympathetic neurons to develop in the fetal period and to be maintained throughout life. NGF is also found in the cortex and hippocampus, as well as in the forebrain cholinergic neurons. BDNF supports outgrowth of axons from both dopamine and Ach neurons. Higher levels of neuronal activity stimulate release of BDNF. Mice that cannot produce BDNF die within a few weeks of birth, and animals who are living in high-stress environments produce lower levels of BDNF; these animals also show a shrinking of their hippocampi. These "brain-nurturing" chemicals are further examined in Chapter 11 on stress and anxiety disorders.

SUMMARY

This chapter has shown where some of the major neurotransmitter systems are located. We also glimpsed how the various neurotransmitter systems operate. In the next three chapters, I take up specific behaviors. Chapter 5 looks at motor behavior, as well as how we respond to rewarding stimuli. Chapter 6 discusses memory and emotion, and Chapter 7 examines language, attention, and executive function. Then, in Part II, we see how these functions might be disturbed in mental disorders.

REFERENCES

Agren, H., Mefford, I. N., Rudorfer, M. V., Linnoila, M., & Potter, W. Z. (1986). Interacting neurotransmitter systems: A non-experimental approach to the 5-HIAA-HVA correlation in human CSF. *Journal of Psychiatric Research, 20,* 175–193.

Anisman, H., Zaharia, M. D., Meaney, M. J., & Merali, Z. (1998). Do early-life events permanently alter behavioral and hormonal responses to stressors? *International Journal of Developmental Neuroscience, 16,* 149–164.

Arnsten, A. F. T. (1998). Catecholamine modulation of prefrontal cortical cognitive function. *Trends in Cognitive Sciences, 2,* 436–447.

Aston-Jones, G., Rajkowski, J., & Cohen, J. (1999). Role of locus coeruleus in attention and behavioral flexibility. *Biological Psychiatry, 46,* 1309–1320.

Caldji, C., Francis, D., Sharma, S., Plotsky, P. M., & Meaney, M. J. (2000). The effects of early rearing environment on the development of $GABA_A$ and central benzodiazepine receptor levels and novelty-induced fearfulness in the rat. *Neuropsychopharmacology, 22,* 219–229.

Carmichael, C. M., Warburton, V. L., Dixen, J., & Davidson, J. M. (1994). Relationships among cardiovascular, muscular and oxytocin responses during human sexual activity. *Archives of Sexual Behavior, 23,* 59–77.

Dingledine, R., & McBain, C. J. (1999). Glutamate and aspartate. In G. J. Siegel, B. W. Agranoff, R. W. Albers, S. K. Fisher, & M. D. Uhler (Eds.), *Basic neurochemistry: Molecular, cellular and medical aspects* (6th ed., pp. 315–334). Philadelphia: Lippincott Williams & Wilkins.

Francis, D. D., Caldji, C., Champagne, F., Plotsky, P. M., & Meaney, M. J. (1999). The role of corticotropin-releasing factor-norepinephrine systems in mediating the effects of early experience on the development of behavioral and endocrine responses to stress. *Biological Psychiatry, 46,* 1153–1166.

Francis, D. D., Champagne, F. A., Liu, D., & Meaney, M. J. (1999). Maternal care, gene expression, and the development of individual differences in stress reactivity. *Annals of the New York Academy of Sciences, 896,* 66–84.

Francis, D. D., & Meaney, M. J. (1999). Maternal care and the development of stress responses. *Current Opinion in Neurobiology, 9,* 128–134.

Frazer, A. & Hensler, J. G. (1999). Serotonin. In G. J. Siegel (Ed.), *Basic neurochemistry: Molecular, cellular and medical aspects* (6th ed., pp. 263–292). Philadelphia: Lippincott Williams & Wilkins.

Gray, J. A. (2000). *The neuropsychology of anxiety: An enquiry into the functions of the septo-hippocampal system* (2nd ed.). New York: Oxford University Press.

Hough, L. B. (1999). Histamine. In G. J. Siegel (Ed.), *Basic neurochemistry: Molecular, cellular and medical aspects* (6th ed., pp. 293–314). Philadelphia: Lippincott Williams & Wilkins.

Jacobs, B. L. (1990). Locus coerulus neuronal activity in behaving animals. In D. J. Heal & C. A. Marsden (Eds.), *The pharmacology of noradrenaline in the central nervous system* (pp. 248–265). Oxford, UK: Oxford Medical Press.

Kramer, M. S., Cutler, N., Feighner, J., Shrivastava, R., Carman, J., Sramek, J. J., et al. (1998). Distinct mechanism for antidepressant activity by blockade of central substance p receptors. *Science, 281,* 1640–1645.

Kuhar, M. J., Couceyro, P. R., & Lambert, P. D. (1999). Catecholamines. In G. J. Siegel (Ed.), *Basic neurochemistry: Molecular, cellular and medical aspects* (6th ed., pp. 243–262). Philadelphia: Lippincott Williams & Wilkins.

Lewis, D. A. (2001). The catecholamine innervation of primate cerebral cortex. In M. V. Solanto, A. F. T. Arnsten, & F. X. Castellanos (Eds.), *Stimulant drugs and ADHD basic and clinical neuroscience* (pp. 77–103). New York: Oxford University Press.

Lieberman, J. A., Mailman, R. B., Duncan, G., Sikich, L., Chakos, M., Nichols, D. E., & Kraus, J. E. (1998). Serotonergic basis of antipsychotic drug effects in schizophrenia. *Biological Psychiatry, 44,* 1099–1117.

Mansour, A., Meador-Woodruff, J. H., Lopez, J. F., & Watson, S. J. (1998). Biochemical anatomy: Insights into the cell biology and pharmacology of the dopamine and serotonin systems in the brain. In A. F. Schatzberg & C. B. Nemeroff (Eds.), *Psychopharmacology* (2nd ed., pp. 55–74). Washington, DC: American Psychiatric Press.

Nieuwenhuys, R. (1985). *Chemoarchitecture of the brain.* New York: Springer-Verlag.

Olsen, R. W., & DeLorey, T. M. (1999). GABA and glycine. In G. J. Siegel, B. W. Agranoff, R. W. Albers, S. K. Fisher, & M. D. Uhler (Eds.), *Basic neurochemistry: Molecular, cellular and medical aspects* (6th ed., pp. 335–346). Philadelphia: Lippincott Williams & Wilkins.

Penny, J. B. (1996). Neurochemical neuroanatomy. In B. S. Fogel, R. B. Schiffer,

& S. M. Rao (Eds.), *Neuropsychiatry* (pp. 145–171). Baltimore: Williams & Wilkins.

Pliszka, S. R. (2001). Comparing the effects of stimulant and non-stimulant agents on catecholamine function: Implications for theories of ADHD. In M. V. Solanto, A. F. T. Arnsten, & F. X. Castellanos (Eds.), *Stimulant drugs and ADHD basic and clinical neuroscience* (pp. 332–352). New York: Oxford University Press.

Smith, G. S., Dewey, S. L., Brodie, J. D., Logan, J., Vitkun, S. A., Simkowitz, P., et al. (1997). Serotonergic modulation of dopamine measured with (11C) raclopride and PET in normal human subjects. *American Journal of Psychiatry, 154*, 490–496.

Soubrie, P. (1986). Reconciling the role of central serotonin neurons in human and animal behavior. *Behavioral and Brain Sciences, 9*, 319–364.

Spoont, M. R. (1992). Modulatory role of serotonin in neural information processing: Implications for human psychopathology. *Psychological Bulletin, 112*, 330–350.

Squire, L. R. (1992). Memory and the hippocampus: A synthesis from findings with rats, monkeys, and humans. *Psychological Review, 99*, 195–231.

Squire, L. R., & Kandel, E. R. (1999). *Memory: From mind to molecules.* New York: Freeman.

Taylor, P., & Brown, J. H. (1999). Acetylcholine. In G. J. Siegel, B. W. Agranoff, R. W. Albers, S. K. Fisher, & M. D. Uhler (Eds.), *Basic neurochemistry: Molecular cellular and medical aspects* (6th ed., pp. 213–242). Philadelphia: Lippincott Williams & Wilkins.

Usher, M., Cohen, J. D., Servan-Schreiber, D., Rajkowski, J., & Aston-Jones, G. (1999). The role of locus coeruleus in the regulation of cognitive performance. *Science, 283*, 549–554.

Zubieta, J., Smith, Y. R., Bueller, J. A., Xu, Y., Kilbourn, M. R., Jewett, D. M., et al. (2001). Regional mu opioid receptor regulation of sensory and affective dimensions of pain. *Science, 293*, 311–315.

5

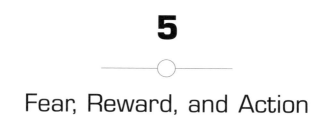

Fear, Reward, and Action

We move about our environment to get or produce the things we need, principally food, clothing, shelter, and sex. We also move to avoid discomfort and danger; humans can be both prey and predator. Out of these primitive needs evolved a complex system for governing motor behavior. We must be motivated to meet our basic needs. We have the drives of thirst, hunger, and sex, and when we satisfy these needs we experience pleasure. If we are to avoid that which is dangerous, we must recognize it and be motivated to flee from it. Thus brain systems evolved to produce both fear and pleasure; disturbances in these systems may be related to a wide variety of mental disorders. I discuss how the amygdala and hippocampus are involved in these emotions, but it is impossible to do so without a basic understanding of how motor behavior itself is managed by the brain.

UNDERSTANDING MOTOR BEHAVIOR

Nearly all brain structures are involved in the production of motor movement, but I focus here on the interactions of the neocortex, the basal ganglia, and the cerebellum. The neocortex, particularly the premotor and prefrontal cortex, is involved in conceptualizing the motor acts that are to be performed. The precentral gyrus, as was discussed in Chapter 2, has neurons that project all the way to the spinal cord. These neurons are probably involved in fine adjustments to motor movements. Virtually every area of the cortex except the primary visual and auditory cortex projects to the caudate and putamen of the basal ganglia. The caudate receives input from multimodality association cortices, whereas the putamen receives relatively more input from primary somatosensory areas, as well as secondary auditory and visual areas. This division of input suggests that the caudate deals more with the cognitive information involved in initiating motor action, whereas the putamen processes information about the sensory context in which that movement occurs. This circuitry between the neocortex and the basal ganglia is involved in the planning, initiation, and termination of motor movements. Interestingly, this circuit is silent during the actual *performance* of the movement. Accurate performance of a movement involves the circuitry between the neocortex and the cerebellum, as I show later.

First, let's examine how the basal ganglia are involved in initiating and terminating movements. Figure 5.1 revisits Step 10 (Figure 2.10) in Chapter 2. Examine the "motor loop" part of the figure on the right. (I discuss the left side of the figure in the next section.) Note the connections between the neocortex and the ventral anterior (VA) and ventral lateral (VL) thalamus—these structures exchange information via excitatory glutamate neurons. The cortex also sends such input to the

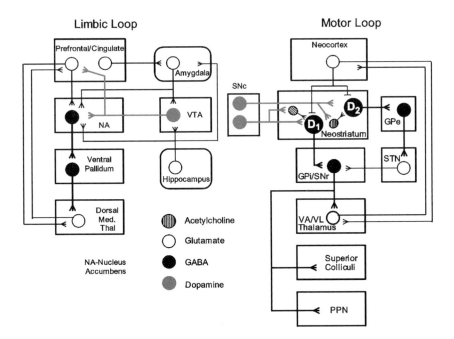

FIGURE 5.1. The motor pathways

neostriatum. Neostriatal neurons use GABA as their neurotransmitter, and they receive dopamine input from the substantia nigra compacta (SNc). The GABA neurons of the neostriatum project to the globus pallidus interna (GPi) and the substantia nigra reticulata (SNr). Both these structures contain GABA neurons that complete the loop by projecting to the VA/VL thalamus. The SNr's projections to the superior colliculi and pedunculopontine nuclei (PPN) influence eye movements and truncal muscles, respectively. Recall that earlier I showed that the SNr is tonically active, meaning that GABA is continuously released onto these structures, inhibiting them. The body is at rest. The first step in motor behavior is a plan, generated in the frontal cortex. Glutamate outflow stimulates GABA neurons in the neostriatum that project to and inhibit the GPi/SNr such that they no longer release GABA onto the thalamus and other structures. In particular, the VA/VL cortical loop is freed from inhibition and begins to run. A new motor behavior is initiated. Notice that the neocortex sends information to a second set of GABA neurons in the neostriatum. These GABA neurons terminate in the globus pallidus externa (GPe). The GPe projects to an intermediate structure, the subthalamic nucleus (STN), which contains glutamate neurons. Notice that when the striatal neurons inhibit the GPe, the GPe no longer can inhibit the STN. STN releases glutamate into the GPi/SNr, stimulating it, which is the opposite effect of the *direct* pathway described previously. This *indirect* pathway through the STN thus serves a braking function. Stroke patients who sustain damage to the STN on one side of the body develop a condition called "hemiballism." When they try to move a limb, it may suddenly fly out of control. This happens because the disruption in the circuitry of the indirect pathway has removed its steadying influence.

The input from the cortex to the neostriatum alone is usually not strong enough to shut down the tonic inhibitory influence of the GPi/SNr. Thus dopamine is a critical neurotransmitter in this regard, and its actions are complex. Dopamine from the SNc further stimulates neostriatal neurons projecting to the GPi/SNr (via D_1 receptors), but it inhibits neostriatal GABA neurons headed to the GPe (via D_2 receptors). Normally, therefore, dopamine enhances the action of glutamate on the direct pathway, but it inhibits the effect of glutamate on the indirect pathway. The direct pathway now even more strongly inhibits the GPi/SNr, and with even less GABA in the thalamus the VA/VL nuclei are even more likely to fire (i.e., initiate a movement). Next, if the GABA striatal neurons in the indirect pathway are inhibited (through the D_2 receptors), then the GPe becomes more active (because it experiences less GABA). The more active GPe GABA neuron inhibits the STN, so less excitatory glutamate is released in the GPi/SNr. Thus dopamine converts the antagonist effects of the direct and indirect pathways into dual facilitatory effects, enhancing movement. Patients with Parkinson's disease (slow movements, stiffness, tremors), who lose dopamine in the substantia nigra, find themselves unable to move because of the excessive outflow from the GPi/SNr, in spite of input from the cortically stimulated neostriatal neurons. This excessive GABA outflow prevents initiation of new movements. Older antipsychotic drugs such as haloperidol have as one of their main mechanisms the blocking of dopamine receptors. Thus their main side effects are symptoms very similar to those of Parkinson's disease, termed "extrapyramidal symptoms" (EPS). These symptoms can be removed by giving an anticholinergic agent. How does this work? Remember the small acetylcholine (Ach) interneurons in the neostriatum. As shown in the figure, they are positioned between the dopamine and neostriatal GABA neurons. At least some of the time Ach inhibits the neostriatal GABA neurons. In Parkinson's, there is already a decline in outflow from the neostriatum; the Ach neurons worsen this decline. By using an anticholinergic drug, the inhibitory effect of Ach on the neostriatum is blocked, and the neostriatal GABA neurons can increase their firing, reversing the excessive output of the GPi/SNr.

As stated, the previously described circuitry will initiate a new behavior. Figure 5.2 shows the role of the cerebellum in monitoring ongoing motor performance. The motor association areas of the frontal lobe and the sensory association areas of the parietal lobe send information

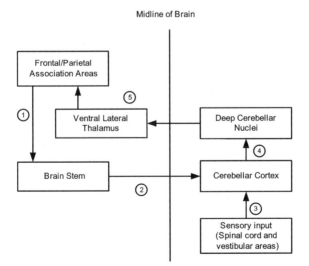

FIGURE 5.2. The role of the cerebellum in motor behavior

about the motor movements to the cerebellum (1). This input is arranged in such a way that the body surface is mapped onto the cerebellum. Information from the visual association cortex involved in processing motion is particularly important. This data is first relayed to the brain stem on the same side of the brain; it then crosses over to the cerebellar cortex on the other side (2). The cerebellum also receives direct sensory input from the spinal cord, particularly data about the position of various body parts in space (3). The cerebellar cortex integrates information from the neocortex about the intent, context, and nature of the motor movement with the sensory data about how well the motor movement is being performed. A "corrective" signal is generated, and the deep cerebellar nuclei transfer this data back to the original side of the brain (4). The thalamus receives this information, and it is relayed back to the motor cortex. Here, new motor programs can be initiated to adjust the action according to environmental circumstances.

THE LIMBIC STRIATUM

Now examine the left side of Figure 5.1. Notice that the limbic loop has a parallel circuitry to the motor loop. Imagine that the motor loop (sensory–motor striatum) is engaged in some routine motor action. Parallel to this action, the limbic loop (limbic striatum) is operating. The prefrontal cortex is involved in long-term planning and in inhibiting inappropriate motor actions. This information is conveyed via the prefrontal–dorsal medial thalamus loop. As with the motor loop, new behavior can be initiated with the help of dopamine inputs, but the inputs come from the ventral tegmental area (VTA) rather than the SNc. Dopamine inhibits the neurons of the nucleus accumbens (NA; part of the ventral striatum). The tonic output of the ventral pallidum (analogous to the GPi/SNr) is inhibited, and a motor program can be initiated.

How is this different from what the motor loop does? Notice that two structures, the amygdala and the hippocampus, have input to the VTA and NA. Whereas the motor loop previously described plays a critical role in initiating routine motor behaviors, the limbic loop plays a crucial role in initiating actions related to the survival of the organism. The limbic striatal loop, together with the amygdala and hippocampus, helps determine our responsiveness to stimuli in the environment, particularly when the stimuli evoke fear or are related to reward. It governs our responses to signals showing the presence of food when we are hungry, to signs of threat, and to sexual stimuli. It may well create the drive we feel to pursue desirable stimuli and to flee from or fight dangerous stimuli. The role of both dopamine and the ventral striatum (or NA) in movement and the processing of rewarding stimuli is shown in two recent PET studies with human volunteers. M. J. Koepp and his colleagues had eight men undergo PET scanning at baseline and while playing video games. They administered the radiochemical raclopride, which binds to the dopamine receptors, as noted in Chapter 4. During the video-game PET study, less raclopride bound to the striatum; this implies that more dopamine was being released during the game. Furthermore, the participants' performances correlated strongly with the amount of dopamine released in the *ventral* striatum. Before discussing the limbic circuit further, however, let us look at the amygdala in more detail.

THE AMYGDALA

Go back to Step 8 (Figure 2.8) in Chapter 2 to review the position of the amygdala. It sits just anterior to the hippocampus. The studies of Joseph LeDoux, Michael Davis, and others have shown the amygdala to be a critical structure in formulating an emotional response, particularly fear. Classical conditioning, by which an individual reacts with fear to a harmless stimuli that has been repeatedly paired with a noxious stimuli, does not occur if the amygdala is damaged. Monkeys in whom the amygdala is removed bilaterally lose all sense of fear. They become hypersexual in a strange way: Male monkeys no longer can recognize when a female is receptive, and they will engage in sexual behavior with inanimate objects. They lose the ability to recognize food and will put inedible objects into their mouths. This phenomena has been termed "psychic blindness" because it is not due to any sensory deficit per se; rather, the animal loses the ability to recognize the biological significance of stimuli.

The function of the amygdala can be better understood by examining Figure 5.3. The amygdala area receives information from the olfactory bulb (the most primitive sense), as well as from structures that inform the amygdala about the physical state of the body. The hypothalamus and the nucleus tractus solitarius (NTS) report data on blood volume, on sugar level in the bloodstream, on concentration of the plasma, and so forth. The amygdala thus has information about the body's physical needs. It contains receptors for sex hormones. If certain parts of the amygdala are simulated via an electrode, the animal begins to smack its lips, salivate, and chew. The parasympathetic system is activated, with emptying of the bladder and rectum. Other inputs to the amygdala are quite different. They come from the higher brain areas: the prefrontal cortex and temporal lobe in particular. If the basal and lateral nuclei are stimulated with an electrode, the animal becomes attentive; the sym-

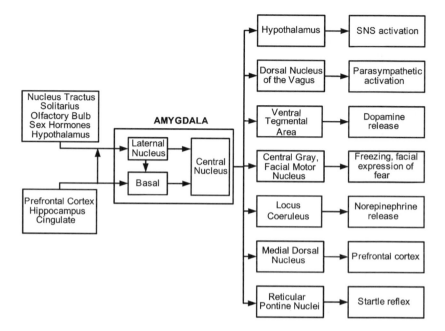

FIGURE 5.3. The amygdala and its connections

pathetic nervous system is activated. The animal becomes aroused and fearful and may become aggressive. During brain surgery with anesthetized but awake humans, stimulation of the amygdala produces *déjà vu*-like hallucinations and is experienced as unpleasant and anxiety provoking.

It appears that the amygdala is the place in which the perception of stimuli is matched to information about its biological significance. The temporal lobe, for instance, is important in visual perception. An assembly of neurons in the temporal lobe may recognize that an object is round, red, and has a stem on the top, but the basolateral amygdala integrates the smell of the object with memories of it being eaten, and we recognize it as an apple. Furthermore, if we are hungry and signals of food deprivation are reaching the amygdala via the corticomedial area, the amygdala will set up a drive to eat. The motor programs needed to obtain the apple and consume it are more likely to be set in motion. The output of the amygdala is shown in Figure 5.3 as well. The central nucleus of the amygdala is the interface with various output systems. The amygdala issues commands to the hypothalamus to activate the parasympathetic or sympathetic nervous system, depending on the demands of the situation. It projects to the locus coerulus and ventral tegmental area to control the release of norepinephrine and dopamine. It can also directly produce facial expression (baring the teeth, etc.) and freezing. The startle reflex is greatly increased. Thus the amygdala helps us recognize the things we need for survival (food, sexual partners), alerts us to things that may harm us (predators), and helps provide the motivation for behaviors we need to gratify our needs or escape harm (flight or fight).

Taketosh Ono and Hisao Nishijo reviewed studies that examined the activity of amygdaloid neurons in awake, behaving monkeys. Electrodes were inserted into these neurons, and the animals were trained to perform various tasks. Amygdala neurons fired strongly when the animals saw a preferred food (an orange) but not when they saw a more mundane food. The amygdala was active when the monkeys saw a model of a spider but not a role of tape. The activity of amygdala neurons varied according to the need state of the animal. When the monkeys were thirsty, the sight of their water bottles elicited strong amygdaloid activity, but it did not after the monkeys drank their fill. On the other hand, the juice bottles always elicited amygdala activity, even when the monkeys were not thirsty. The reason is most likely that the juice was so tasty that the amygdala signaled its desirability even when the animal's thirst was quenched. This is consistent with human experience. When we are full, we may ignore unappealing food, but we may consume a favorite dish even if we have eaten recently.

There are very few injuries or diseases in humans that specifically damage the amygdala and leave all other areas of the brain intact. Examinations of the few patients in whom this has happened have shown that they lose the ability to become fearful after exposure to a an aversive stimuli. Several studies have demonstrated the role of the amygdala in the experience of fear. J. S. Morris and his colleagues in Cambridge, England, showed healthy volunteers pictures of either happy or fearful faces while they underwent a PET scan that assessed blood flow to various regions of the brain. Blood flow is highly correlated with brain activity. When contrasting the blood flow increases for each type of face, they found that the fearful faces caused an increase in blood flow in the left amygdala. Paul Whalen and colleagues at Harvard Medical School also showed pictures of faces to volunteers undergoing functional magnetic resonance imaging (fMRI), which assesses the degree of blood oxygenation in brain regions, also a measure of brain activity. This study used a "backward masking" technique. Participants looked at neutral, happy, or fearful faces. The happy and fearful faces were presented so quickly (33 milliseconds [msec]) that the participants were not consciously aware of the face having been presented. The emotional face was followed by a neutral face that was on the screen for 167 msec. When asked afterward, the participants had no awareness of having seen angry or happy faces, yet the right amygdala was strongly activated by the fearful faces relative to the happy faces. Thus the amygdala not only processes the emotional content of faces but it may also do so at an unconscious level.

Recently Kevin LaBar and his colleagues performed a similar experiment. Eighteen college students volunteered to be part of a fear conditioning study. They underwent an fMRI scan while they were shown two different visual stimuli. After one stimulus, they received a mild electric shock; whereas after the other stimulus, they did not. The scan measured brain activity in response to both stimuli, and the activity during the nonshock scans was subtracted from that during the shock scans to see what areas of the brain were activated by fear. The right amygdala was specifically activated by the visual cue linked to shock; interestingly, it was also linked to extinction. As the shock was omitted, the amygdala appeared to play a role in recognizing that a painful experience was no longer coming. The investigators also measured changes in skin sweating (a measure of autonomic activation and a common fear response). The amount of sweating correlated very strongly with amygdala activation. Finally, the amygdala has also been found to process linguistic threat. N. Isenberg and colleagues at Cornell University presented various words on a video monitor to human volunteers undergoing PET scan. Some of the words were neutral ("dial," "bookcase"), whereas others were fear provoking ("kill," "abuse," or "steal"). Compared with the neutral words, the threatening words activated the amygdala bilaterally.

COMPLETING THE CIRCUIT

Now let us return to Figure 5.1. The amygdala and hippocampus both provide input to the VTA, thus influencing the dopamine released in the NA. P. O'Donnell and Anthony Grace have studied the relative effects of the amygdala and hippocampus on the NA. The hippocampus facilitates the flow of information from the prefrontal cortex to the NA and then on to the ventral pallidum. Grace proposes that the hippocampus increases the ability of the organism to stay "on task," that is, to execute the behavior according to a long-term plan. The amygdala also facilitates the flow of information from cortex to NA, but in a very different fashion. The amygdala can facilitate information flow only 30–40 msec after it has been stimulated from elsewhere in brain. Grace has used a "bear and butterflies" paradigm to describe the relative contributions of the hippocampus and amygdala to motor action. He gives an example of a man in the forest searching for butterflies. As he walks, he scans the area for butterflies, and, if he sees one he wishes to add to his collection, he sweeps it up with his net. The hippocampus is critical in driving this type of "context-dependent" behavior. The man must keep in mind the type of butterfly he wants, scan intently for it, remember where he is likely to find it, and so on. The hippocampus facilitates activity in the limbic loop conducive to this behavior and increases resistance to distracting stimuli. (I examine how the hippocampus does this in Chapter 6.) The motor striatal loop initiates and maintains the specific motor behaviors (looking, reaching, swinging the net, etc.) Now imagine that a bear suddenly emerges from the forest. It is not in the man's interest to ignore the bear. As the bear is perceived, the amygdala is informed and its recognizes a predator. The amygdala activates the fear response and initiates an "affective override of current task focus." That is, the man drops his net and runs. To expand Grace's analogy, suppose that a bear does not appear but that the man works hard all morning collecting his butterflies. Around noon, he becomes hungry. The amygdala begins to respond. Suddenly the man notices apples hanging from the trees that he had not paid attention to all morning. Again, the amygdala may interrupt the current task to initiate behaviors such as climbing the tree to pick the apple.

The VTA dopamine input to the NA has a pronounced effect on which type of influence, amygdaloid or hippocampal, predominates in this structure. The greater the dopamine input, the more the affect-laden inputs of the amygdala will take control. As I said earlier, activity in the VTA-NA pathway is clearly experienced by the animal as pleasurable. This is nature's way of reinforcing us for doing the things necessary for survival, such as eating, procreating, or fleeing from or attacking predators. Brian Knutson, Charles Adams, Grace Fong, and Daniel Hommer (all of the National Institute on Alcohol Abuse and Alcoholism) measured activity in the NA using fMRI with normal volunteers while they played video games. In some trials, the volunteers earned money for a good performance, whereas on other trials they were punished for poor performance by a loss of money. Being punished did not activate the NA, but as the monetary reward increased, the NA became more active, and the participants' self-ratings of happiness correlated with this activation.

Freud, as part of his psychic apparatus, proposed the *id*, a hypothetical structure that embodied the biological drives for water, food, sex, and comfort. The id operated on the pleasure principle, that is, it required immediate gratification. It many ways, the actions of the amygdala, VTA, and NA are quite close to this formulation. They respond to the physical needs of the body and are activated by the presence of rewarding or threatening stimuli. The role of dopamine is critical in modulating this process. I return to these structures in Chapter 10 when discussing pathological aggression and substance abuse.

REFERENCES

Alexander, G. E., DeLong, M. R., & Strick, P. L. (1986). Parallel organization of functionally segregated circuits linking basal ganglia and cortex. *Annual Review of Neuroscience, 9,* 357–381.

Brodal, P. (1992). *The central nervous system: Structure and function.* New York: Oxford University Press.

Chevalier, G., & Deniau, J. M. (1990). Disinhibition as a basic process in the expression of striatal functions. *Trends in Neuroscience, 13,* 277–280.

Davis, M. (1992). The role of the amygdala in fear-potentiated startle: Implications for animal models of anxiety. *Trends in Neuroscience, 13,* 35–40.

Davis, M. (1997). Neurobiology of fear responses: The role of the amygdala. In S. Salloway, P. Malloy, & J. L. Cummings (Eds.), *The neuropsychiatry of limbic and subcortical disorders* (pp. 71–94). Washington, DC: American Psychiatric Press.

Gerfen, C. R. (1992a). D1 and D2 dopamine receptor regulation of striatonigral and striatopallidal neurons. *Seminars in the Neurosciences, 4,* 109–118.

Gerfen, C. R. (1992b). The neostriatal mosaic: Multiple levels of compartmental organization in the basal ganglia. *Annual Review of Neuroscience, 15,* 285–320.

Grace, A. A. (1991). Phasic versus tonic dopamine release and the modulation of dopamine system responsivity: A hypothesis for the etiology of schizophrenia. *Neuroscience, 41,* 1–24.

Grace, A. A. (1995). The tonic/phasic model of dopamine system regulation: Its relevance for understanding how stimulant abuse can alter basal ganglia function. *Drug and Alcohol Dependence, 37,* 111–129.

Grace, A. A. (2001). Psychostimulant actions on dopamine and limbic system function: Relevance-related behavior and impulsivity. In M. V. Solanto, A. F. T. Arnsten, & F. X. Castellanos (Eds.), *Stimulant drugs and ADHD: Basic and clinical neuroscience* (pp. 134–157). New York: Oxford University Press.

Knutson, B., Adams, C. M., Fong, G. W., & Hommer, D. (2001). Anticipation of increasing monetary reward selectively recruits nucleus accumbens. *Neuroscience, 21,* 1–5.

Koepp, M. J., Gunn, R. N., Lawrence, A. D., Cunningham, V. J., Dagher, A., Jones, T., et al. (1998). Evidence for striatal dopamine release during a video game. *Nature, 393,* 266–268.

LaBar, K. S., Gatenby, J. C., Gore, J. C., LeDoux, J. E., & Phelps, E. A. (1998). Human amygdala activation during conditioned fear acquisition and extinction: A mixed-trial fMRI study. *Neuron, 20,* 937–945.

LeDoux, J. (1996). *The emotional brain: The mysterious underpinnings of emotional life.* New York: Simon & Schuster.

Morris, J. S., Friston, K. J., Buchel, C., Frith, C. D., Young, A. W., Calder, A. J., & Dolan, R. J. (1998). A neuromodulatory role for the human amygdala in processing emotional facial expressions. *Brain, 121,* 47–57.

O'Donnell, P., & Grace, A. A. (1994). Tonic D2-mediated attenuation of cortical excitation in nucleus accumbens neurons recorded *in vitro. Brain Research, 634,* 105–112.

O'Donnell, P., & Grace, A. A. (1995). Synaptic interactions among excitatory afferents to nucleus accumbens neurons: Hippocampal gating of prefrontal cortical input. *Journal of Neuroscience, 15,* 3622–3639.

O'Donnell, P., & Grace, A. A. (1996). Hippocampal gating of cortical through-put in the nucleus accumbens: Modulation by dopamine. *Biological Psychiatry, 39,* 632.

Ono, T., & Nishijo, H. (2000). Neurophysiological basis of emotion in primates: Neuronal responses in the monkey amygdala and anterior cingulate cortex. In M. S. Gazzaniga (Ed.), *The new cognitive neurosciences* (2nd ed., pp. 1099–1114). Cambridge, MA: MIT Press.

Purves, D., Augustine, G. J., Fitzpatrick, D., Katz, L. C., LaMantia, A. S., & McNamara, J. O. (1997). *Neuroscience.* Durham, NC: Sinauer Associates, Inc.

Whalen, P. J., Rauch, S. L., Etcoff, N. L., McInerney, S. C., Lee, M. B., & Jenike, M. A. (1998). Masked presentations of emotional facial expressions modulate amygdala activity without explicit knowledge. *Journal of Neuroscience, 18,* 411–418.

Wilson, C. J. (1998). Basal ganglia. In G. M. Shepherd (Ed.), *The synaptic organization of the brain* (pp. 329–375). New York: Oxford University Press.

6

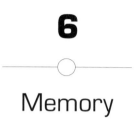

Memory

Recently I was in New York for a meeting and went out for a stroll. While walking down Fifth Avenue in Manhattan, I happened on the main branch of the New York City Public Library, with its well-known lions. Almost immediately, the film *Ghostbusters* came to mind, and with the memory of the film, the soundtrack, unbidden, began to run through my head. Next came thoughts of Dan Aykroyd and Bill Murray and memories of watching *Saturday Night Live* in the late 1970s with friends from medical school, some of whom I had not seen or thought of in over a decade. This vignette illustrates some of the peculiar aspects of human memory. It is not organized like an encyclopedia. There is not one place in the brain in which memories, say, of fourth grade are stored right next to fifth-grade memories. Human memory is quite different from that of the hard drive of a computer. On a computer, each piece of information is stored at a specific location on the drive; each document has an address that the computer uses to locate the file when instructed to do so. When we open a file, the computer searches the hard drive until it finds the file. The immense speed of the processing unit of the computer allows this task to be quickly executed. Neuronal transmission is far too slow to use such a method. Imagine if, whenever we had to recall our phone number, our brains had to go through all our memories to locate the information. The brain would never finish the task in time to make a phone call. The method of storing and retrieving memories in the brain must use a completely different paradigm.

The other interesting aspect of memory is that it is highly contextual. Being in a particular place quickly triggers associations to other places and events. It is often very easy to remind us of things from our past; an odor, a particular sunset, an old movie on TV, any of these will quickly allow us to access memories from years ago. When we do remember, our minds are not like a video recorder, playing back events exactly as they occurred. Instead, the event is recreated in our minds. Our grandparents retell stories from their youth; we hear them several times over, and we notice that the story is slightly different each time. Rarely do two people remember an event in exactly the same way. Brain injuries do not selectively remove memories from a particular point in our lives, and only the most severe brain injury will wipe out long-term memories.

In recent years there has been an explosion of knowledge about the mechanisms of memory. Much of the data come from animal studies, but these animal studies have been complemented by clinical work with amnesic human beings, as well as by neuroimaging studies of memory in normal volunteers. This chapter moves from the cellular level to the neuroimaging of the human brain itself. Figure 6.1 illustrates the phenomenon of kindling and long-term potentiation (LTP). The upper part of the figure demonstrates kindling. If neuron A fires only sporadically, then neuron B is never sufficiently depolarized to fire. This corresponds to example 1 in the upper figure. If, on the other hand, neuron A fires a

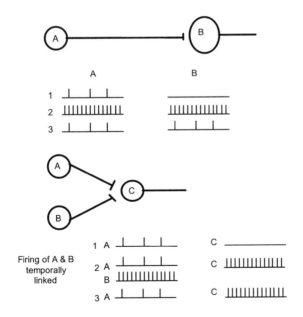

FIGURE 6.1. Neuronal activity is modified by experience

train of action potentials, then neuron B does fire (2). If neuron A repeatedly depolarizes neuron B, neuron B will become sensitized. Changes will occur postsynaptically in neuron B such that it now requires only a modest input from neuron A to fire. This state is shown in example 3 of the upper figure.

Long-term potentiation is shown in the lower part of Figure 6.1. Neurons A and B both stimulate neuron C. Neuron A fires sporadically, which is insufficient to depolarize neuron C and generate an action potential (example 1 in lower figure). Neuron B strongly stimulates neuron C, producing an action potential. Now consider the situation in which the firing of A and B are temporally linked (example 2). A modest input from neuron A is always followed by a strong train of impulses from neuron B. The impulses from neuron B cause a depolarization. If this association (if A, then B) is repeated consistently enough, then neuron C learns this relationship. From this point forward, it now fires in response only to the input from A (example 3). D. O. Hebb in 1949 first hypothesized this ability of neurons to alter their firing properties in response to experience and to "learn" relationships. Before examining the role of LTP in memory, we need to examine the structure of the hippocampus in more detail.

THE HIPPOCAMPUS

Review Step 9 (Figure 2.9) in Chapter 2, which showed you where the hippocampus is located in the brain. The top panel of Figure 6.2 shows the hippocampus still attached to the medial temporal lobes. The hippocampus consists of two sheets of neurons, which are illustrated in the middle panel. One sheet is the dentate gyrus, and the other is the cornu ammonis (CA). If the hippocampus is flattened out, you can see how these two sheets of neurons are rolled into semicircles and interdigitated. Now if a cross-section of the hippocampus (bottom panel) is viewed head-on, one can see how the hippocampus perches on the temporal lobe, as well as how the dentate and CA are positioned with respect to each other. Figure 6.3 is a schematic that shows the internal circuitry of the hippocampus. Information flows from the medial temporal lobe to the entorhinal cortex (this area of the brain is close to the olfactory bulbs, hence the name, from Latin for "around the nose") via the "perforant path," synapsing on the neuron of the dentate gyrus. Glutamate stimulates the neurons of the dentate gyrus.

Axons from the dentate project to the CA3, one of the subdivisions of the CA. These axons are referred to as mossy fibers due to their appearance under the microscope. Glutamate is released onto the CA3

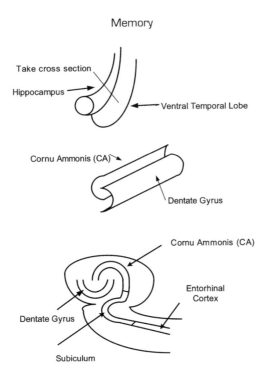

FIGURE 6.2. The structure of the hippocampus

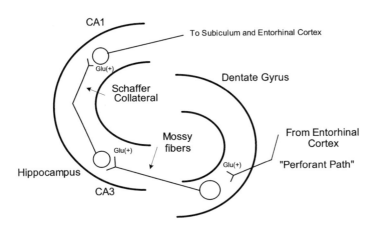

FIGURE 6.3. The circuitry of the hippocampus

neurons, which in turn fire and stimulate the CA1 neurons. The pathway from CA1 to CA3 is referred to as the "Schaffer collaterals." Finally, the neurons of CA3 project to the subiculum of the hippocampus, as well as back to the entorhinal cortex. Neurons of CA1 and CA3 can undergo long-term potentiation (LTP).

The critical step to understanding memory involves grasping how the hippocampal circuit just described fits into the Papez circuit discussed earlier in Step 9 of Chapter 2 (Figure 2.9). This is shown in Figure 6.4. Let's imagine a simple act of remembering. Suppose a person you don't know makes a remark of no consequence to you. You will perceive

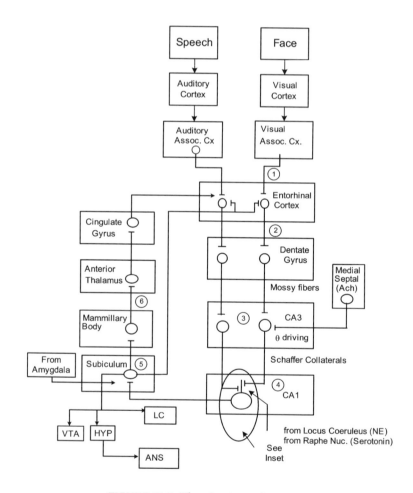

FIGURE 6.4. The circuitry of memory

both the person and his remarks at the time they occur. This perception is represented by the two boxes at the top of the figure. Your visual association cortex will assemble the attributes of the person's face, while your auditory cortex and language processing areas will decode the person's speech. If, in fact, what the person says is truly of no consequence, you will soon move on and forget the incident. After a half-hour or so, you may even forget that you ever saw the individual. Now suppose the person says something of great relevance to you. He says you've just won the lottery and are a multimillionaire. You may well remember this individual for the rest of your life. What processes in the brain might underlie this phenomenon? First, let's look at the circuit.

Both the auditory (what the man said) and the visual (the man's face) input are transmitted to the entorhinal cortex (1). From here the information is transferred to the dentate gyrus (2), then onto CA3 (3) and CA1 (4). Processing in CA1, involving LTP, is critical to memory information, as is shown in the next figure. After processing in CA1, information moves on to the subiculum (5), from which it is sent in diverse directions. Note that from the subiculum, the hippocampus can influence the output of the ventral tegmental area and locus coeruleus, influencing dopaminergic and noradrenergic tone, respectively. The hippocampus can influence the hypothalamus, which in turn will govern the output of the ANS (flight-or-flight reaction). Before completing the circuit, let's examine the inset to see how LTP works and how it is involved in memory.

Panel 1 of Figure 6.5 shows a dendrite of a CA3 neuron. Note that it is receiving input from neurons carrying information about the person's face and what he is saying. Panel 1 represents the situation in which what is said is of no consequence. Neuronal firing is at a low level, releasing some glutamate onto the CA3. This glutamate binds to some AMPA/kainate receptors, but not enough to depolarize the neuron. Recall from Chapter 3 that if the neuron does not become depolarized, magnesium continues to block the calcium channel associated with the NMDA receptor. Thus, even if glutamate managed to stimulate an NMDA receptor, the magnesium block would prevent any calcium from entering through the channel.

Panel 2 represents the situation is which you have just been awarded several million dollars. Such an announcement would be highly arousing; the neurons carrying the auditory information would be firing vigorously, releasing large amounts of glutamate onto the CA3 neuron. The AMPA/kainate receptors are stimulated, and their Na/K channels open, depolarizing the neuron. This depolarization removes the magnesium blockade. Now the rather modest release of glutamate induced by the visual (facial) input binds to NMDA receptors and opens the channel. Now the main event of LTP and memory formation begins. Calcium

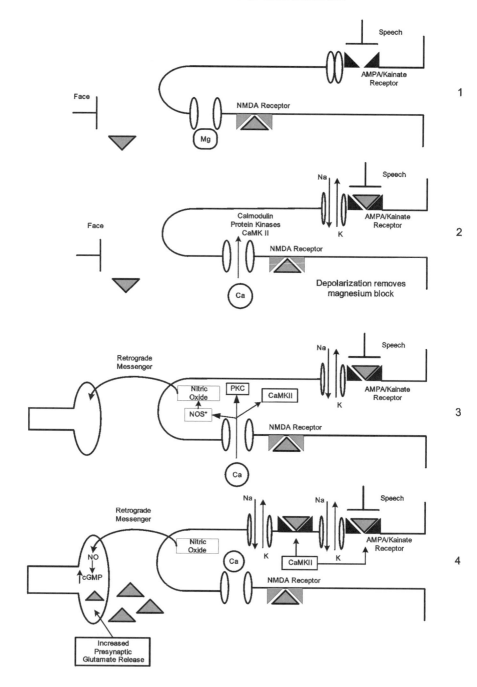

FIGURE 6.5. The mechanism of long-term potentiation

flows into the neuron, activating a number of enzymes. These include calmodulin, which in turn activates calmodulin kinase II (CaMKII). The influx of calcium also activates various protein kinases, which phosphorylate and thus activate a number of cellular proteins.

Panel 3 shows how the influx of Ca activates nitric oxide synthase (NOS). NOS produces the gas nitric oxide (NO), not to be confused with nitrous oxide (N_2O), or "laughing gas." NO becomes a retrograde messenger; it diffuses back to the presynaptic neuron. The final stage of LTP is shown in Panel 4. When NO enters the presynaptic neuron, it stimulates enzymes that increase the production of cyclic guanylyl monophosphate (cGMP). Cyclic GMP, in turn, stimulates enzymes that will ultimately cause increased presynaptic release of glutamate. CaMKII will activate processes that will increase the number of postsynaptic AMPA/kainate receptors, enhancing postsynaptic sensitivity.

What does this mean for memory? Now any reminder of the person's face will trigger an increased release of glutamate presynaptically. The postsynaptic membrane has been made more sensitive, so that any appearance (or thought) of the person's face will trigger the same perceptions as the announcement that you just won a million dollars. The hippocampus has written the association of the major event (winning a million dollars) with the appearance of the person who announced it to you. A critical point here is that the hippocampus does not store the memory of winning a million dollars or of the appearance of your benefactor but of the association between the two.

Now let us return to Figure 6.4. Suppose, many years later, you are walking through an airport and you notice the face of the person who announced that you had become a millionaire. When you see him, the visual input enters the hippocampal circuits. Because the CA3 connections have strengthened as described, CA3 neurons fire more easily. This information moves on to the subiculum and then into the Papez circuit (6). The information moves through the mammillary bodies and the anterior thalamus, on to the cingulate gyrus, and back to the entorhinal cortex. What is happening here? The information about the current state of the world (seeing the face in an airport) is being quickly shunted through the cingulate gyrus, which can access past memories (particularly those that carry heavy emotional baggage). Quickly the association is recognized—this is the person who told you that you were a millionaire—and all the happiness of that moment is also triggered. Because the subiculum has access to the locus coeruleus, the VTA, and the ANS, an emotional reaction is triggered. You again feel elated; you rush up to the person and tell him how happy you are to see him.

Some things we remember for only a few hours, whereas other memories last a lifetime. The effect of LTP, mediated through the

NMDA receptors, lasts only hours to weeks. Other processes are important in maintaining a memory for months or years. Returning to Figure 6.4 momentarily, you will notice that acetylcholine neurons from the septal nucleus project to the hippocampus. The cholinergic neurons help set a particular firing rate of the hippocampus neurons, referred to as the "theta rhythm." Jonathan Winson of Rockefeller University found that theta rhythm appears at different times in different species of animals. In the cat, it occurs during hunting, in the rabbit it arises during apprehension (freezing), and in the rat it is seen during active exploration. The consistent feature of theta rhythm is that it appears when the animal is engaged in specific behaviors that are critical to the animal's survival. During such times, it would make sense that memory systems are activated. Winson and his colleagues also found that LTP is much more easily induced in the hippocampus at each peak of the theta rhythm, presumably when the cell had again been further depolarized. Theta rhythm is also present during rapid eye movement (REM) sleep, which is discussed later.

Figure 6.6 shows that, to maintain LTP (and memory) over the long term, other factors involving the nucleus must be brought into play. Processes inducing LTP via the NMDA receptor are again shown in the dendrite. Notice the norepinephrine and serotonin receptors at the top of the neuron; this noradrenergic input comes from the locus coeruleus (LC), whereas the serotonergic input is from the raphe. When NE stimulates the β receptor, G proteins are activated, which lead to the production of cAMP, which in turn stimulates protein kinase A (PKA). The 5HT1A receptors on the hippocampus also activate PKA; CaMKII, which was activated in the induction phase of LTP, can further stimulate PKA. PKA will phosphorylate the K channels, which, as you recall from Chapter 2, will decrease the outflow of K during the hyperpolarization stage. This will make the neuron less refractory to firing again. The more often the neuron is depolarized, the longer the magnesium block of the NMDA receptor calcium channel remains relieved. This means a greater influx of calcium and even more LTP. PKA can also translocate to the nucleus, and this is where the processes most critical to LTP maintenance are involved. PKA activates the CREB (CRE-binding element) protein. In the figure, two types of CREB are shown. CREB-1 binds to the CRE and enhances the transcription of DNA into messenger RNA. Messenger RNA then guides the expression of multiple proteins, leading to neuronal growth, the sprouting of new dendrites, and strengthening of the synapses. These processes lead to physical changes in the neuron that hardwire the association between events into the brain. In addition to NE, other factors can affect the maintenance of LTP. CREB-2 actually inhibits the development of the processes previously described. PKA will

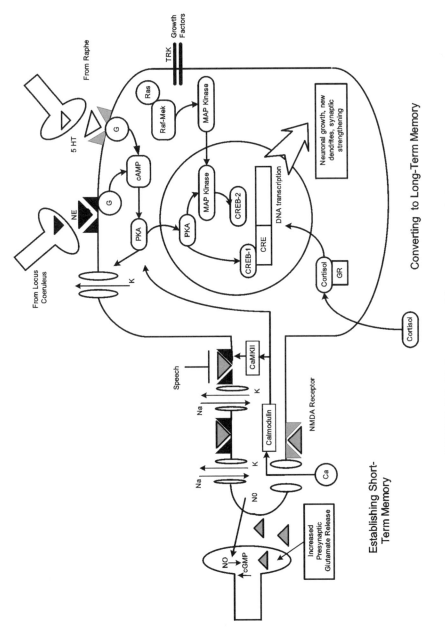

FIGURE 6.6. Maintenance of long-term potentiation

inhibit the binding (via the microtubule-associated protein [MAP] kinases) of CREB-2 to CRE, enhancing the effects of CREB-1. These MAP kinases are also influenced by the growth factors, such as brain-derived neurotrophic factor (BDNF), that activate them via the tyrosine kinase receptor system. Finally, cortisol, released in response to stress, binds to a free-floating receptor molecule that enters the nucleus and also influences DNA transcription.

The LC activates in response to new stimuli. Stress influences the release of cortisol and growth factors, so it is easy to see how stress has an effect on memory. Painful and stressful events are particularly well remembered. Many people can still recall exactly where they were the day they heard President John F. Kennedy had been killed in November 1963 or where they were on September 11, 2001. In posttraumatic stress disorder, patients suffer from intrusive and unwanted memories of the traumatic event; it is possible that the high levels of arousal at the time of these painful events cause the very potent induction and maintenance of LTP. Continual activation of this hippocampal circuitry may be injurious to the brain tissue itself, as I show in Chapter 11.

The mechanisms of LTP have largely been worked out in animal studies, but there is strong evidence from human studies that the hippocampus is important in memory. In Chapter 1, I introduced patient H. M., who had his medial temporal lobes, which included the hippocampi, removed bilaterally. H. M. lost the ability to form any new long-term memories, although his short-term memory remained intact. He also suffered from retrograde amnesia; that is, in addition to being unable to form new long-term memories (anterograde amnesia), he also could not recall people or events from several years before the surgery. Interestingly, he could recall his childhood and early adult years. Thus at some point it is clear that retrieving memories becomes independent of the hippocampus. Years later, another patient, R. B., suffered a stroke in which the CA1 cells of the hippocampus were damaged. He had a loss of memory very similar to that of H. M.

Animal and lesion studies thus suggest that the hippocampus (and the associated medial temporal cortex) would be strongly activated in neuroimaging studies of memory. In 1992 Larry Squire and colleagues performed PET scans in normal volunteers. Participants studied a list of words and then had to complete word stems while being scanned. (For instance, they would memorize the word "strong" and then repeat that word is response to the cue "str-.") This task caused the right hippocampus (as well as the right prefrontal cortex) in the participants to activate. It was assumed that the right hippocampus was activated because the visual nature of the word stems evoked the right side of the brain, even though the left hemisphere generally performs language tasks. In a follow-up study, participants were shown whole words (rather than just stems) and asked if the words had been on a list that they had memorized earlier. When recalling the words in this task, the left hippocampus was activated. Haxby and colleagues found that the right hippocampus was activated when participants performed a facial recognition task, suggesting that the right hippocampus is specialized for nonverbal, visual–spatial memory, whereas the left hippocampus is more prominent in verbal memory.

It is important to emphasize again that memories are not stored in the hippocampus. For instance, if a person undergoes a PET scan and is told to visualize his house, he will activate the same areas of the brain as if he stood in front of his house and actually saw it. The brain calls up our memories by using the same mechanisms by which we perceive the world. For instance, suppose you take a trip to Seattle and have a cup of coffee at a quaint shop. The Space Needle is on the horizon, a mist hangs over the city. All of these sights and sounds stimulate the appropriate areas of your brain. Your visual association cortex assembles the skyline, your auditory cortex perceives the sound of foghorns, and your gustatory and olfactory cortexes are aware of the taste and smell of your coffee. There is no one place in the brain in which these separate aspects of the experience are assembled into the experience "coffee in Seattle." Rather, neurons from different areas are all simultaneously active and communicating with each other; from this a coherent experience emerges.

Many months later, you buy the same brand of coffee and prepare it in your kitchen. As the coffeepot percolates, the aroma of the coffee stimulates your olfactory cortex, which sends the information to the entorhinal cortex and into the hippocampal circuit. What is stored in the hippocampus is the key to the connections. The output of the hippocampus activities the diverse cortical areas, visual and auditory, and a mental image of your trip to Seattle appears in your mind—an image, like the original perception, created by the simultaneous activation of the multiple cortical areas, each adding a piece to the image. Because this image is created anew, it may be slightly different from what actually transpired that day, but the emotional aspects of the memory will be clear.

THE FRONTAL LOBES IN MEMORY

It is clear, however, that other areas of the brain besides the hippocampus are involved in memory processes, particularly the frontal lobes. In interpreting these studies, it is critical to distinguish between memory formation (referred to as "encoding") and memory retrieval. Neuroimaging studies of these processes have led to a model called "hemispheric encoding retrieval asymmetry," or HERA, first proposed by E. Tulving and colleagues in 1994. HERA suggests that encoding processes are mediated by the left dorsal prefrontal cortex, whereas the right dorsolateral prefrontal cortex is more active when retrieving previously learned material. The degree of activation of the left dorsolateral appears to be related to the complexity of the encoding process. Kapur and colleagues performed PET studies in which participants had to remember lists of words. In the simple condition, participants had to remember only if the word contained the letter "A." In the complex encoding condition, the participants had to remember whether the word represented an animate or an inanimate object. Participants showed better recall of the words in the complex condition relative to the simple condition, and the former condition resulted in much greater activation of the *left* dorsolateral cortex. Several imaging studies have now been performed that have compared the brain activations for words that the participant would later either remember or forget. Those words that would later be remembered showed much greater left dorsolateral prefrontal activation during the memorizing process than the words that would be forgotten. When participants actively recall the words they have memorized, they activate the *right* dorsolateral cortex. A left-hemisphere location for encoding may not be absolute, however, and may be related to the verbal nature of the stimuli used in these studies. W. M. Kelley and colleagues had participants memorize and then recall both words and pictures of faces. The faces either were unfamiliar to the participants or were the faces of famous persons. Consistent with prior studies, encoding of words activated the left dorsolateral prefrontal cortex. When the participants had to encode the unfamiliar faces, the *right* dorsolateral prefrontal cortex was activated. When the participants were memorizing famous faces, the left and right prefrontal cortices were activated bilaterally. When the faces were unfamiliar, the nonverbal processes of the right hemisphere were called on to do the encoding. If, however, the face was famous (i.e., already stored in memory), then the left hemisphere could carry out the encoding. If some sort of verbal cue was associated with the famous face, the stronger left hemisphere effect returned. Thus the type of material (verbal vs. nonverbal) and the type of cognitive activity (encoding vs. retrieval) may interact to determine which prefrontal hemisphere is activated during memory functions.

So how do the medial temporal areas (where the hippocampus is located) interact with the prefrontal areas in memory formation and retrieval? This question remains to be worked out, but the hippocampus participates when memories dependent on a cue in the environment (such as the coffee in the previous example) are critical to forming or retrieving the memory. In contrast, in tasks such as word or face memorizing, which call up no past memory, the hippocampus and medial temporal structures may not be so critical. The amygdala is also highly involved in memory, particularly when the material is emotionally laden. LTP can occur in the amygdala, as well as the hippocampus, and NE released into the amygdala during stress enhances LTP as it does in the hippocampus. The amygdala is not the storage site for fearful memories, as lesions of the amygdala do not always impair fear conditioning. Figure 6.6 shows how stress hormones enhance LTP in the hippocampus. If the amygdala is lesioned, this enhancement of memory by stress hormone does not occur. L. Cahill and colleagues performed a PET study on normal volunteers. Participants viewed videotapes that were either emotionally arousing or neutral. After 3 weeks, the participants were asked to recall scenes from the video. This was a "pop quiz"; participants had not been told at the time of viewing the video that they would ever be asked to recall the material. There was a very strong correlation between the amount of activity in the right amygdala and the number of film clips recalled. Thus, although it is a something of a simplification, memory may be distributed among numerous brain systems. The frontal lobes encode and retrieve basic information, whereas the role of the hippocampus may be to recall memories within a temporal or spatial context. The amygdala helps encode the emotional significance of those memories.

SLEEP AND DREAMING

It behooves us to examine sleep and dreaming in this chapter because the role that dreaming may play in memory, or at least in the consolidation of knowledge. Dreams have long held significance for humans. In ancient times, dreams were thought to predict the future; for Freud they were the "royal road to the unconscious," and psychotherapy relies heavily on dream interpretation. In spite of this, we do not fully understand why we sleep or dream. All mammals sleep, and it seems quite odd to spend a third of one's life unconscious, vulnerable to predators, yet sleep is as great a necessity as food and water. Dolphins sleep one cerebral hemisphere at a time, in order that they can continue swimming. Humans cannot go for more than 96 hours without sleep, or severe delirium and psychosis will set in. Sleep has a very predictable pattern. It is divided into rapid-eye-movement (REM) and non-REM (NREM) sleep. NREM sleep has four stages, each progressively deeper. We begin the night in NREM sleep, and when we descend into Stage 4 of NREM, we are virtually comatose, unresponsive to external stimuli. If awakened during NREM, people are groggy and disoriented, rarely report dreams, and fall back asleep quickly. During NREM sleep, cortical and brain stem neuronal activity fall by 50%, as does cerebral blood flow. Electroencephalograph (EEG) waves become slow and synchronous. Cholinergic, noradrenergic, and serotonergic inputs to the cortex cease.

About 90 minutes into sleep, we enter our first episode of REM sleep. Abruptly, the cholinergic neurons become active, stimulating the visual cortex and limbic areas of the brain. Indeed, the brain stem begins to strongly stimulate the cortex. The body remains unresponsive to external stimuli, and the motor neurons of the spinal cord are paralyzed, but the brain stem produces ponto-geniculo-occipit (PGO) waves. Neurons from the brain stem stimulate the geniculate nuclei (a visual relay station that normally carries information from the retinas). The geniculate nuclei in turn stimulate the visual cortex, producing images. Our eyes move in response to these images; hence the term "rapid eye movement." If a person is awakened during this period, he or she will invariably report a dream. After about 10 minutes, the first REM period ends, and we return to Stage 1 NREM sleep, again descending to Stages 3 and 4. In this second phase, we do not descend as deeply into NREM. Then we enter another phase of REM, then cycle back to NREM. People run through 2 to 5 cycles of sleep in this manner. It doesn't seem to hurt if every REM cycle is interrupted and people are prevented from dreaming. Other than feeling tired, they do fine the following day, although subtle memory deficits may emerge. The following night, however, they will experience "REM rebound"—engaging in twice as much REM as normal to make up for what was lost.

During REM sleep, while the cholinergic system is active, the NE and serotonin systems remain quiescent. The cortical EEG strongly activates, appearing similar to the EEG of an awake person. The prefrontal cortex, which during our waking hours helps us plan our long-term behavior, remains turned off. The amygdala, the organ of one's deepest fears and desires, is online, however, and this probably accounts for the highly emotional content of dreams. We have been able to work out the circuitry of dreams, but this has not brought us any closer to understanding *why* we dream. Infants spend nearly all of their sleep in REM. The proportion of sleep time that we spend in REM falls as we get older, so that by the age of 50 we spend less than 2 hours in REM sleep every night.

Francis Crick and Graeme Mitchison have proposed that dreaming is the mechanism for purging unwanted material from the brain. The NE and serotonin systems are not active during REM, and these systems are critical to LTP. We remember only our dreams from the last phase of REM, before we wake up; dreams from earlier in the night are lost forever. But why, then, do infants spend so much time in REM? Surely they do not have very much material to purge. Jonathan Winson proposed the opposite hypothesis: that dreaming is a critical aspect of consolidating long-term memory. Winson noted a curious fact when he compared the brains of live-bearing mammals to those of egg-laying mammals, such as the spiny anteater (echidna). The echidna has a larger prefrontal cortex, proportional to its body, that any other mammal, including humans. Because it is clear that we are smarter than the spiny anteater or the platypus, some "paradigm shift" must have occurred during evolution to make storage of information more efficient. Mammals engage in REM sleep; the egg-laying mammals do not. Winson proposes that without the evolution of REM, brains would have had to get larger and larger to store more information. Brain size might well have exceeded the capacity of the skull. In Winson's view, REM, and hence dreaming, is part of the brain's system for enhancing long-term memory. As Winson states, "Dreams may reflect a fundamental aspect of mammalian memory processing. Crucial information acquired during the waking state may be reprocessed during sleep" (p. 94). Pierre Maquet and his research group performed PET scans on two groups of participants: one group was trained in a motor task, the other was not. The participants in both groups were scanned while sleeping. During REM sleep, the trained participants activated the same areas of the brain that they had activated while learning the task. Performance on the task improved after the participants had "slept on it," suggesting that sleep did play a role in memory consolidation. Sleep may have multiple functions, but it seems highly likely that sleep and dreaming play a major role in memory. A cautionary note is in order, however. Many facts, as reviewed by Jerome Siegel, are not consistent with the role of sleep in learning. Antidepressant medications, which decrease REM sleep, do not affect memory. Humans with brain lesions that disrupt REM do not show memory deficits, and time spent in REM sleep is not correlated with learning ability. The role of sleep and dreaming in our lives remains something of a mystery.

REFERENCES

Buckner, R. L. (2000). Neuroimaging of memory. In M. S. Gazzaniga (Ed.), *The new cognitive neurosciences* (2nd ed., pp. 817–828). Cambridge, MA: MIT Press.

Cahill, L. (1996). The neurobiology of memory for emotional events: Converging evidence from infra-human and human studies. In *Function and dysfunction in the nervous system* (pp. 259–264). Cold Spring Harbor, NY: Cold Spring Harbor Press.

Crick, F., & Mitchison, G. (1983). The function of dream sleep. *Nature, 304,* 111–114.

Fletcher, P. C., & Henson, R. N. (2001). Frontal lobes and human memory: insights from functional neuroimaging. *Brain, 124,* 849–881.

Frith, C. D., & Frith, U. (1999). Interacting minds: A biological basis. *Science, 286,* 1692–1695.

Gazzaniga, M. S., Ivry, R. B., & Mangun, G. R. (1998). *Cognitive neuroscience: The biology of the mind.* New York: Norton.

Haxby, J., Ungerleider, L., Horwitz, B., Maisog, J., Ropoport, S., & Grady, C. (1996). Face encoding and recognition in the human brain. *Proceedings of the National Academy of Sciences USA, 93,* 927.

Hebb, D. O. (1949). *The organization of behavior.* New York: Wiley Interscience.

Kapur, S., Craik, F. I., Tulving, E., Wilson, A., Houle, S., & Brown, G. (1994). Neuroanatomical correlates of encoding in episodic memory. *Proceedings of the National Academy of Sciences USA, 91,* 2008–2011.

Kelley, W. M., Buckner, R. L., Miezin, F. M., Cohen, N. J., & Raichle, M. E. (1998). Encoding of famous and nonfamous faces using fMRI. *Society of Neuroscience Abstracts, 24,* 760.

Kelley, W. M., Miezin, F. M., & McDermott, B. (1998). Hemispheric specialization in human dorsal frontal cortex and medial temporal lobe for verbal and non-verbal encoding. *Neuron, 20,* 927–936.

Maquet, P. (2001). The role of sleep in learning and memory. *Science, 294,* 1048–1052.

Maquet, P., Laureys, S., Peigneux, P., Fuchs, S., Petiau, C., Phillips, C., et al. (2000). Experience-dependent changes in cerebral activation during human REM sleep. *Nature Neuroscience, 3,* 831–836.

McGaugh, J. L., Roozendaal, B., & Cahill, L. (2000). Modulation of memory storage by stress hormones and the amygdaloid complex. In M. S. Gazzaniga (Ed.), *The new cognitive neurosciences* (2nd ed., pp. 1081–1098). Cambridge, MA: MIT Press.

Siegel, J. M. (2001). The REM sleep-memory consolidation hypothesis. *Science, 294,* 1058–1063.

Smith, E. E., & Jonides, J. (1999). Storage and executive processes in the frontal lobes. *Science, 283,* 1657–1661.

Squire, L. R., & Kandel, E. R. (1999). *Memory: From mind to molecules.* New York: Freeman.

Squire, L. R., Ojemann, J. G., Miezin, F. M., Petersen, S. E., Videen, T. O., & Raichle, M. E. (1992). Activation of the hippocampus in normal humans: A functional anatomical study of memory. *Proceedings of the National Academy of Sciences USA, 89,* 1837–1841.

Tulving, E., Kapur, S., Craik, F. I., Moscovitch, M., & Houle, S. (1994). Hemispheric encoding/retrieval asymmetry in episodic memory: Positron emission tomography findings. *Proceedings of the National Academy of Sciences USA, 91,* 2016–2020.

Winson, J. (1990). The meaning of dreams. *Scientific American, 263,* 86–96.

7

An Overview of Cortical Function

Looking at a photograph of the cortex is a little overwhelming. Yet the locations of the functions that clinicians are most interested in can be better understood with a simple schematic, as shown in Figure 7.1. From Chapter 2 you will recall the location of the frontal, temporal, and parietal lobes, which are shown in the upper panel of the figure. Note the central sulcus with the primary motor and somatosensory areas on each side. In the lower panel, I have labeled a number of the important gyri, as well as defined some critical functional areas of the cortex. Let's start in the temporal lobe by drawing a line just below and parallel to the lateral fissure. This is the superior temporal gyrus. Draw two semicircles at the end of the lateral fissure and the superior temporal gyrus; these define the supramarginal and angular gyri. These areas are involved in auditory perception and language comprehension. In the inferior part of the frontal lobe, just anterior to the primary motor area, draw an upside-down U with a line down the middle—this represents Broca's area, a region critical for speech production and understanding grammar. Next, we will subdivide the frontal lobe. Just anterior to the precentral gyrus are the supplemental motor area (SMA) and premotor cortex, the former being more dorsal than the latter. These areas become active just before any type of motor movement, they are also activated during PET studies if a participant simply images a motor act without actually moving a muscle. Anterior to the SMA are the frontal eye fields, which govern eye movements. The prefrontal cortex encompasses the largest part of the frontal lobe, and is subdivided into the dorsolateral prefrontal cortex (DLPFC) and the ventromedial (or orbitofrontal) PFC. When looking at the brain from a lateral view, one mostly sees the DLPFC. The small inset in the bottom of the lower panel of the figure

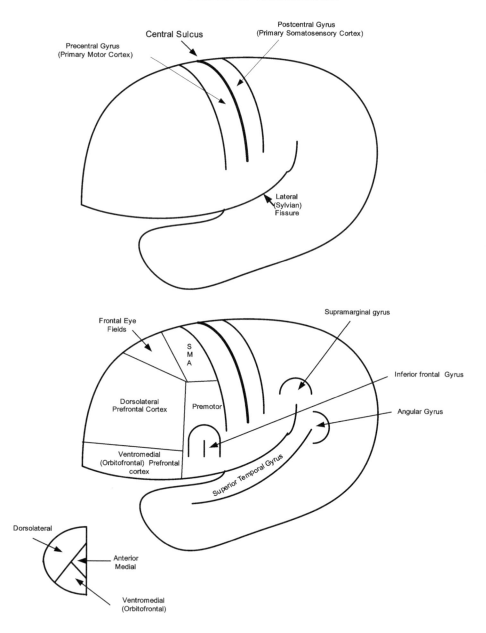

FIGURE 7.1. Overview of the cortex

shows a head-on view of the right frontal cortex (from an anterior view). This allows you to see how these two parts of the PFC are partitioned at an angle. The anterior medial part of the PFC cannot be seen from a lateral view of the intact brain.

Figure 7.2 shows the frontal lobe from the medial view of a sagittal section. The gray structure is the corpus callosum; wrapped around it is the cingulate gyrus. I have already discussed the cingulate gyrus in relation to memory. Here it is subdivided into its anterior and posterior regions. The anterior cingulate, although not structurally part of the frontal lobe, is strongly related to it functionally. The anterior cingulate is a key structure in emotional regulation and attention.

Figure 7.3 is an overview of key cortical functions and is the road map for this chapter. The predominant functions of the right and left hemisphere are shown. The phrases "left-brain" and "right-brain" have found their way into popular culture to designate verbal, highly logical pursuits on the one hand and artistic, intuitive behavior on the other. This distinction, although overly simplistic in many ways, nonetheless is backed up by a significant body of work in both pathology and neuroimaging. I examine cortical functions in terms of language, visual–spatial skills, attention, and, finally, executive functions, which also entail the regulation of emotion.

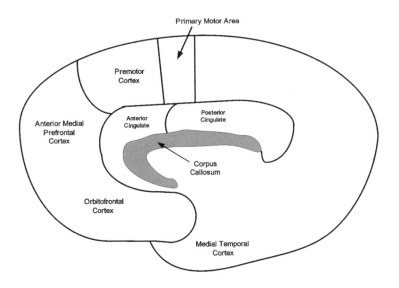

FIGURE 7.2. Medial view of the cortex

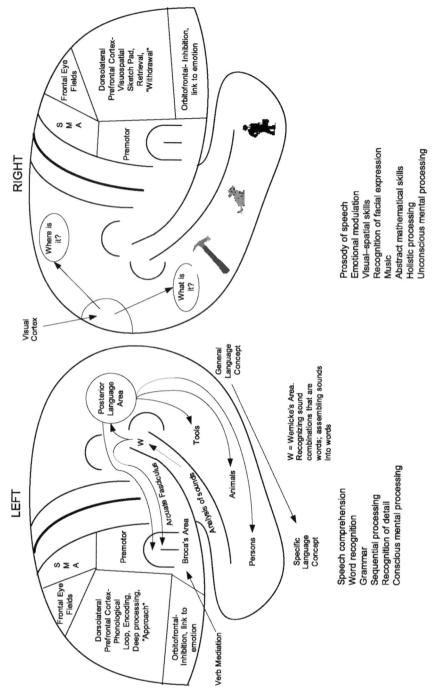

FIGURE 7.3. Hemispheric "division of labor" in the cortex

LANGUAGE

The primary auditory processing areas are in the superior temporal gyrus bilaterally. Speech sounds are quite different from the many other sounds we encounter in our daily life. Speech is extraordinary if you think about for a moment. Our vocal cords are two strips of tissue in the larynx. On command, they beat together as we breathe out, setting the air in vibration. This creates sound waves, and as these sound waves travel through our throats and mouths, the motions of our palates, tongues, and lips shape them. This complex sound wave travels to another individual's ear and sets the eardrum in motion. As the eardrum beats, the small bones of the middle ear transmit the frequency, amplitude, and pattern of these vibrations to the fluid of the cochlea of the inner ear. The movement of the fluid causes the hair cells of the cochlea to bend; this sets off neuronal firing, and information about the sound is carried first to the brain stem, then on to the primary auditory area in the superior temporal gyrus.

Take the word "baby." If we hear this word, what must the brain do to give it meaning? Two sounds make up the word: "bay" and "bee." What is key is that the two sounds must be sequential and follow each other very rapidly. The primary auditory area recognizes the two sounds, but this information must then be sent to a region at the very posterior end of the superior temporal gyrus. This region is named for its discoverer, Carl Wernicke. Wernicke's area contains the memories of the sequences of sounds that form words. For instance, Wernicke's area recognizes that the sound "ooo-ba" is not a word, that the sound "bay" by itself is the word "bay," and that a "bay" sound followed immediately by the "bee" sound is "baby." Wernicke's area does not, however, attach meaning to the word. This is the role of the posterior language area, which is located in the supramarginal and angular gyri. The posterior language area has extensive connections to all areas of the cortex, but particularly to the left temporal lobe. Thus the posterior language area ties the sound of the word to what it represents. Recent work by Hanna and Antonio Damasio and others have yielded insights into how the brain compartmentalizes word meanings. As shown in Figure 7.3, the tip of the temporal lobe seems to contain word meanings for people; animals are represented in the middle of the temporal lobe; and nouns for tools are found in the more posterior part of the temporal lobe. Stroke patients with lesions in the temporal lobe may have difficulty finding the word for a particular object, depending on where the damage is. A patient with an anterior temporal lobe lesion may not be able to name a picture of a person, even though he recognizes who or what the person is. For instance, if shown a picture of a policeman, he may say, "Oh, that's a guy, he has a gun, he stops the traffic, but I don't know what he is . . . ". The same patient, however, may have no trouble naming a hammer.

Notice that Wernicke's area has two outputs, one to the posterior language area just described and another that travels anterior through the arcuate fasciculus to Broca's area. Broca's area receives another input directly from the posterior language area; this is also shown in the figure. Broca's area contains the memories of the motor movements necessary to produce speech sounds. It also is critical in the use of grammar. Although the meanings of nouns appear to be located in the temporal lobe, the meanings of verbs appear to be accessed through an area in the inferior frontal lobe intimately associated with Broca's area. Persons who suffer a lesion in Broca's area (*Broca's aphasia*) comprehend most aspects of language but have pronounced articulation deficits. Like the patients with lesions in temporal lobe mentioned previously, they cannot name objects. The patients with temporal lobe lesions had difficulty only in naming a particular class of objects; the rest of their speech was fluent. Patients with Broca's aphasia cannot articulate any words very well and cannot name a wide variety of objects because the motor programs that activate the sequence of lip, tongue, and mouth movements to produce the word are lost. Patients with Broca's aphasia also suffer "agrammatism." Verbs are most likely to be left out. If a patient with Broca's aphasia is asked to describe a picture that shows a car crashing into a wall, he or she will say something like, "The car . . . car . . . there . . . the car and . . . the wall." The patient is unable to produce the verb "crash" at all, and each word is pronounced very haltingly. The patient can be shown two pictures, one of a boy hitting a girl and another of a girl hitting a boy. If he is asked to point to the picture in which "the boy hit the girl," he will get it right. But if he is told to point to the picture in which "the boy was hit by the girl," an error is much more likely. Broca's area appears key to understanding the grammatical construction of more complex sentences.

Patients with *Wernicke's aphasia* have very different language deficits from those with Broca's. These patients are completely fluent in their speech, but their speech makes no sense. They cannot comprehend speech and thus cannot follow commands unless nonverbal cues attend them. The speech output of a Wernicke's patient might sound as follows: "Well, food is happening last night I went mooing, then he told is no good. Mary I don't know she righting the house and well, it just pessing." Curiously, the patient is unaware that anything is wrong. Each time the examiner asks a question, the patient responds with gibberish. In Wernicke's aphasia, not only is Wernicke's area itself damaged, but so is the posterior language area. When the patient hears words, Wernicke's area no longer recognizes them as words. With the posterior language area destroyed, the brain can longer attach a word to a concept. Thus what is sent forward to Broca's area is meaningless (as in the computer jargon, "garbage in, garbage out"). The fact that the patient is unaware that anything is wrong raises interesting philosophical questions about language and consciousness.

When a stroke is less severe, only the posterior language area may be damaged, leaving Wernicke's area intact. This causes *transcortical sensory aphasia*. These patients also do not comprehend what is said to them, yet they will repeat what they hear said around them. How is this possible? The sounds are processed in the primary auditory area, sent to Wernicke's area in which they are recognized as words, and then sent directly to Broca's area, in which they can be repeated. Because the posterior language area is damaged, however, the patient does not have access to the word's meaning. So although the patient repeats what she hears, she cannot understand it. *Conduction aphasia* is the opposite of this condition. The patient comprehends language and is fluent but cannot repeat things on command. Here the direct connection between Wernicke's area and Broca's area (the arcuate fasciculus) is damaged. The sounds the patient hears move normally from the primary auditory cortex to Wernicke's area to the posterior language area. Speech is thus comprehended, and because the posterior language area can still communicate with Broca's area, speech production is not impaired. The patient cannot, however, articulate a simple repetition because the direct route from Wernicke's area to Broca's area is disrupted. This direct pathway, called the "phonological loop," does not require us to know the meaning of a word. We use this loop when saying a word in a foreign language that we do not understand or when saying a "pseudoword"(a pronounceable set of letters that does not form a word, such as "wuzzo"). When normal adults are asked to memorize a set of pseudowords, PET scans show activation in both Wernicke's area and Broca's area simultaneously, documenting the presence of this phonological loop.

In reading, many of the same processes are involved. When we see a word, the left visual areas in the occipital–parietal visual association cortex are activated. There is an interaction of the visual areas containing the representation of the letter with the posterior language area and Wernicke's area. The letter symbols must be mapped onto the sounds they represent, a process referred to as phonemic analysis. In word recognition, more is involved than *phonemic analysis*, however. Take the words "threw" and "through." The first word can be perceived through phonemic analysis: the "th" and "rew" combination of letters each stand for separate sounds. The brain needs only to decode them and recognize that, together, they form "threw," which means to have launched a projectile. In contrast, phonemic analysis is not helpful in decoding the word "through." English speakers must simply memorize the fact that the letter combination "ough" has been arbitrarily assigned to represent an "ew" or an "oh" sound, depending on which letters proceed it ("thr-ough" or "thor-ough"). What is amazing is that the brain can keep track of all this. It does so by having two systems for analysis of the written word—phonemic analysis and whole-word recognition—and it can flexibly move back and forth between the two as we read.

The foregoing processes can be seen in the live brain via PET scanning. Plate 2 (opposite p. 121) shows the results of a study by S. E. Petersen, Peter Fox, Michael Posner, and others. Participants were given PET scans while performing four tasks: passively viewing a word, listening to words, reading words from a monitor, and, finally, generating a verb to go with a noun. If the participant sees a picture of a car, he or she might say "drive." As can be seen, when a person is simply viewing words, the visual association cortex in the occipital–temporal area is activated. When he or she is hearing words, the auditory cortex and parietal–temporal junction (in which Wernicke's and the posterior language area reside) light up. Passively speaking words activates the primary motor area, but Broca's area is not strongly activated until the person actively uses language, that is, generates the verb.

Plate 3 (opposite p. 121) shows the results of a PET study done while normal participants view different types of reading stimuli. In the far-left panel, participants are viewing "false fonts," small geometric shapes the size of letters. Note the right-hemisphere activation. The next panel shows brain activation caused by strings of consonants such as "VSFFHT." Compare this to the third panel, in which the person is viewing pseudowords, combinations of vowels and consonants that could be pronounced, such as "WOBBY." Note the stronger left-cortex activation compared with the letter-string condition. The amount of activation is the same as in the presentation of real words, shown in the far-right panel. This left-sided activation probably represents the brain accessing the posterior language area in response to a visual stimulus (words or pseudowords) that might be meaningful to an English-speaking person. Consistent with this advantage of the left hemisphere for language, the superior part of the temporal lobe, called the "planum temporale," is larger on the left than on the right in most persons. Over 95% of right-handers have language functions localized to the left hemisphere, but so do approximately 70% of left-handers.

VISUAL–SPATIAL SKILLS

The right hemisphere has only the most rudimentary language capacity; it concerns itself with nonverbal, visual–spatial functions. Note in Figure 7.3 that there are two "streams" of information flow from the visual cortex. The ventral stream flows into the temporal lobe, in which representation of objects is the principal function. Assemblies of neurons activate when certain objects, animals, or persons are present. Unlike the left hemisphere, the right hemisphere produces primarily nonverbal, conceptual representations of the object or persons. Patients in whom strokes have damaged the right temporal lobe are more likely than those with left-temporal-lobe lesions to experience *prosopagnosia*, that is, an inability to recognize faces. Indeed, patients with right-sided lesions are more likely to exhibit *agnosia* (lack of knowing) about many objects, whereas the patients with left-sided lesions tend to exhibit *anomia* (inability to name the object). A patient with a right-sided lesion, when shown a hammer, may state that he or she does not know what it is; when asked to demonstrate how to use it, he or she will fail to accurately do so. In contrast, the patient with a left-sided lesion will make pounding motions with his or her hands but be unable to access the correct word for the item.

The dorsal stream feeds visual information into the dorsal parietal lobe, in which it is integrated with other data (principally auditory) to determine where the object is in space. The parietal area deals both with the position of objects in space and our sense of our own bodies. Right–left discrimination is a critical part of this ability. Patients with right parietal strokes develop an array of interesting deficits. They often lose their sense of geography and are no longer able to navigate around their home or city. In severe cases, they may develop *hemineglect*, a failure to recognize the left sides of their own bodies or the left side of their world. Asked to draw a picture of a clock, they draw only a semicircle, the right side of the clock. They may fail to wash their left hands or comb their hair on the left side. The right hemisphere appears predominant for a wide variety of visual–spatial functions. Whereas rote arithmetic seems more the province of the left hemisphere, the right hemisphere may handle more complex mathematical concepts, such as geometry and algebra, which makes sense given the visual–spatial nature of these studies. Persons with very high levels of mathematical ability are more likely to be left-handed. Zatorre and colleagues showed in 1994 that music activates the right hemisphere and that patients with right-hemisphere damage have impaired music perception.

The right hemisphere plays a critical role in recognition of emotion. Patients with right-hemisphere damage show, for the most part, normal language comprehension, and they have fluent speech. Right-hemisphere mechanisms control prosody, the changes in intonation and emphasis in speech that convey emotion or meaning. For instance, the difference in the meaning of the sentences "Joe got a raise," and "Joe got a raise?" are conveyed by tone of voice. In the former, the tone of voice is even throughout the sentence, but in the latter, the voice rises at the end to indicate a question rather than a statement. Patients with damage to the right hemisphere have difficulties making such distinctions, and their speech takes on a flat, nonemotional tone.

More broadly, right and left have different styles of processing information. The left hemisphere is more language based, uses conscious processing, and is logical and rule based. In contrast, the right hemisphere is more abstract in its functioning, and its processing is unconscious. The left hemisphere concerns itself with details of stimuli in the world; the right interprets the global pattern. These differences can be seen most clearly in Figure 7.4. Participants are asked to draw figures that consist of small stimuli embedded in larger stimuli. For instance, the large letter "A" is made up of small "X's." Normal persons have no difficulty including both the detail and the overall pattern. As the figure illustrates, patients with right-hemisphere damage lose the overall pattern, and patients with left-hemisphere damage lose sight of the detail.

FRONTAL LOBES AND EXECUTIVE FUNCTION

In the previous sections, I concentrated on specific functions, such as language and object recognition. To successfully carry out tasks, we must clearly perceive the world accurately and be able to communicate

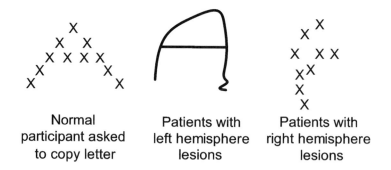

| Normal participant asked to copy letter | Patients with left hemisphere lesions | Patients with right hemisphere lesions |

FIGURE 7.4. Stimuli requiring attention to both the fine details and the overall pattern that are processed differently by the right and left hemispheres

our desires and intentions. No matter how skilled the cortex is in performing these functions, our behavior is not adaptive unless we carry out our actions according to a long-term plan, and we must have the capacity to wait to respond to stimuli in our environment until it is appropriate to do so. After we perceive information, we must hold those data in our minds, manipulate, ponder what they mean, and select a behavioral response. Many eminent scientists, working with both humans and animals, have studied these *executive functions* and the degree to which the prefrontal cortex (PFC) controls them. These individuals include Patricia Goldman-Rakic, who studied the activity of PFC neurons in monkeys. Joaquim Fuster has focused on the role of the PFC in the temporal organization of memory, and Antonio Damasio has discussed the role of the PFC (particularly the orbitomedial areas) in allowing emotion to mediate current behavior. Amy Arnsten and colleagues have studied how the catecholamine input to the frontal lobes influences executive functions. The discussion here draws on all these theories. Executive functions, and therefore the PFC circuitry, are impaired in a wide variety of mental disorders.

As Figure 7.2 showed, the frontal lobe is divided into three functional areas; the DLPFC, the orbitofrontal PFC, and the anterior cingulate. I take up the DLPFC and the concept of *working memory* first. Take the following word problem:

> "Sally was walking down the street, carrying 5 apples. She walked 5 blocks north and met her friend. She gave her friend 2 apples, then walked 4 blocks west. She ate an apple and then walked one block south to her home. How many apples did she have left?"

Several cognitive functions are critical for solving this problem. Most obviously, language areas must be intact to understand all the elements of the problem; arithmetic skills are required as well. More than this is required to be successful, however. As you listen, you must keep track of the number of apples exchanging hands, and you must realize that the number of blocks walked is not relevant to the problem. This active, mental manipulation of information is done in working memory, and the DLPFC is a key structure. Goldman-Rakic and colleagues showed this process in monkeys using a simple task. A monkey is shown a morsel of food, which is then placed in one of two wells. Both wells are covered, and then a screen is lowered in front of the wells. After a delay, the screen is lifted, and the monkey must lift the cover of the well to find the food. Monkeys with DLPFC lesions have great difficulty doing this task. Goldman-Rakic then had the monkeys do a slightly different task. The covers of the wells had different symbols on them (a circle and a cross), and the food morsel was always placed under one of the symbols. After several trials, the monkeys learned which cover to lift. DLPFC lesions did not affect this skill. This result tells us that long-term memory (associating the correct well with the symbol) was not impaired by frontal lobe damage. When the monkeys must hold the location of the well in their minds, however, the DLPFC is critical. The same task can be performed with monkeys who have indwelling electrodes in their frontal lobes. When the screen was lowered, particular DLPFC neurons fired during the delay, but they stopped once the response was made. Thus the DLPFC is critical for online processing of information.

In Figure 7.3, slightly different executive functions are ascribed to the right and left PFC. The left PFC controls verbal working memory, which includes the "phonological loop" discussed earlier. Here language information, such as the word problem previously presented, is placed in a "mental buffer" and manipulated. Recall from Chapter 6 that the DLPFC also is active during the encoding (remembering) portion of a memory task and whenever a deeper level of processing is required. (Recall that when the participants in a PET study had to say whether a word represented an object that was alive or not, the DLPFC was active compared with the condition in which they merely had to say whether the word contained a particular letter.) The right DLPFC contains the "visuospatial sketchpad," which manipulates objects in space. This area would be active when a person is thinking about a geometry problem or, more practically, trying to remember the directions to a place he or she has not often been to. The right DLPFC is also active during the retrieval portions of memory tasks.

Patients with lesions in the DLPFC are quite different from those with lesions in the temporal or parietal lobes. They rarely exhibit overt language problems and they recognize objects easily; indeed, in the initial conversation, they may appear quite normal. When tested, however, subtle impairments are detected. If given the problem described previously, they confuse the number of blocks with the number of apples. If a patient with a right parietal lesion and one with a DLPFC lesion are both given a maze to complete, they both have difficulties, but for different reasons. The patient with the parietal lesion, having lost his geographic sense, will fail to comprehend the task altogether. Instead of guiding the pencil through the maze, he makes stray marks on the paper that bear no relationship to the path. He finally just gives up, saying, "I can't do it, I don't understand." The patient with the DLPFC lesion will voice understanding, eagerly grab the pencil, and plow through the maze, taking the first path without sitting back and considering routes that might be more successful. When at a dead end in the maze, she may simply keep drawing, ignoring the rule to stay within the walls.

A variety of tests have been used to assess working memory functions. One that has been widely used in studies of psychiatric patients is the Wisconsin Card Sort Test (WCST). This test is illustrated in Figure 7.5. The examiner places three cards on the table in front of the participant. The cards contain objects of different shapes and colors and have varying numbers of the objects on them. The patient is told to guess by what rule the cards are to be sorted. For instance, if the cards are to be sorted by color, the patient should put the card on the middle stack. If they are to be sorted by shape, the card will go on the right stack, and if they are to be sorted by number of objects, the card goes on the left stack. If the participant guesses wrong, she is told to try again until she succeeds. Then a second card is presented, and because the person has learned the rule, she usually places it on the correct stack on her first try. Let's say the rule is to sort by number. She does so for several tries; then the examiner changes the rule without telling the participant, and she must guess again and then sort by the new rule (for instance, color instead of shape). Patients with DLPFC damage make a large number of preservative errors when the rule changes—they continue to sort the card by the previous rule even though the examiner tells them this is wrong. When neuroimaging methods such as PET are used to study normal volunteers doing the WCST, the DLPFC is strongly activated.

In Chapter 6 I discussed memory for discrete events, such as recalling a face associated with a significant life event. Working memory has another dimension to it, however—a temporal one. When performing a complex task, we must remember the sequence of actions to take. Although the sequences of routine motor acts, such as tying one's shoes, ultimately do not involve PFC input, complex motor acts require a knowledge of the order of steps to take. When changing the oil in your car for the first time, you must jack the car up, locate the oil filter, loosen the bolts, drain the old oil, and so on. Joaquim Fuster proposed that the DLPFC encoded the temporal aspects of behavior, thus giving us the ability to reflect on past events (retrospection) and the ability to antici-

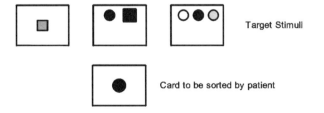

FIGURE 7.5. Stimuli used in the Wisconsin Card Sort Task

pate how our actions might turn out in the future (prospective function). B. Milner showed patients with DLPFC lesions a series of cards with objects presented on each card. After several cards were presented, participants were shown a target card with two objects on it and asked to pick the one they had seen most recently. Compared with both controls and patients with temporal lobe lesions, the patients with frontal lesions had great difficulty recalling which objects they had seen most recently.

The orbitofrontal PFC plays a lesser role in working memory. Patients with lesions in this area do not show severe deficits on the WCST. On initial examination, they also appear intact cognitively, but a review of their behavior often shows distinct deficits in social behavior. The effects of orbitofrontal damage have been most famously shown by the case of Phineas Gage, a railway worker in the mid-nineteenth century. An accidental explosion drove a railway spike up through his cheek and orbitofrontal cortex. Amazingly, he survived, but although intellectually intact, he underwent a major personality change. Before the injury, he had been responsible and hardworking; afterward he became impulsive, impatient, and rude. He no longer could follow a long-term plan of action. In his book *Descartes' Error*, Antonio Damasio described a patient he called a "modern Phineas Gage." The patient was a professional in his thirties who developed a brain tumor (a meningioma) that damaged his orbitofrontal cortex. The tumor was removed, but the orbitofrontal areas did not recover. Like Phineas Gage before him, the patient could no longer hold a job. He spent money foolishly and began to collect meaningless pieces of junk. He divorced his wife of many years and married impulsively.

These two cases show the critical role of the orbitofrontal cortex in social behavior. This area is key in *behavioral inhibition*, the ability to withhold a response. Inhibition allows working memory to do its job, to consider all the options and to execute the behavior with regard to the long-term plan. The orbitofrontal areas have input to the amygdala, and inhibit the amygdala's tendency to react in response to immediate needs. D. Dougherty and colleagues had healthy men read scripts that were anger inducing while they received PET scans. Compared with a neutral script, the anger-laden script induced higher blood flow in the left orbitofrontal cortex. In another study, by Blair and colleagues, participants underwent PET scans while looking at angry faces; this induced activity in the right orbitofrontal cortex. Again, we see that processing of verbal and nonverbal stimuli are segregated to the left and right hemispheres. In both studies, it was felt that the orbitofrontal cortex increased its activity in order to inhibit the aggression engendered by the stimuli. Recently, a study used neuroimaging to examine individuals who read a script in which a stranger attacked their mothers. In one sce-

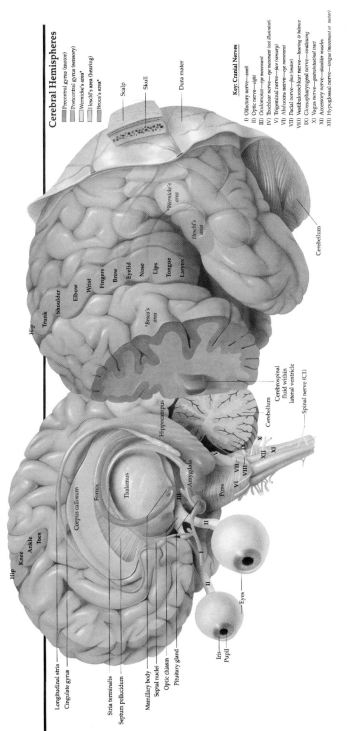

Cerebral Hemispheres

- Precentral gyrus (motor)
- Postcentral gyrus (sensory)
- Wernicke's area*
- Heschl's area (hearing)
- Broca's area*

Scalp
Skull

Dura mater

Key: Cranial Nerves

I) Olfactory nerve—*smell*
II) Optic nerve—*sight*
III) Oculomotor—*eye movement*
IV) Trochlear nerve—*eye movement (not illustrated)*
V) Trigeminal nerve—*face (sensory)*
VI) Abducens nerve—*eye movement*
VII) Facial nerve—*face (motor)*
VIII) Vestibulocochlear nerve—*hearing & balance*
IX) Glossopharyngeal nerve—*swallowing*
X) Vagus nerve—*gastrointestinal tract*
XI) Accessory nerve—*shoulder muscles*
XII) Hypoglossal nerve—*tongue (movement or motor)*

Hip
Trunk
Shoulder
Elbow
Wrist
Fingers
Brow
Eyelid
Nose
Lips
Tongue
Larynx
"Broca's area"

Wernicke's area
Heschl's area

Cerebellum

Hip
Knee
Ankle
Toes

Longitudinal stria
Cingulate gyrus
Stria terminalis
Septum pellucidum
Mamillary body
Septal nuclei
Optic chiasm
Pituitary gland

Corpus callosum
Fornix
Thalamus
Amygdala
Hippocampus

Cerebrospinal fluid within lateral ventricle
Cerebellum
Spinal nerve (C1)

Pons

Iris
Pupil
Eyes

PLATE 1. Anatomy of the brain. Created by the Anatomical Chart Company. Copyright Lippincott Williams & Wilkins. Reproduced by permission.

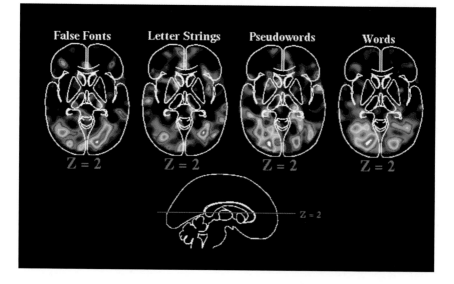

PLATE 2. PET studies of language processing. Reprinted by permission from Peterson et al. (1998), Positron emission tomography studies of the cortical anatomy of single word processing. *Nature, 331, 585–589.* Copyright 1998 by Nature Publishing Group.

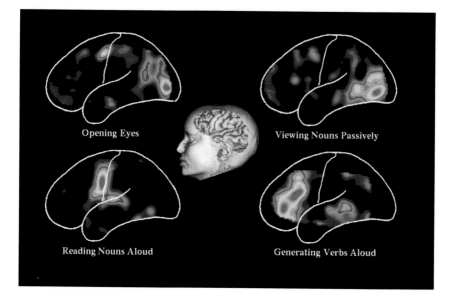

PLATE 3. PET studies of the processing of the visual presentation of false fonts, letters, and words. Reprinted by permission from Petersen et al. (1990), Activation of extrastriate and frontal cortical areas by visual words and word-like stimuli. *Science, 249, 1041–1044.* Copyright 1990 by the American Association for the Advancement of Science.

nario, they had to imagine just standing by, and in the other scenario, they imagined physically attacking the stranger. When the patients imagined restraining themselves, blood flow *increased* in inferior frontal lobes; but when they imagined actually fighting the attacker, blood flow in these regions *decreased*. Thus we can see why patients become aggressive or impulsive when the orbitofrontal areas are damaged. The orbitofrontal areas are no longer online to inhibit aggressive or impulsive responding. I return to this theme in Chapter 10.

I have discussed the right and left hemispheres in terms of the processing of verbal and nonverbal information, but the two hemispheres, particularly in the frontal region, may govern different types of emotions. Richard Davidson, Nathan Fox, and their colleagues have preformed an elegant series of studies examining right and left frontal activation in both positive and negative mood states. Their studies utilize electroencephalograms (EEG). EEG in the awake individual varies in its rhythm from the slower alpha (8–13 Hz) to the faster beta (greater than 13 Hz) waves. Alpha rhythm indicates less activation of particular area of the brain, though EEG is far less precise than PET scan in determining the source of brain activity. By calculating the amount of alpha in an EEG epoch, a measure of hemispheric activation can be obtained. Davidson and colleagues first found that when normal adults were watching movie clips, happy periods of the films were associated with more left-sided frontal EEG activation, whereas negative films induced more right-sided activation. Next, participants played a computer game in which on some trials they could earn a reward, whereas on other trials they were punished (fined money) for an incorrect response. When the participants were anticipating a punishment, they showed significantly more right-frontal activation.

Davidson and colleagues noted that, at baseline, adults differed in the asymmetry of frontal activation and that this trait was very stable within individuals. They divided participants into those with high amounts of left-sided versus right-sided frontal activation. Those with more right-sided activation reported much more intense feelings of disgust in response to films with gory content, whereas those with left-sided activation showed more pleasurable reaction to films with happier content. On rating scales, those with more right-sided activation reported more negative mood in their lives generally. These findings were found to hold even in infants and preschoolers. Infants with more right-sided frontal EEG activation cried more intensely in response to maternal separation than those with left-sided activation. Davidson and colleagues then examined a large group of preschool children, dividing them into a shy, inhibited group, an uninhibited, outgoing group, and a "middle" group of children who were intermediate on this dimension. Consistent with the adult studies, the inhibited children had more right-sided EEG frontal activation, whereas the uninhibited children had more left-sided activation. Davidson suggests that the right frontal lobe governs "withdrawal" functions and plays a greater role in negative emotion, whereas the left frontal lobe governs "approach" functions, which are associated with more positive emotions. From an evolutionary, perspective this makes sense; if there is something out there that we need to withdraw from, a negative mood will make us more likely to do so. Temperamentally, people may be divided into "approachers" and "withdrawers" based on their relative amounts of right or left frontal activation. Whether such frontal lobe differences are innate or a result of experience is in need of further study. One fact is well known, however—brain tumors or strokes that damage the right frontal lobe are far more likely than left-sided lesions to produce a manic episode as a sequelae. Taking the right frontal lobe offline appears to allow an abnormally positive and expansive mood to emerge.

THE ANTERIOR CINGULATE AND ATTENTION

Although it is not part of the frontal lobe structure, the anterior cingulate is discussed along with the frontal lobe because of its role in what is termed "executive attention." In PET studies, the anterior cingulate becomes active in a number of tasks. It was active, in addition to Broca's area, when participants had to think of a verb in response to a noun in the study mentioned previously. It is strongly activated by the Stroop test. In this test, participants are shown words that name colors, and most the time the word is printed in a color of ink that is compatible with the written word. For instance, the word "red" is printed in red ink. The person is told to name the color of the ink. On some of the trials, the ink is a different color from the word. For instance, the word "blue" is printed in brown ink. Because the participant must give the color of the ink, he or she must resist the temptation to read the word and say "blue" but must instead say "brown." When the PET trials taken during this "incompatible" condition are subtracted from the trials in which the ink matched the color of the word, the results show strong activation in the anterior cingulate. When participants must scan a list of nouns and count the number of animal words, anterior cingulate activity increases as the number of words in the list increases. All this suggests that the cingulate is involved in active attention. In the verb-generation task, the anterior cingulate may help choose among several options. During the Stroop test, it helps inhibit the participant's tendency to read the word first and then to examine the color. Finally, in the word-scanning task, it brings working memory online to help store the words in the buffer so that each may be examined. In Chapter 11, I explore the role of the cingulate in mood regulation.

Studies have revealed that the cingulate is part of one of two systems of attention, as shown in Figure 7.6. Michael Posner and colleagues have elaborated on this model. The posterior attention system governs the intake of information (particularly visual) and is distributed over three structures. In the right parietal lobe, there appears to be an area that specifically controls the process of disengaging from the current stimulus that has the focus. The superior colliculus then governs the movement of attention to the new focus. Finally, the pulvinar, a part of the thalamus, enhances the focus on the new stimulus. All of these areas are strongly innervated by the noradrenergic system, which becomes active when novel stimuli appear in the environment.

In contrast, the anterior cingulate forms the anterior or executive attention system. Once the information has been read in by the posterior attention system, the executive system brings working memory online to begin processing the information and selecting a response. The anterior

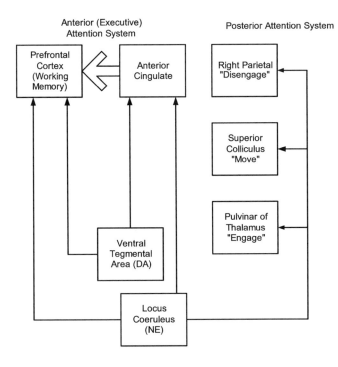

FIGURE 7.6. The anterior and posterior executive systems

cingulate, like the PFC itself, receives input from both dopaminergic and noradrenergic structures. Thus both catecholamines are critical to attention and working memory.

Amy Arnsten has reviewed research regarding the role of both NE and dopamine (DA) in PFC functioning. Depletion of both NE and DA from the PFC of animals results in cognitive impairments as severe as those in animals in which the PFC was ablated. Arnsten's summary of how NE and DA affect PFC neurons is shown in Figure 7.7. In the figure, a PFC neuron has input from a glutamate neuron carrying information (either from the brain stem or another location in the cortex). This neuron synapses on a glutamate receptor on the trunk of the dendrite. An NE neuron from the locus coeruleus releases its neurotransmitter onto a postsynaptic α_2 receptor on the PFC neuron, as well as onto a presynaptic receptor on the glutamate neuron. The α_2 receptors are much more sensitive than the α_1 receptors, as the latter are activated only at high levels of stress, when large amounts of NE are released from the locus coeruleus. Stimulation of the α_2 receptors appears to enhance working memory in animals, possibly by inhibiting the production of cAMP and thus decreasing the activity of protein kinase A (PKA). When monkeys are given guanfacine, a drug that stimulates α_2 receptors in the brain, PFC activity increases. In contrast, α_1 receptors activate the PIP_2 cascade, and this has the effect of increasing the amount of glutamate released onto the PFC neuron. In animals, drugs that act at the α_1 receptor impair working memory, possibly because the increased glutamate produces "noise" in the system, decreasing the efficiency of the PFC neuron.

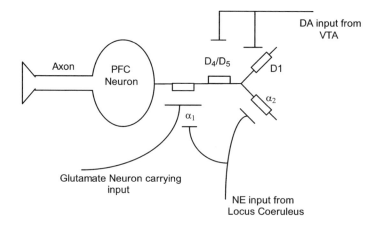

FIGURE 7.7. Dopaminergic and noradrenergic modulation of a prefrontal cortex neuron

DA effects on PFC functioning are complex. As shown in the figure, DA is released onto the spines of the dendrites, stimulating D_1 receptors. In moderate amounts, this stimulation enhances PFC functioning. Either very low or very high amounts of D_1 stimulation impair working memory functioning, however. Stimulation of D_4/D_5 receptors on the trunk of the dendrite may also impair the PFC neuron functioning by disrupting the transfer of information from the dendritic spines to the neuron. Thus effective working memory depends not only on an intact PFC but also on exquisite modulation by NE and DA. This is important in the discussion of attention-deficit/hyperactivity disorder (ADHD) in Chapter 9.

SUMMARY OF PART I

In the first part of this book, I have examined the basic neuroanatomy of the brain, examined many of its neurotransmitters, and developed an understanding of the brain circuitry involved in specific cognitive processes and behavior. You have taken a tour of the higher cortical functions, such as language, attention, visual–spatial skills, and executive functions. In Part II, I use these principles to explore the common mental disorders. The goal is not only to see how neurobiological factors figure in the etiology of mental illness but also to understand how treatments, both pharmacological and psychological, may act within the brain.

REFERENCES

Arnsten, A. F. T. (2001). Dopaminergic and noradrenergic influences on cognitive functions mediated by prefrontal cortex. In M. V. Solanto, A. F. T. Arnsten, & F. X. Castellanos (Eds.), *Stimulant drugs and ADHD: Basic and clinical neuroscience* (pp. 185–208). New York: Oxford University Press.

Blair, R. J. R., Morris, J. S., Frith, C. D., Perett, D. I., & Dolan, R. J. (1999). Dissociable neural responses to facial expressions of sadness and anger. *Brain, 122,* 883–893.

Carlson, N. R. (1998). *Physiology of behavior* (6th ed.). Boston: Allyn & Bacon.

Damasio, A. R. (1994). *Descartes' error: Emotion, reason, and the human brain.* New York: Putnam.

Davidson, R. J. (1992). Anterior asymmetry and the nature of emotion. *Brain and Cognition, 20,* 125–151.

Davidson, R. J. (1994). Temperament, affective style, and frontal lobe asymmetry. In G. Dawson & K. W. Fischer (Eds.), *Human behavior and the developing brain* (pp. 518–536). New York: Guilford Press.

Davidson, R. J., & Fox, N. A. (1982). Asymmetrical brain activity discriminates between positive versus negative affective stimuli in human infants. *Science, 218,* 1235–1237.

Davidson, R. J., Wheeler, R. E., & Kinney, L. (1992). Psychometric properties of resting anterior EEG asymmetry: Temporal stability and internal consistency. *Psychophysiology, 29,* 576–592.

Dougherty, D. D., Shin, L. M., Alpert, N. M., Pitman, R. K., Orr, S. P., Lasko, M., & Mackin, M. L. (1999). Anger in healthy men: A PET study using script driven imagery. *Biological Psychiatry, 46,* 466–472.

Fox, N. A. (1989). Psychophysiological correlates of emotional reactivity during the first year of life. *Developmental Psychology, 25,* 364–372.

Fox, N. A., & Davidson, R. J. (1986). Taste-elicited changes in facial signs of emotion and the asymmetry of brain electrical activity in human newborns. *Neuropsychologia, 24,* 417–422.

Fox, N. A., & Davidson, R. J. (1988). Patterns of brain electrical activity during facial signs of emotion in ten-month-old infants. *Developmental Psychology, 24,* 230–236.

Fuster, J. M. (1989). *The prefrontal cortex.* New York: Raven Press.

Fuster, J. M. (2001). The prefrontal cortex—an update: Time is of the essence. *Neuron, 30,* 319–333.

Goldman-Rakic, P. S. (1992). Working memory and the mind. *Scientific American, 267,* 110–117.

Goldman-Rakic, P. S. (1995). Architecture of the prefrontal cortex and the central executive. *Annals of the New York Academy of Sciences, 769,* 71–83.

Milner, B., Corsi, B., & Leonard, G. (1991). Frontal lobe contributions to recency judgements. *Neuropsychologia, 29,* 601–618.

Petersen, S. E., Fox, P. T., Posner, M., Mintun, M., & Raichle, M. E. (1988). Positron emission tomographic studies of the cortical anatomy of single-word processing. *Nature, 331,* 585–589.

Petersen, S. E., Fox, P. T., Synder, A. Z., & Raichle, M. E. (1990). Activation of extrastriate and frontal cortical areas by visual words and word-like stimuli. *Science, 249,* 1041–1044.

Pietrini, P., Guazzelli, M., Jaffe, K., & Grafman, J. (2000). Neural correlates of imaginal aggressive behavior assessed by positron emission tomography in healthy subjects. *American Journal of Psychiatry, 157,* 1772–1781.

Posner, M., & Petersen, S. E. (1990). The attention system of the brain. *Annual Review of Neuroscience, 13,* 25–42.

Posner, M. I., & Raichle, M. E. (1994). *Images of mind.* New York: Freeman.

Walsh, K., & Darby, D. (1999). *Neuropsychology: A clinical approach* (4th ed.) Edinburgh, UK: Churchill Livingstone.

Wheeler, R. E., Davidson, R. J., & Tomarken, A. J. (1993). Frontal brain asymmetry and emotional reactivity: A biological substrate of affective style. *Psychophysiology, 30,* 82–89.

Zatorre, R. J., Evans, A. C., & Meyer, E. (1994). Neural mechanisms underlying melodic perception and memory for pitch. *Journal of Neuroscience, 14,* 1908–1919.

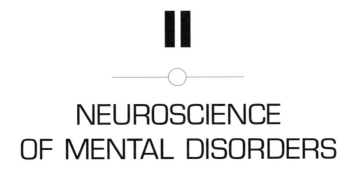

NEUROSCIENCE
OF MENTAL DISORDERS

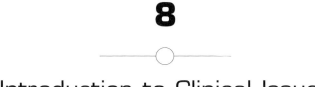

8

Introduction to Clinical Issues

AN OVERVIEW OF MENTAL DISORDERS

Before delving into the neurobiology of specific mental disorders, I present an overview of the major mental disorders and how they relate to each other. This is important because it is unlikely that brain mechanisms map in a direct fashion to mental disorders as we currently define them. That is, it is unlikely that we will find one gene specifically for depression or for attention-deficit/hyperactivity disorder (ADHD). Similarly, dysfunction in a particular area of the brain such as the prefrontal cortex (PFC) may be associated with several different mental disorders. I divide the mental disorders laid out by the fourth edition of the *Diagnostic and Statistical Manual of Mental Disorders* (DSM-IV) into the following categories: behavioral disorders, mood and anxiety disorders, tic disorders, pervasive developmental disorders (PDDs), schizophreniform disorders, cognitive disorders, and substance abuse disorders. These disorders are listed in Table 8.1; Figure 8.1 shows their developmental course and interrelatedness.

The best known of the behavioral disorders is ADHD, which affects up to 5% of school-age children. Also included in this category are oppositional defiant disorder (ODD) and conduct disorder (CD). These three disorders are often viewed as falling along a spectrum. Symptoms of ADHD include maladaptive inattentiveness, impulsivity, and/or hyperactivity; those of ODD include temper outbursts, excessive stubbornness, rule breaking, and socially offensive behavior toward others. Symptoms of CD, in contrast, are antisocial behavior, particularly aggressiveness toward people and property; stealing; lying; and sexual of-

TABLE 8.1. An Overview of DSM-IV Diagnoses

Behavioral disorders
    Attention-deficit/hyperactivity disorder (ADHD)
    Oppositional defiant/conduct disorders (ODD/CD)
    Cluster "B" personality disorders
        Antisocial, borderline, histrionic, and narcissistic personality

Mood and anxiety disorders
    Unipolar depression
        Major depressive episode and dysthymia
    Bipolar disorder
        Mania, cyclothymia, hypomania
    Panic attacks/panic disorder/agoraphobia
    Obsessive–compulsive disorder (OCD)
    Phobias
    Posttraumatic stress disorder (PTSD)
    Generalized anxiety disorder

Tic disorders

Pervasive developmental disorders (PDDs)
    Autism, Asperger's, other PDDs

Cognitive disorders
    Developmental cognitive disorders
        Reading, mathematics, language, speech disorders
    Cognitive disorders of senescence (dementia)
        Alzheimer's disease
        Dementia due to other medical conditions

Alcohol/substance abuse/dependence disorders

fenses. ADHD, ODD and CD all must begin in childhood. Figure 8.1 shows that, by adulthood, some children with ADHD no longer meet criteria for the disorder (i.e., their symptoms improve), so that the size of the ADHD circle shrinks. Oppositional defiant disorder and conduct disorder are not diagnosed in adults. Some of these youths desist in their maladaptive behavior, whereas others develop personality disorders (PD), particularly those in the DSM-IV "cluster B" category: antisocial, borderline, histrionic, or narcissistic.

Depressive and anxiety disorders can begin in childhood, with the latter being more common than the former. Figure 8.1 shows that, by adulthood, the prevalence of these disorders increases substantially, such that the lifetime rates of affective and anxiety disorders (any subtype) number 10% of the adult population. There is considerable controversy regarding the diagnosis of bipolar disorder (BP) in childhood, but it is considerably rarer at this time than depressive or anxiety disorders. Note that during childhood, bipolar disorder is highly *comorbid*, that is, it al-

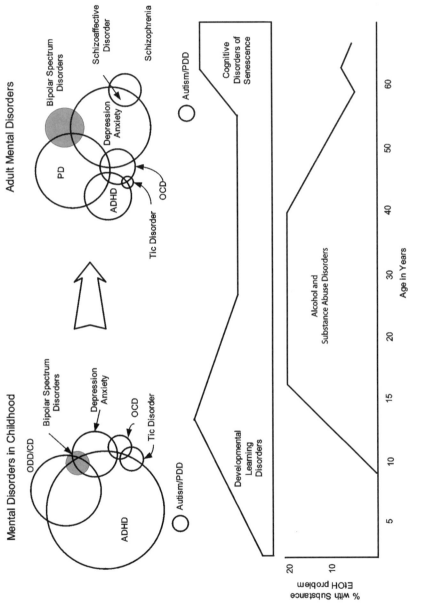

FIGURE 8.1. Life course of comorbidity of psychiatric disorders

most always co-occurs with ADHD, other mood disorders, or ODD/CD. By adulthood, BP becomes more common (at least 1% lifetime prevalence for the adult population); furthermore, BP is more often found in the absence of other disorders. Adult BP remains heterogenous, however. The 1% figure applies to bipolar I disorder, which comprises a distinct episode of abnormal euphoric mood, increased energy, activity and sexual activity, grandiosity, and disturbances of thought. Bipolar II consists of milder episodes of hypomania alternating with depressive episodes. Hagop Akiskal and his colleagues have described a spectrum of mood disturbances in between classic BP I and BP II; when these "softer" cases of BP are considered, the lifetime prevalence of the disorder may be as high as 5–8%. Furthermore, as shown in the figure, BP spectrum disorders may overlap with the cluster B personality disorders.

The schizophreniform disorders comprise schizophrenia itself and other psychotic disorders. These are quite rare in childhood and have an adult lifetime prevalence of about 1.5%. The line between schizophrenia and other disorders is not clear-cut, however, and an undetermined number of patients will fit into the overlapping condition of schizoaffective disorder, showing symptoms of both schizophrenia and affective disorder. Autism and other PDDs stand apart from the other disorders and remain fairly consistent in their prevalence over the life span. Finally, tic disorders appear in childhood but fall in prevalence as the population ages. During childhood, OCD is rare (and frequently overlaps with tic disorders), but the prevalence of OCD rises during adulthood. OCD may have neurobiological correlates distinct from those of the other anxiety disorders.

The lower part of Figure 8.1 shows the life course of the cognitive and alcohol–substance abuse disorders. A patient with any of the mental disorders just discussed may also have one of these disorders. During childhood, there is a rise of the prevalence of reading disorder, mathematics disorder, and any of the disorders of language and speech. These frequently impair educational performance. Some of these individuals with learning disabilities improve (with maturity or treatment), and thus the prevalence of these disorders falls by young adulthood. In late adulthood, disorders such as Alzheimer's disease, as well as other medical disorders, begin to take their toll on a wide range of cognitive functions, although it is important to understand that the majority of adults will live out their lives without suffering dementia.

Alcohol and substance abuse begin to emerge in early adolescence and peak by young adulthood. They remain at a fairly consistent prevalence through the young adult years and then begin to decline in prevalence in late adulthood. The reason is not only that many alcoholics or addicts achieve abstinence but also that some patients die early due to the toxic side effects of excessive alcohol or illegal drugs. Particularly for alcohol, usage increases again in later life. Almost every major mental disorder carries with it a risk of substance or alcohol abuse, and often it is difficult to tell whether the substance abuse disorder is secondary to the mental disorder or whether the abuse of substances leads to the mental disorder. For instance, a patient who develops depression may abuse drugs to "self-medicate" the depression, whereas another patient may first develop a substance abuse disorder and later become depressed because of the effects of the substance (or its withdrawal) on mood. For yet others, a single set of etiological factors may drive both the primary mental illness and the substance abuse disorder. Researchers in clinical neuroscience must carefully disentangle these multiple effects.

Chapters 9 and 10 focus on the behavioral disorders, examining the neurobiology of ADHD, ODD/CD, and personality disorders. The neurobiology of aggression and substance abuse is a major focus in these chapters. Chapter 11 examines the mood and anxiety disorders, and Chapter 12 focuses on schizophrenia and pervasive developmental disorders. The cognitive disorders are covered in Chapter 13.

For each disorder, I explore the following issues: (1) any known genetic underpinning, (2) results of neuroimaging or neurochemical studies of the disorder, (3) impact of specific psychosocial factors, and (4) mechanisms by which treatments might operate. Cutting across these four points is the theme of how three factors in mental disorders interact: genetic predisposition, early experiences (prenatal insult or abuse and neglect), and psychosocial factors.

Some analogies to well-known medical disorders are helpful in understanding the upcoming approach. Consider cancer and hypertension (high blood pressure). Cancers may differ their severity, but it is always abnormal to have malignant cancer cells in one's body. Cancer is qualitatively different from the normal state. In contrast, hypertension is defined quantitatively. In an adult, a blood pressure of 110/80 is clearly within the normal range, 130/100 is borderline high, and 180/120 is abnormal and would be a cause for alarm. The exact place to set the cutoff for high blood pressure is somewhat arbitrary. In both cancer and hypertension, genetics and environmental factors (diet, exposure to toxins, stress, smoking) play a role in causation. Some psychiatric disorders, such as autism, are like cancer in that they represent a disturbance that is qualitatively different from the normal state. Other disorders, such as ADHD, are defined quantitatively—the behaviors become abnormal when they are present in such excessive amounts as to be maladaptive.

BASIC PRINCIPLES OF GENETICS

Humans have anywhere from 30,000 to 70,000 genes distributed over 23 pairs of chromosomes (22 autosomal chromosomes and 1 pair of sex chromosomes). For each gene, we have one allele on each chromosome. Disorders such as cystic fibrosis are caused by single genes. If a child inherits two disease alleles, he will develop the disorder. The pattern of inheritance follows Mendel's laws. Most psychiatric disorders are polygenetic in nature. Multiple genes work together to convey a risk for a disorder. For instance, a disorder might involve 10 different genes. For each gene, it would be necessary to identify which allele conveyed the risk for the disorder and which did not (the "wild" type). A person with all 10 wild-type alleles would have no genetic risk for the disorder. A disorder could then express itself depending on how many of the disease alleles the individual had. A disorder could have a threshold. People with five or six disease alleles do not have the disorder, but a person with 5 out of 10 of the disease alleles would. Alternatively, a person with 4 out of 10 disease alleles might have a moderate risk for the disease (or a mild form of the disorder), whereas those with 8 out of 10 disease alleles would have a very high risk or would develop a severe form of the disorder. Genetics can interact with environmental factors to complicate the picture, as shown in Figure 8.2.

Assume that there is a disorder in which genetic factors are thought to be involved. The solid line represents individuals with this risk; those without such risk are represented by the dotted line. The y-axis shows the probability of developing the disorder or the severity of the disorder when it is expressed. The x-axis represents the severity of a psychosocial factor (to the right, more severe). In the left panel, the genetic factors predominate. Those at high genetic risk will develop the disorder even at very low levels of psychosocial adversity, whereas those without genetic

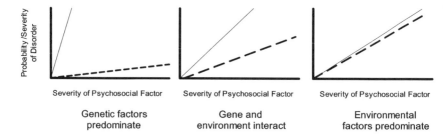

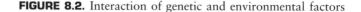

FIGURE 8.2. Interaction of genetic and environmental factors

risk rarely develop the disorder, even at very high levels of adversity. The middle panel shows the situation in which gene and environment interact. Both groups have a higher rate of the disorder as psychosocial adversity increases, but those with the high genetic risk will develop the disorder at lower levels of adversity than those without genetic risk. Finally, in the right panel, genetics is irrelevant to the overall risk of the disorder; only the degree of psychosocial adversity is related to disease expression.

Heritability has been used in many studies of mental disorders. Heritability (h^2) is a measure of how much of the *variance* of a trait can be attributed to genetics. Take the example of human height. Imagine a third-world village in which nutrition is quite poor. We go to the village and measure the height of every adult person, and we find a typical bell curve; but the mean height of the population is lower than that in the Western world, as shown in Figure 8.3. A generation later, we come back and measure the adult heights of the children of the first generation and find that the mean height of the population has not changed. We find that the relatively shorter people in generation 1 have had the rela-

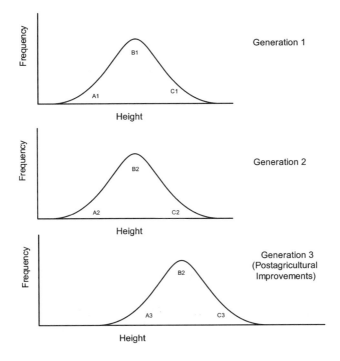

FIGURE 8.3. Understanding heritability

tively shorter children in generation 2. Thus the offspring of individuals A1, B1, and C1 occupy the same relative positions in the second generation as their parents did (A2, B2, and C2).

Now suppose that agricultural improvements are introduced for the next generation. When we measure the height of the grandchildren, we find that the mean height of the population has risen. When we look at the heights of the individuals, however, we find that the relative position within the population of the offspring is similar to that of the previous generation. Although all the offspring are taller than their parents, the relatively shorter parent (A2) still has the relatively shorter children (A3); similarly, the tallest parents (C2) still have the taller children (C3). When heritability for a trait is high, the amount of variance in the trait (i.e., the point within the population at which the individual falls) is determined by genetics. Heritability does not say anything about the point at which the mean of the population will fall, nor does high heritability preclude the effects of environment, as is seen after the introduction of agricultural improvements. In humans, heritability is calculated from twin studies and ranges from 0 (no effect of genetics on variance) to 1.0 (genetics governs all the variance). What kind of trait has a heritability of 0? Consider the width of men's ties. If we measured tie width in the 1950s, we would find a very small mean, but there still would be a variance in the widths. Some men might like ties one-half inch wide, others would wear ties 1½ inches wide. If we examined the tie width of their sons in the 1970s, mean tie width would have expanded. Some men, again, would like the widest 5-inch tie, whereas others prefer a mere 2 inches. But unlike height, there would be no correlation between the width of tie worn by fathers and sons because there is no gene governing choice of tie width. Because heritability is zero, the environment can determine all the variance: We may decree that everyone will wear exactly the same width tie. With height, no matter how we adjust the environment, even to the point of making everyone eat the same thing everyday, we cannot make everyone the same height. Heights will always fall along a bell curve, and genes will govern an individual's relative position within the bell curve.

MOLECULAR GENETICS

Twin and adoption studies can only take us so far. If heritability is high for a trait, or if adopted-away children develop the illnesses of their biological parents, then we know genetics plays a role, but we do not know which genes are involved. Thanks to advances in molecular genetics, studies to identify possible genes (or regions of chromosomes) involved in mental disorders are progressing. Thus it is important to have a basic understanding of these techniques. Chromosomes consist of long strands of DNA, made up of the four bases: thymine (T), guanine (G), adenine (A), and cytosine (C). In Figure 8.4, only one strand of the DNA is shown, one should bear in mind that the complementary strand has an adenine for every thymine and a cytosine for every guanine. In between the actual genes lay stretches of "nonsense" DNA. This DNA is never transcribed into messenger RNA (or translated into protein). Because it appears to do little, mutations in it have no effect on human functions. Thus over many generations we acquire many mutations in this area of genome to the point that our nonsense DNA is unique. This forms the basis of DNA fingerprinting. When an area of DNA is unique, we refer to it as a "marker." People can have very different sequences of DNA at these markers; these are referred to as "polymorphisms." There are two major types of molecular genetic studies: association and linkage.

First, let's examine association studies. We may, through good fortune, already know where a gene important to brain function is located in the genome. For instance, we know that the gene for the dopamine

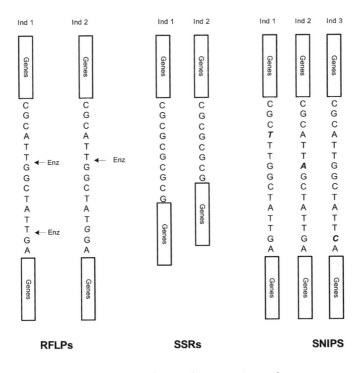

FIGURE 8.4. Understanding genetic markers

transporter, which governs the termination of the dopamine signal by taking dopamine back into the neuron, is on chromosome 5. We might perform an *association* study. We gather blood from both patients and controls, who are unrelated to each other. We want to know if the DNA in the region of the transporter gene is different in patients than in controls; that is, we wish to know if certain polymorphisms are found in the patients that are not found in the controls. One of the simpler forms of polymorphisms is shown on the left of Figure 8.4. These are called restriction length fragment polymorphisms (RLFPs). There are enzymes that cut DNA at certain base sequences. In the figure, the enzyme cut the DNA only at the sequence ATT. In Individual 2, a mutation has changed a T into a G and removed one of the enzyme cutting sites. If DNA from these two individuals are exposed to the enzyme, this region of DNA will produce three short fragments in Individual 1 and two long ones in Individual 2. When the fragmented DNA is placed on gel and exposed to an electric field ("electrophoresis"), the short fragments will travel further on the gel. By examining the patterns of gels from the two individuals, we can see that they have different polymorphisms. If the patients have a statistically significantly greater likelihood of having a particular polymorphism, then we conclude that one of the genes near that marker may be involved in the disease. If we already that know a gene of interest is there (for instance, the dopamine transporter), then we have reason to believe that our "candidate gene" is involved in the disease. We have not proved it, however. We must sequence the gene in both the patients and controls and show that the gene functions differently in the two groups.

Most of the time, we are not so well informed as to the location of the gene of interest. We know only that the polymorphisms at a particular marker are different in the patients and the controls, but we have no idea what genes are around that marker. If we do, we don't know which of the hundreds of genes are the ones involved in the disorder of interest. When we compare unrelated patients and controls, we must take great care to match the groups ethnically, because the nonsense DNA varies by ethnic group. The possibly of chance error in an association study is high, and they require many replications before these studies can be accepted.

Another approach is the linkage study. Stephen Faraone and his colleagues used an example that clearly illustrates this type of endeavor. Early studies of bipolar disorder had shown that some families showed no transmission of the illness from father to son, suggesting a X-linked factor in bipolar disorder. It was already known that a gene on the X chromosome caused color blindness. Many members of families with bipolar were examined for both BP and color blindness. Within one set of families (illustrated by Family 1 in Figure 8.5), those with BP were al-

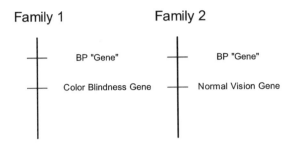

FIGURE 8.5. Linkage of bipolar illness and color blindness

most always color-blind. The reason is that the two genes (for BP and for color-blindness) are linked. If you had an ancestor with color-blindness who experienced a mutation and now had the BP-causing allele, that ancestor would pass both traits onto his progeny. In contrast, if the mutation occurred in a person with normal vision who had the mutation in the bipolar gene, the affective illness would almost always be associated with normal vision. From this pattern of inheritance, we conclude that a bipolar gene and color blindness are linked, that is, close to each other on the chromosome. As I discuss in Chapter 11, many other genes contribute to the risk of BP, but this gives you an idea of how linkage studies work.

There are very few observable human traits such as color blindness that can be used in linkage studies. Instead, scientists try to link the psychiatric illness to a marker whose location on a chromosome is known. A linkage study requires access to many patients and their family members, preferably over several generations. This is often not easy. Fortunately, a type of linkage study has been developed, called the "affected sib-pair" design. DNA is obtained from families who have two children with the illness of interest. The parent's DNA is examined for many different markers. Imagine a set of parents (all of whom have two affected children) who are heterozygous for a marker at the region of interest. Thus one parent has allele A on one chromosome and allele B on the other chromosome (AB). Assume that the other parent is heterogenous for two different alleles, C and D (CD). If these alleles have nothing to do with the illness, they will segregate by chance. This segregation is shown in the upper half of Table 8.2. Each cell contains two sibs, and the table represents all the possible progeny of AB and CD parents: 25% share both alleles, 50% share one allele, and 25% share no alleles. Now suppose the marker is linked to the disease. The findings would deviate from this pattern, as shown in the lower half of the table. The likelihood is more than chance that the affected sibs will share alleles; thus it is

TABLE 8.2. Segregation of Alleles in Affected Sib Pair Design

No linkage of marker with illness:

AC *AC*	*AD* AC	BC AC	**BD** AC
AC *AD*	*AD* AD	**BC** **AD**	BD AD
AC *BC*	**AD** **BC**	*BC* *BC*	BD BC
AC **BD**	*AD* BC	BC BD	*BD* *BD*

Italicized share both alleles (25%); **bold** share no alleles (25%); the rest share one allele (25%).

Linkage of marker with illness:

AC *AC*	*AD* AC	BC AC	**BD** **AC**
AC *AD*	BD *AD*	BC AC	BD AD
AC *BC*	BD BC	*BC* *BC*	BD BC
AD AC	*AD* *AD*	*BD* *BD*	*BD* *BD*

Italicized share both alleles (31.25%); **bold** share no alleles (6.25%); the rest share 1 allele (62.5%).

more likely that the marker is linked to the disease. A gene involved in the disorder may be near to the marker.

RFLPs are limited in number in the DNA. With advancing sensitivity of techniques, more subtle polymorphisms can be detected. Simple sequence repeats (SSRs) are shown in the middle section of Figure 8.4. Here the nonsense DNA consists of the bases "CG" repeated over and over. One individual has more repeats than the other; the DNA fragments with more repeats will not migrate as far. Modern electrophoresis gels can distinguish fragments different by as few as two base pairs. Finally, techniques have been developed that can distinguish single nucleotide polymorphisms (SNPs or "Snips"). Thus three individuals can be distinguished as shown on the right-hand side of Figure 8.4. Thus we can detect many more markers throughout the genome. The more markers we look for, the greater the chance that we will find one that is linked with the disorder of interest.

Linkage and association studies have different strengths and weaknesses. Linkage studies are systematic, but they can miss genes that have only small effects. In contrast, association studies can detect genes with small effects on a disorder, but they are prone to false positives, particularly if groups are not matched precisely on ethnic variables. Two new advances are increasing the power of association studies: within family association studies and "whole genome scans." An example of the former is the transmission disequilibrium test (TDT). Here sib pairs that are discordant for an illness are studied, along with their parents. Although an association study ordinarily uses normal controls, they are not needed in TDT study. The study checks to see if certain alleles go to the unaffected siblings while others tend to be transmitted to the ill siblings. This suggests that the illness is associated with the marker. Ethnic matching is automatic, as the study is done within families. Finally, the whole-genome scan takes advantage of the explosion of markers that have been developed, as described previously. No candidate gene is required; rather, thousands of markers are screened to see which ones are associated with a disorder. Such techniques may be ideal for psychiatric disorders, which are highly polygenetic in nature.

Throughout the remaining chapters, you will encounter the statement, "A polymorphism at a certain chromosome _____ has been linked (or associated) with illness X." It is important to bear in mind two facts about all such statements in this book. First, they are preliminary and require replication. Second, the statement does not mean that a gene for a psychiatric disorder has been identified. For some of these findings, I discuss interesting candidate genes near the implicated regions and how they might be involved in the pathophysiology of the disorder. As exciting as these discussions are, they remain preliminary. Most of our discussions will center on the 22 autosomal chromosomes and the two sex chromosomes, but there is also a separate genome in our mitochondria, the small organelles in the cytoplasm that produce the cell's energy. We inherit these genes solely from our mothers, and there is now evidence that this mitochrondrial genome may be involved in several psychiatric and developmental disorders. I also discuss other departures from Mendelian genetics, such as imprinting, by which a gene produces different effects depending on whether it is inherited from one's mother or father.

REFERENCES

Akiskal, H. S., Bourgeosis, M. L., Angst, J., Post, R., Hans-Jurgen, M., & Hirschfield, R. (2000). Re-evaluating the prevalence of and diagnostic comparison within the broad clinical spectrum. *Journal of Affective Disorders*, 59, S5–S30.

Faraone, S. V., Tsuang, M. T., & Tsuang, D. W. (1999). *Genetics of mental disorders: A guide for students, clinicians, and researchers.* New York: Guilford Press.

Ott, P. J., Tarter, R. E., & Ammerman, R. T. (1999). *Source book on substance abuse: Etiology, epidemiology, assessment and treatment.* Boston: Allyn & Bacon.

Pliszka, S. R., Carlson, C. L., & Swanson, J. M. (1999). *ADHD with comorbid disorders: Clinical assessment and management.* New York: Guilford Press.

Plomin, R., DeFries, J. C., McClearn, G. E., & McGuffin, P. (2000). *Behavioral genetics.* New York: Worth.

Regier, D. A., & Burke, J. D., Jr. (2000). Epidemiology. In B.J.Sadock & V. A. Sadock (Eds.), *Comprehensive textbook of psychiatry* (7th ed., pp. 500–522). Philadelphia: Lippincott Williams & Wilkins.

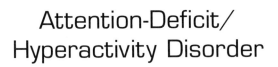

9

Attention-Deficit/ Hyperactivity Disorder

Attention-deficit/hyperactivity disorder (ADHD) consists of developmentally inappropriate levels of inattention, impulsivity, and/or hyperactivity that produce impairment of function in the person's everyday life. It is widely treated with stimulant medication, and this fact has made it one of the more controversial psychiatric conditions. All too often, ADHD is thought of as a "modern" condition, yet the hypothesis that behavioral disturbances of childhood might involve disturbances in brain mechanisms goes back nearly 100 years. (Keith Conners has recently described the history of the concept of ADHD.) In 1902, the British pediatrician George Still published a description of 20 children in his practice who showed deficits in self-control and attention span. He distinguished these children from those with mental retardation and noted that males were more affected; he also noted the co-occurrence of learning problems and aggressive/defiant behavior. In 1918 there was a worldwide epidemic of encephalitis (Von Economo's encephalitis). Children who contracted this infection developed (after recovering from the acute phase of the illness) a syndrome of hyperactivity and severe impulsivity very much like the one that Still had described.

In 1937, the psychiatrist Charles Bradley was working at the Emma Pendleton Bradley Home for Children, a residential facility for brain-injured children. As was standard practice at the time, children received a pneumoencephalogram as part of the diagnostic procedure. In this procedure, a small amount of air was entered into the spinal fluid; it floated up into the brain, and an X ray was taken. The air outlined the cerebral ventricles on the X ray, allowing the radiologist to see if any space-occupying lesion was present. This procedure caused severe headache. Bradley decided to use the amphetamine Benzedrine in an attempt to ameliorate the pain. When given the Benzedrine, the children showed immediate improvements in behavior. Bradley noted increases in academic performance, better self-control, and improved attention to task.

Bradley used amphetamines in behaviorally disturbed children for over two decades. He published a paper summarizing his experience in 1950 and observed that children with hyperactivity, moodiness, and impulsivity were most likely to respond. In the early 1960s the first double-blind placebo controlled trials of dextroamphetamine (the right-handed isomer of amphetamine) and methylphenidate (Ritalin) were performed, confirming Bradley's observation. Over the past four decades, hundreds of studies have been performed comparing these stimulant mediations to placebo. In a typical stimulant study, about 75% of participants receiving the stimulant show marked improvement in behavior and academic performance, whereas perhaps only 25% (and sometimes none) of the participants in the placebo group show such improvement.

There still remained the question as to what diagnosis these children should be given. As Conners describes it, in 1962, Sam Clements and John Peters referred to the syndrome as "minimal brain dysfunction" (MBD). In this, they fell back on the knowledge gained from Von Economo's encephalitis—that injury to the brain produced behavioral difficulties. It was also well known that severe head injury at birth could produce such a syndrome. Most children presenting with behavior problems, however, did not have clear-cut evidence of central nervous system (CNS) dysfunction. Their neurological exams were normal or were abnormal in mild and nonspecific ways, and they had no history of perinatal trauma, head injury, or CNS infection. Yet because they showed the kind of behavioral difficulties that many patients with CNS injury displayed, it was concluded that the brain damage must be there, and because it could not be detected by neurological examination, it was deemed "minimal."

The MBD label was unsatisfactory to most scientists. They objected to its circular nature: If the child was hyperactive, he or she must be brain damaged. How do we know he or she is brain damaged? Because he or she is hyperactive. In the 1970s Virginia Douglas and her colleagues at McGill University in Canada extensively studied hyperactive children and found that these children exhibited a variety of cognitive deficits, in addition to increased motor activity. Douglas proposed four key features of the syndrome of "hyperactivity": (1) difficulty maintaining attention and effort, (2) failure to inhibit impulsive responding, (3) inability to modulate arousal to appropriate levels for the situation (i.e., becoming overexcited in some situations, but lacking motivation in others), and (4) a strong inclination to seek immediate reinforcement (inability to delay gratification). In Douglas's model, hyperactivity is viewed as secondary to these deficits.

Douglas's work strongly influenced the American Psychiatric Association, which changed the name of the disorder to attention-deficit disorder (ADD) in DSM-III, published in 1980. This conception viewed the disorder as having three core symptoms: inattention, impulsivity, and hyperactivity. Patients were required to be *both* abnormally inattentive and impulsive, but being hyperactive was optional, forming the subtypes ADD "with and without hyperactivity." More research and clinical observations showed, however, that many children displayed significant inattentiveness without being impulsive. However, it was rare that children were abnormally hyperactive without also being impulsive. Put another way, when children were rated by parents or teachers with regard to hyperactivity and impulsivity, these ratings were positively correlated, such that children who were impulsive were hyperactive and vice versa. Hence DSM-IV in 1994 created two lists of symptoms: one of inattention and another of impulsivity–hyperactivity. Patients could meet criteria for three subtypes of ADHD: predominantly inattentive subtype, predominately hyperactive–impulsive subtype, and the combined subtype. Children with ADHD, combined type, are probably most similar to the long line of children treated since the days of Bradley. Epidemiological studies show a prevalence for the combined type of ADHD to be about 5% of the school-age population. Most neurobiological research has been conducted with this subgroup. ADHD, inattentive type, may be as common as the combined type, but it is less well researched, and, although it is treated with stimulants, it may have a different neurobiological underpinning than the combined type.

With the advent of DSM-III and DSM-IV, the field moved away from vaguely defined concepts such as MBD and hyperkinesis and produced a specific list of symptoms. Over the years, rating scales have been devised based on the DSM symptoms that give us a very good idea of the prevalence of these symptoms in the general population of children, as rated by both parents and children. Thus by comparing the patient's score on a rating scale to those of a group of children who are the same age and gender, it becomes clear how disturbed the child is relative to the general population. Yet have we really made any progress from the days of MBD? How do we know that ADHD is a neurobiological disorder? Genetic studies make a strong contribution in this regard. ADHD runs in families. If a parent has ADHD, a child has a more than 50% chance of also having ADHD; for siblings of a child with ADHD, the risk is

32%. Identical twins are far more likely to be concordant (i.e., both have the disorder) for ADHD than fraternal twins are. In these studies (see Figure 9.1) heritability can be shown to average about 0.80. Thus, possibly 80% of the variance of traits such as inattentiveness, impulsivity, and hyperactivity is the result of genetic factors. Twin studies also divide environmental influences into shared and nonshared effects. Shared effects are those life events that the twins have in common (socioeconomic status, parent's discipline style), and nonshared effects are things the twins do not have in common (i.e., having different teachers). Surprisingly, shared environmental effects account for very little (0–6%) of the variance of ADHD symptoms, whereas nonshared effects have somewhat more influence (9–20%). As Russell Barkley has stated, shared environmental effects such as social class, family educational background, general home environment, family nutrition habits, toxins in the environment, and child-rearing characteristics of the family play very little role, if any, in the etiology of ADHD. Nonshared characteristics that might be relevant in ADHD are head injury, infection, or *individual* exposure to toxins, rather than global cultural or environmental effects.

ADHD most likely has a polygenetic nature. If the genetic effect on ADHD is so strong, then where is the best place to look for "ADHD

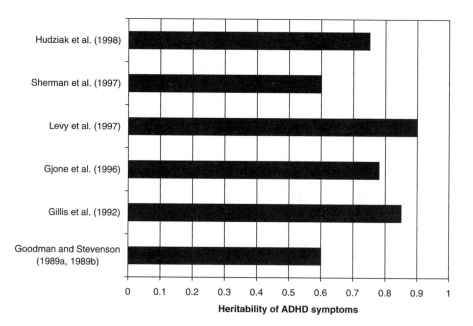

FIGURE 9.1. Heritability of ADHD symptoms

genes"? Fortunately, we have a clue in the mechanism of action of the medications used to treat the condition. The stimulant medications, such as methylphenidate (Ritalin, Metadate, Concerta) or amphetamine (Adderall, Dexedrine), have pronounced effects on the catecholamine systems, norepinephrine (NE) and dopamine (DA). At the end of this chapter, I discuss the therapeutic effects of the medication in more detail. Drugs that do not affect these systems do not seem to be helpful for ADHD. Thus genes that govern the DA and NE systems are a logical place to begin.

Most of the genetic work has concerned genes that govern the dopamine system, as shown in the lower panel of Figure 9.2. We discussed the

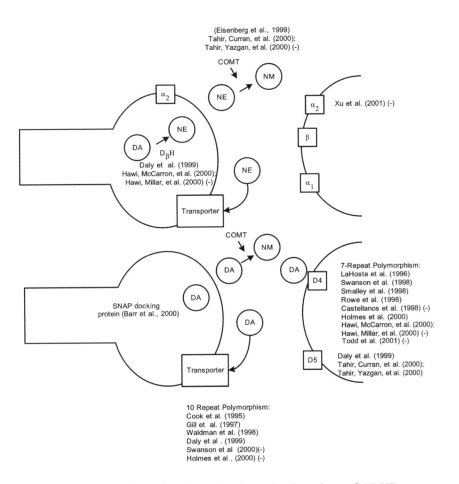

FIGURE 9.2. Genes implicated in the pathophysiology of ADHD

dopamine receptor subtypes in previous chapters. The D_1 and D_2 receptors do not appear to be involved in ADHD, but several studies have implicated a variant of the D_4 receptor, termed the "7-repeat." The D_4 receptor structure is shown in Figure 9.3. The amino acid chain forming the receptor protein is folded over on itself several times, spanning the neuronal membrane. Part of the amino acid chain faces the cytoplasm of the cell. The part of the gene that codes for this section of the receptor amino acid chain has a segment that can be repeated two, four, or seven times. The 2- and 4-repeats are the most common in the general population. The 7-repeat allele has been associated with the personality trait of "novelty seeking" in some but not all studies. That is, normal adults with the 7-repeat rate themselves to be more impulsive, exploratory, and excitable—traits that children with ADHD share. G. Lahoste and James Swanson at the University of California at Irvine first found an association with the 7-repeat D_4 gene and ADHD. The studies shown in Figure 9.2 find, for the most part, that children with ADHD are more likely to have the 7-repeat. The effect is modest; in the positive studies, about 25–30% of the ADHD sample will have the 7-repeat allele compared with about 10–15% of the controls. So having the 7-repeat gene alone is neither necessary nor sufficient to produce ADHD. Furthermore, as the fig-

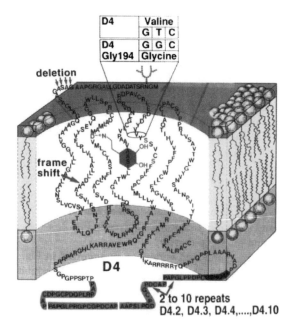

FIGURE 9.3. The dopamine 4 receptor

ure shows, there have been negative studies. To a degree, this is to be expected with a gene that has only a modest effect. It is also important to note how studies have varied from country to country. Positive studies more often have been done in North America; studies in Ireland, Israel, and Turkey have been more negative. Again, this is not surprising for a polygenetic condition. If many genes govern impulse control, then variations in different genes can lead to the same conditions in separated populations. More generally, at one time in evolution it may have been advantageous to have a certain number of impulsive people in the population; natural selection would have favored whichever genetic variations produced this trait.

The 7-repeat allele of the D_4 receptor may be subsensitive to DA; thus when activated by DA, the receptor is less likely to inhibit adenylyl cyclase. The 2-, 4-, and 7-repeat alleles vary considerably among different ethnic groups. Worldwide, about 64% of people have at least one 4-repeat, with the 7-repeat occurring in about 21% of individuals. The frequency of 7-repeat appears similar in Africans and Europeans, but it is only about 1% among the Japanese. Two studies have found a particular variant of the D_5 receptor to be more common among probands with ADHD, although whether this variant effects the function of the D_5 receptor is unclear at this point.

The dopamine transporter (DAT) has been another focus of genetic research in ADHD. The DAT governs the reuptake of DA into the neuron, which is the prime method by which the effect of DA is terminated. The gene for the DAT is found on chromosome 5. Edwin Cook at the University of Chicago first examined areas of the DAT gene in which repeats of nucleotides occurred, as in the case of the D_4 receptors. When a segment of the DNA is repeated 10 times, the allele is 480 base pairs long; when it is repeated 9 times, it is 440 base pairs long. In patients with ADHD, 86% had the 10-repeat, whereas 14% had the 9-repeat. In controls, 68% had the 10-repeat, and the remainder (32%) had the 9-repeat. Thus having the 10-repeat conveyed a slightly higher risk of ADHD. This finding has been replicated by three other groups of researchers, though two studies did not confirm it. Caution is required, however, because a recent neuroimaging study by Diana Martinez and colleagues did not find people with 9- and 10-repeat polymorphisms of the DAT gene to have differences in DA release or DAT density.

The enzyme dopamine β-hydroxylase (DBH) catalyzes the transformation of DA into NE within the NE neurons. There is a suggestion from one study that a variant in this gene could be associated with ADHD. When NE is released from the neuron, its action is also terminated by reuptake into the neuron, but there is an enzymatic method of doing this as well. The extracellular enzyme catechol-O-methyltransferase (COMT) catalyzes the breakdown of DA and NE into inactive metabolites. Eisenberg and colleagues studied a variant of the enzyme in which one amino acid, valine, was substituted for methionine. Persons who are homozygous for the valine substitution have very high levels of COMT activity, those homozygous for methionine have low levels of COMT activity, and heterozygotes have intermediate levels of enzyme activity. Parents were more likely to transmit the valine allele to a child with ADHD, and those children with ADHD with a valine allele made many more impulsive errors on a computer test of attention than those children homozygous for the methionine allele. One could speculate that having higher levels of COMT activity would also lead to early termination of NE or DA action. (I again examine COMT in our study of schizophrenia.) Other studies, however, have not shown a relationship of COMT to ADHD. NE can affect frontal lobe functioning via postsynaptic α_{2A} receptors. Chun Xu and colleagues examined a polymorphism located in the promotor region of the α_{2A} gene but found no linkage of it with ADHD. Recently, C. L. Barr and colleagues studied "synaptosomal-associated protein of 25 kilo-Daltons" (SNAP-25) protein, which is a key component of docking the vesicle to the membrane and inducing neurotransmitter release. Barr and colleagues found a particular variant of the gene for SNAP-25 to be associated with ADHD. Finally, a recent study from China found a marker near a gene for monoamine oxidase (MAO) to be associated with ADHD. MAO is an enzyme that breaks down DA and NE after it is taken back up into the neuron. Amphetamine, in addition to blocking the reuptake of DA and NE, inhibits MAO, further increasing supplies of these neurotransmitters. More genes are certain to be involved in ADHD than the ones studied thus far.

STRUCTURAL NEUROIMAGING

With the advent of magnetic resonance imaging (MRI), it became possible to study the volume of brain structures thought to be involved in psychopathology more precisely. In working with children, MRI was a particularly important development because it did not involve radiation, making the use of normal control groups possible. Three areas of the brain have been shown to differ in children with ADHD relative to controls: the frontal lobes, the caudate nuclei, and the cerebellum. Given that children with ADHD have marked difficulty with impulsivity and social judgment, it comes as no surprise that there might be problems in the frontal lobe. In normal individuals, the right frontal lobe is somewhat larger than the right; four studies have shown that children with

ADHD tend to have slightly smaller right frontal lobes, such that the right and left frontal lobes are more symmetrical. In Chapter 7, the right frontal lobe was described as being involved in the "withdrawal" behavioral function and as being more active when aversive stimuli were present. Individuals with ADHD are well known for their tendency to rush in and to ignore possible negative consequences. Whereas boys show a decrease in volume in the right frontal region, a recent study by Castellanos and colleagues of girls with ADHD found bilateral decreases in frontal lobe volume relative to controls.

I showed in Chapter 5 how the caudate nuclei participate in the initiation of motor behavior. The caudates of children with ADHD have been found to differ from those of controls, although the studies disagree on the nature of the difference. Xavier Castellanos and colleagues found that normal children had larger right caudates relative to the left but that the children with ADHD had smaller right caudates. Two other groups, led by George Hynd and Pauline Filipek, found normal children to have larger left than right caudates and children with ADHD to have smaller left caudates. Margaret Semrud-Clikeman also found that children with a left > right asymmetry of the caudate head did better on the Stroop task, which, as explained in Chapter 7, measures inhibitory control. Castellanos found that children with ADHD had smaller cerebellar volumes, with the midline structure of the cerebellum, called the vermis, being reduced in its posterior aspect. The vermis is the only part of the cerebellum that receives DA input. It, like the whole cerebellum, also receives NE input. The vermis also has output to both the ventral tegmental area and locus coeruleus; thus it also plays a role in governing the output of the dopaminergic and noradrenergic systems.

FUNCTIONAL IMAGING

In 1990, Alan Zametkin and colleagues showed via positron emission tomography (PET) that total brain glucose metabolism was reduced in adults with ADHD relative to controls. Zametkin and his colleague Monique Ernst several year later found total glucose metabolism to be decreased in girls with ADHD relative to girls without ADHD, but boys with and without ADHD did not differ in this regard. These early studies showed that there are developmental differences in brain functioning in people with ADHD; furthermore, males and females are likely to also have different neurobiological mechanisms at work in the disorder. Because PET does involve radiation, it is rarely used in young children as a research tool. In functional MRI (fMRI), techniques are used that assess blood oxygenation in the brain, giving a measure of brain activity while the participant performs a task. Chandan Vaidya at Stanford University performed one of the first fMRI studies of ADHD. Ten normal children and 10 with ADHD did the go/no go task while being scanned twice, once while on placebo and a second time while on methylphenidate. On placebo, the children with ADHD had less activity in the heads of the caudate than the controls. On methylphenidate, both the groups improved their performances on the go/no go task but had different patterns of brain activity. Caudate activity increased in the ADHD children but declined in the controls. In the frontal lobes, the level of brain activity depended on the rate at which the task was presented. When the letters appeared every 1.5 seconds, there were no differences between the groups in frontal lobe activity, and methylphenidate increased this activity equally in children with ADHD and controls. When the rate was slower, the frontal lobe activity was *higher* in the group with ADHD than in the controls. Thus interpreting functional imaging studies is not straightforward; results will depend on the type of task the patient performs during their scan as well as medication status.

Gordon Logan developed the stop signal task, a simple test in which the person presses one of two buttons depending on which letter (for instance, *A* or *B*) appears on the screen. On about a quarter of the trials, a letter *S* appears after the *A* or *B*. On these trials, the participant must inhibit his or her button press. This task is very good for assessing inhibitory control because the participant must stop a movement that has already been activated. In 1999, Katya Rubia and colleagues studied adolescents with ADHD, comparing them with teenagers without ADHD using fMRI. During the portion of the task that required stopping, the control group adolescents strongly activated their right inferior frontal lobes; the teenagers with ADHD showed much less activation of this area. Also of interest in view of the caudate structural findings, the controls more strongly activated the left caudate compared with the adolescents with ADHD. (All the participants were right-handed.) Along with my colleagues Mario Liotti and Marty Woldorf, I used the stop signal task in a study with event-related potentials (ERPs). In ERP, an EEG is obtained while the participant does the task many times. The EEG is averaged, canceling out random brain activity and leaving an EEG tracing that represents the brain's response to the stimuli of the task. We found that when the stop signal was presented, the normal children produced a large, negative EEG wave over their right inferior scalp; this wave was much reduced in the children with ADHD, as shown in Figure 9.4. Thus there are three bodies of data that are highly consistent with each other: The right frontal lobes modulate withdrawal and negative affect; the right frontal lobe may be smaller in persons with ADHD; and, when doing an inhibitory task, persons with ADHD evidence less right frontal

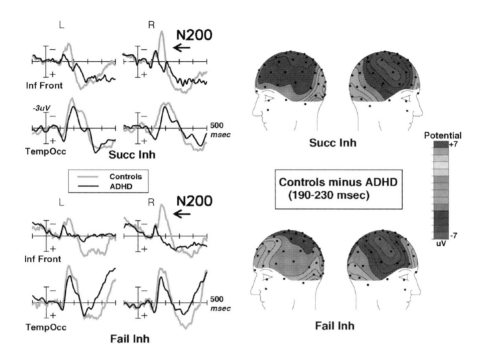

FIGURE 9.4. Event-related potential findings in children with ADHD implicating dysfunction in the right frontal lobe. From Pliszka et al. (2000). Reprinted by permission of Elsevier Science

lobe activation. Neuroscientist George Bush has done fMRI with adults (both with and without ADHD) while they performed the Stroop test. Only the controls showed an increased activation of the anterior cingulate during the incompatible condition. This suggests impairment of the executive attention system in people with ADHD.

Other neuroimaging techniques are beginning to give us a look at neurotransmitter function in live humans. Monique Ernst used PET scanning with the radiochemical 18-fluorodopa that labels NE and DA terminals in the brain. Adults with ADHD had fewer of these terminals in the prefrontal cortex than controls. In adolescents, on the other hand, 18-fluorodopa uptake was increased in the midbrain but not in the cortex. The DAT can be labeled with the radiochemical 123I-Altropane; Dougherty and colleagues showed that adults with ADHD had much higher levels of DAT in their brains than controls, although they studied only a small sample of six men with ADHD. Klaus-Henning Krause and colleagues in Germany replicated these results. Their sample of 10 adults with ADHD had never been treated with medication; after methylphenidate treatment the number of DAT receptors decreased to the levels in the control group.

MECHANISMS OF STIMULANT TREATMENT

As noted, stimulants have a variety of effects on NE and DA. Most important, they block the reuptake of the neurotransmitter into the neuron. Drugs that enhance only the action of DA are generally not effective as treatments for ADHD, whereas drugs that enhance only the effects of NE are better than placebo but not as effective as the stimulants. Thus it seems that it is necessary to effect both NE and DA to fully attenuate the symptoms of ADHD. Can ADHD be viewed as a simple deficit of NE or DA? Do stimulants work by simply "pumping up" the amount of DA and NE in the brain? It clearly is not this straightforward. In 1984, Mary Solanto of Mount Sinai University noted that the doses of stimulants used to reduce hyperactivity are low enough that they might work by inducing the stimulation of presynaptic autoreceptors, thus *decreasing* the amount of DA or NE released. During the 1970s and 1980s many studies were done measuring the metabolites of NE and DA in the urine of children with ADHD before and after treatment with stimulants. Although interpretation of these studies is not straightforward, it does seem that an acute dose of stimulant raises the amount of NE and DA in the synaptic cleft. The NE and DA rapidly stimulate presynaptic autoreceptors and lead to a decrease in firing of the locus coeruleus and DA neurons (VTA and substantia nigra). Xavier Castellanos and colleagues measured the amount of homovanillic acid (HVA, the main metabolite of DA) in the spinal fluid of children with ADHD before they were treated with stimulants. First, the higher the HVA level in the spinal fluid at baseline, the more hyperactive the child was. With stimulant treatment, the HVA level in spinal fluid declined, and those children with the highest baseline HVA had the best response to the stimulant.

In Chapter 5 I discussed Anthony Grace's work on the role of dopamine in balancing the influence of the amygdala and hippocampus on behavior. Grace has also put forward a hypothesis on how stimulants might effect DA and thereby act therapeutically in ADHD. First, Grace distinguishes between phasic and tonic release of DA (upper panel, Figure 9.5). Phasic DA release occurs in response to an action potential in the DA neuron. After release, most of this DA is taken back up into the neuron via the DAT. There is, however, another pool of DA that is left in the cleft. This tonic pool consists of DA not taken back up by the transporter, as well as DA released through the stimulation of "hetero-receptors." These are glutamate receptors on the DA nerve terminals; they stimulate the release of DA that in turn stimulates the DA autoreceptors. *Stimulation of these autoreceptors decreases the phasic release of DA.* Thus the higher the level of tonic DA, the less phasic release, and vice versa. This action is shown in the lower part of Figure 9.5. The baseline level on the *y*-axis represents the tonic release, and the peaks represent the phasic release. In Grace's model, individuals with ADHD are hypothesized to have lower tonic release. Tonic DA is not available to stimulate autoreceptors, such that whenever an action potential reaches the nerve terminal, a very large bolus of DA is released. Recall from Chapter 5 that this would increase the influence of the amygdala on motor action, that is, produce a greater likelihood of an immediate, affect-driven response. Now the stimulant is administered. This causes a small increase in the already large phasic response, but be-

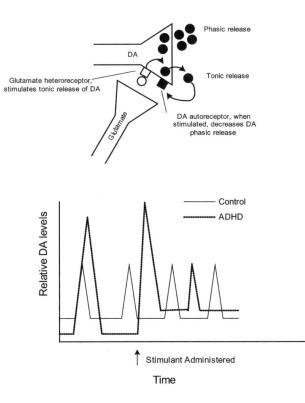

FIGURE 9.5. Grace's (2000) model of stimulant action on dopamine functioning in ADHD

cause this response is "maxed out," the greater influence is on the tonic portion. The rise in tonic DA would lead to autoreceptor stimulation such that the next time the DA neuron fires, the phasic response is smaller. This action would explain why high DA levels are associated with more symptoms of ADHD at baseline but a decline in DA levels is associated with treatment response. Why would the tonic level of DA in ADHD be decreased to begin with? Recall that Dougherty and Krause found higher levels of DAT in adults with ADHD. Perhaps an excessive number of DAT leads to the neuron taking up too much DA, leaving the autoreceptors understimulated and producing an excessive phasic component, although this is purely speculation at this point.

PUTTING IT TOGETHER

Many scientists have contributed to our thinking about ADHD. Russell Barkley suggested that behavioral inhibition, governed particularly by the orbitofrontal cortex, was the prime impairment in ADHD. He theorized that because this basic function was disturbed, other executive functions failed to develop: in particular, working memory (both verbal and nonverbal), regulation of affect, and reconstitution. The latter involves an ability to take behaviors apart and combine them into new repertoires of behavior more adaptive to new situations. As noted, Mary Solanto first proposed that the excessive activity in the DA system might underlie impulsivity. Herbert Quay used the work of Jeffery Gray to develop a theory of ADHD. He suggested that excessive DA activity would lead to inappropriate activation, whereas deficient NE activity might lead to underactivity of a "behavioral inhibition system." Xavier Castellanos's MRI work has focused attention on how deficits in diverse brain regions must be involved in ADHD. Michael Posner's work on the anterior and posterior attention systems has provided a valuable foundation for models of ADHD. James McCracken of the University of California at Los Angeles and I have discussed the interaction of various neurotransmitter systems in the pathophysiology of ADHD. Figure 9.6 summarizes all of these ideas.

Begin with the brain stem. Sensory events (primarily visual, auditory, and tactile) are transmitted to the cerebral cortex, where perception occurs. As shown in (1), diverse sensory events also activate the nucleus paragigantocellularis (PGi). The PGi, in turn, activates the locus coeruleus (LC) and the intermediolateral cell column (IML) of the spinal cord. The LC releases NE throughout the cortex, while the IML activates the sympathetic nervous system (SNS), as I discussed in Chapter 4. In Chapter 4 I also discussed the role of epinephrine (EPI) in the SNS.

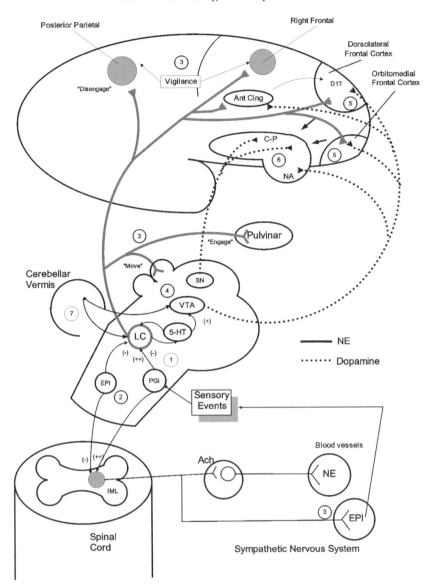

FIGURE 9.6. Interaction of brain systems in ADHD (see text for details)

EPI neurons also exist in the brain stem (2), and stimulants also increase release of central EPI. Note that EPI decreases the activity of the LC and IML, thus perhaps providing important negative feedback on these systems. NE is released into three areas forming the posterior, or orienting attention system (3). The parietal area governs disengagement from the current focus of attention, the superior colliculi influence the movement of attention to the new stimulus, and the pulvinar of the thalamus "reads out" the information into working memory. The NE system influences the entire cortex, however. As shown in Figure 9.6, NE influences the anterior cingulate (part of the executive attention system), as well as the dorsolateral and orbitomedial prefrontal cortex. The posterior attention system governs vigilance, allowing the brain to maintain its focus and allowing it to disengage when the information readout is complete. Note the NE input to the hippocampus, which engages memory but also, according to Anthony Grace's model, helps the prefrontal cortex govern behavior according to long-term goals. Thus deficits in NE functioning could cause a failure of attention at several levels: failure to disengage and attend to new stimuli; failure to remain sufficiently vigilant to read out all the data working memory needs to fully grasp the situation. Meanwhile, the SNS system has been brought online to regulate arousal for the task: Too little activation and the person is bored and unmotivated; too much and he or she is too excited to perform. Persons with ADHD often display both types of arousal deficits.

Now move to the prefrontal cortex (4). The information has arrived in working memory; now the orbitomedial areas provide inhibition so that working memory has time to operate, as well as more fully regulating the affective response. In the dorsolateral cortex, both verbal and nonverbal working memory are processing the data and developing a response. The VTA provides DA input to the amygdala, nucleus accumbens (NA), and prefrontal cortex (5). Through DA influence on the NA, input from the amygdala is given greater weight. This favors an immediate, affectively driven response over a reflective one. Activity in the NA involves the "pleasure circuit"; the greater the DA release, the more the response is seen as pleasurable. Both DA and NE influence the prefrontal cortex and are critical for effective working memory. If, due to genetic factors, DA activity is set at too high a level (see the previous discussion of Grace's hypothesis), the individual is too prone to be governed by immediate needs, the processing of working memory is interrupted, and a response is made prematurely (impulsively). Stimulants may function by improving the "signal to noise" ratio in the NE and DA systems. Tonic levels of NE and DA in the synaptic cleft are reduced; phasic releases, although decreased, are more efficient at transmitting information. The situation is somewhat like that of a car with a leaky carburetor. When the driver steps on the gas, too much fuel floods the engine, and the car stalls. Stimulants, like tuning a carburetor, downregulate the system, thereby allowing NE and DA to play their roles: NE facilitates the intake of information and its processing, DA allows emotion to play a role and permits action to take place.

A final role may be played by the cerebellar vermis (6). As discussed in Chapter 5, the cerebellum is active in ongoing motor activity, enhancing motor coordination. It is also clear that the cerebellum plays a larger role in learning generally. The vermis, however, is a more primitive part of the cerebellum, more involved in affect regulation. Thus it has input to the LC and VTA. Perhaps, just as the cerebellum plays a role in ensuring the accuracy of ongoing motor programs, perhaps the vermis regulates affect as the behavior is performed. For instance, we may start out being angry at someone and initiate a behavior to confront him or her. At some point during the behavior, being angry may no longer be the appropriate affect; we decide that being calm is a more effective way to make the point. The vermis, through its connections with the VTA and LC, is in a position to do this.

I have focused on possible genetic variations in the NE and DA systems that might be involved in ADHD. Other genetic factors might affect the structure of the frontal cortex and neostriatum, disrupting their function. A small number of cases of ADHD can be accounted for by severe perinatal trauma or head injury that disrupt these same circuits.

SUMMARY

Although many in the lay press challenge the validity of the ADHD diagnosis, the neurobiological evidence for its status as a brain disorder is mounting. The genetic effect, based on family and twin studies, is extremely strong and argues against diet, culture, or changes in educational policies as possible causes. Recent increases in the number of persons diagnosed represent increasing recognition of the disorder, as opposed to any increase in ADHD per se. Future research will allow us to take the phenotype of ADHD, break it down into various genotypes, and understand how these genes work together to produce the disorder. This research will open the way for new and more effective treatments that might be targeted at the specific type of genetic deficit the individual has. ADHD does not always stand alone, however; it is frequently comorbid with oppositional defiant or conduct disorders, as well as mood disorders. Thus we turn to personality disorder and aggressive behavior in the next chapter. The scientific challenges are greater, and the political controversies abound.

REFERENCES

Barkley, R. A. (1997). *ADHD and the nature of self control.* New York: Guilford Press.

Barr, C. L., Feng, Y., Wigg, K., Bloom, S., Roberts, W., Malone, M., et al. (2000). Identification of DNA variants in the SNAP-25 gene and linkage study of these polymorphisms and attention-deficit hyperactivity disorder. *Molecular Psychiatry, 5*, 405–409.

Bradley, C. (1937). The behavior of children receiving benzedrine. *American Journal of Psychiatry, 94*, 577–585.

Bush, G., Frazier, J. A., Rauch, S. L., Seidman, L. J., Whalen, P. J., Jenike, M. A., et al. (1999). Anterior cingulate cortex dysfunction in attention-deficit/hyperactivity disorder revealed by fMRI and the Counting Stroop. *Biological Psychiatry, 45*, 1542–1552.

Castellanos, F. X., Elia, J., Kruesi, M. J. P., Marsh, W. L., Gulotta, C. S., Potter, W. Z., et al. (1996). Cerebrospinal homovanillic acid predicts behavioral response to stimulants in 45 boys with attention-deficit hyperactivity disorder. *Neuropsychopharmacology, 14*, 125–137.

Castellanos, F. X., Giedd, J. N., Berquin, P. C., Walter, J. M., Sharp, W., Tran, T., et al. (2001). Quantitative brain magnetic resonance imaging in girls with attention-deficit/hyperactivity disorder. *Archives of General Psychiatry, 58*, 289–295.

Castellanos, F. X., Giedd, J. N., Marsh, W. L., Hamburger, S. D., Vaituzis, A. C., Dickstein, D. P., et al. (1996). Quantitative brain magnetic resonance imaging in attention-deficit hyperactivity disorder. *Archives of General Psychiatry, 53*, 607–616.

Castellanos, F. X., Lau, E., Taybei, N., Lee, P., Giedd, J. N., Sharp, W., et al. (1998). Lack of an association between a dopamine-4 receptor polymorhphism and attention deficit hyperactivity disorder: Genetic and brain morphometric analyses. *Molecular Psychiatry, 3*, 431–434.

Conners, C. K. (2000). Attention-deficit/hyperactivity disorder—Historical development and overview. *Journal of Attention Disorders, 3*, 173–191.

Cook, E. H., Jr., Stein, M. A., Krasowski, M. D., Cox, N. J., Olkon, D. M., Kieffer, J. E., & Leventhal, B. L. (1995). Association of attention-deficit disorder and the dopamine transporter gene. *American Journal of Human Genetics, 56*, 993–998.

Daly, G., Hawi, Z., Fitzgerald, M., & Gill, M. (1999). Mapping susceptibility loci in attention deficit hyperactivity disorder: Preferential transmission of parental alleles at DAT1, DBH and DRD5 to affected children. *Molecular Psychiatry, 4*, 192–196.

Dougherty, D. D., Bonab, A. A., Spencer, T. J., Rauch, S. L., Madras, B. K., & Fischman, A. J. (1999). Dopamine transporter density in patients with attention deficit hyperactivity disorder. *Lancet, 354*, 2132–2133.

Douglas, V. I. (1983). Attentional and cognitive problems. In M. Rutter (Ed.), *Developmental neuropsychiatry* (pp. 280–329). New York: Guilford Press.

Douglas, V. I., & Peters, K. G. (1979). Toward a clearer definition of the attentional deficit of hyperactive children. In G. A. Hale & M. Lewis

(Eds.), *Attention and Cognitive Development* (pp. 173–248). New York: Plenum Press.

Eisenberg, J., Mei-Tal, G., Steinberg, A., Tartakovsky, E., Zohar, A., Gritsenko, I., et al. (1999). Haplotype relative risk study of catechol-O-methyltransferase (COMT) and attention deficit hyperactivity disorder (ADHD): Association of the high-enzyme activity Val allele with ADHD impulsive–hyperactive phenotype. *American Journal of Medical Genetics, 88,* 497–502.

Ernst, M., Zametkin, A. J., Matochik, J. A., Jons, P. H., & Cohen, R. M. (1998). DOPA decarboxylase activity in attention deficit hyperactivity disorder adults: A [fluorine-18]fluorodopa positron emission tomographic study. *Journal of Neuroscience, 18,* 5901–5907.

Ernst, M., Zametkin, A. J., Matochik, J. A., Pascualvaca, D., Jons, P. H., & Cohen, R. M. (1999). High midbrain [18F]DOPA accumulation in children with attention deficit hyperactivity disorder. *American Journal of Psychiatry, 156,* 1209–1215.

Filipek, P. A., Semrud-Clikeman, M., Steingard, R. J., Renshaw, P. F., Kennedy, D. N., & Biederman, J. (1997). Volumetric MRI analysis comparing subjects having attention-deficit hyperactivity disorder with normal controls. *Neurology, 48,* 589–601.

Gill, M., Daly, G., Heron, S., Hawi, Z., & Fitzgerald, M. (1997). Confirmation of association between attention deficit hyperactivity disorder and a dopamine transporter polymorphism. *Molecular Psychiatry, 2,* 311–313.

Gillis, J. J., Gilger, J. W., Pennington, B. F., & DeFries, J. C. (1992). Attention deficit disorder in reading-disabled twins: Evidence for a genetic etiology. *Journal of Abnormal Child Psychology, 20,* 303–315.

Gjone, H., Stevenson, J., & Sundet, J. M. (1996). Genetic influence on parent-reported attention-related problems in a Norwegian general population twin sample. *Journal of the American Academy of Child and Adolescent Psychiatry, 35,* 588–596.

Goodman, R., & Stevenson, J. (1989a). A twin study of hyperactivity: I. An examination of hyperactivity scores and categories derived from Rutter teacher and parent questionnaires. *Journal of Child Psychology and Psychiatry, 30,* 671–689.

Goodman, R., & Stevenson, J. (1989b). A twin study of hyperactivity: II. The aetiological role of genes, family relationships and perinatal adversity. *Journal of Child Psychology and Psychiatry, 30,* 691–709.

Grace, A. A. (2001). Psychostimulant actions on dopamine and limbic system function: Relevance-related behavior and impulsivity. In M. V. Solanto, A. F. T. Arnsten, & F. X. Castellanos (Eds.), *Stimulant drugs and ADHD: Basic and clinical neuroscience* (pp. 134–157). New York: Oxford University Press.

Gray, J. A. (1982). *The neuropsychology of anxiety: An enquiry into the functions of the septo-hippocampal system.* New York: Oxford University Press.

Hawi, Z., McCarron, M., Kirley, A., Daly, G., Fitzgerald, M., & Gill, M. (2000). No association of the dopamine DRD4 receptor (DRD4) gene polymorphism with attention deficit hyperactivity disorder (ADHD) in the Irish population. *American Journal of Medical Genetics, 96,* 268–272.

Hawi, Z., Millar, N., Daly, G., Fitzgerald, M., & Gill, M. (2000). No association between catechol-O-methyltransferase (COMT) gene polymorphism and attention deficit hyperactivity disorder (ADHD) in an Irish sample. *American Journal of Medical Genetics, 96,* 282–284.

Holmes, J., Payton, A., Barrett, J. H., Hever, T., Fitzpatrick, H., Trumper, A. L., et al. (2000). A family-based and case-control association study of the dopamine D4 receptor gene and dopamine transporter gene in attention deficit hyperactivity disorder. *Molecular Psychiatry, 5,* 523–530.

Hudziak, J. J., Heath, A. C., Madden, P. F., Reich, W., Bucholz, K. K., Slutske, W., et al. (1998). Latent class and factor analysis of DSM-IV ADHD: A twin study of female adolescents. *Journal of the American Academy of Child and Adolescent Psychiatry, 37,* 848–857.

Hynd, G. W., Hern, K. L., Novey, E. S., Eliopulos, D., Marshall, R., Gonzalez, J. J., & Voeller, K. K. (1993). Attention deficit-hyperactivity disorder and asymmetry of the caudate nucleus. *Journal of Child Neurology, 8,* 339–347.

Hynd, G. W., Semrud-Clikeman, M., Lorys, A. R., Novey, E. S., & Eliopulos, D. (1990). Brain morphology in developmental dyslexia and attention deficit disorder/hyperactivity. *Archives of Neurology, 47,* 919–926.

Krause, K. H., Dresel, S. H., Krause, J., Kung, H. F., & Tatsch, K. (2000). Increased striatal dopamine transporter in adult patients with attention deficit hyperactivity disorder: Effects of methylphenidate as measured by single photon emission computed tomography. *Neuroscience Letters, 285,* 107–110.

LaHoste, G. J., Swanson, J. M., Wigal, S. B., Glabe, C., Wigal, T., King, N., & Kennedy, J. L. (1996). Dopamine D4 receptor gene polymorphism is associated with attention deficit hyperactivity disorder. *Molecular Psychiatry, 1,* 121–124.

Levy, F., Hay, D. A., McStephen, M., Wood, C., & Waldman, I. (1997). Attention-deficit hyperactivity disorder: A category or a continuum? Genetic analysis of a large-scale twin study. *Journal of the American Academy of Child and Adolescent Psychiatry, 36,* 737–744.

Logan, G. D., Schachar, R. J., & Tannock, R. (1997). Impulsivity and inhibitory control. *Psychological Science, 8,* 60–64.

Martinez, D., Gelernter, J., Abi-Dargham, A., van Dyck, C. H., Kegeles, L., Innis, R. B., & Laruelle, M. (2001). The variable number of tandem repeats polymorphism of the dopamine transporter gene is not associated with significant change in dopamine transporter phenotype in humans. *Neuropsychopharmacology, 24,* 553–560.

McCracken, J. T. (1991). A two-part model of stimulant action on attention-deficit hyperactivity disorder in children. *Journal of Neuropsychiatry and Clinical Neuroscience, 3,* 201–209.

Pliszka, S. R., Liotti, M., & Woldorff, M. G. (2000). Inhibitory control in children with attention deficit/hyperactivity disorder: Event-related potentials identify the processing component and timing of an impaired right-frontal response-inhibition mechanism. *Biological Psychiatry, 48,* 238–246.

Pliszka, S. R., McCracken, J. T., & Maas, J. W. (1996). Catecholamines in attention deficit hyperactivity disorder: Current perspectives. *Journal of the American Academy of Child and Adolescent Psychiatry, 35,* 264–272.

Quay, H. C. (1988). The behavioral reward and inhibition systems in childhood behavior disorders. In L. M. Bloomingdale (Ed.), *Attention deficit disorder (Vol. 3, pp. 176–186). Oxford, UK: Pergamon.*

Rowe, D. C., Stever, C., Giedinghagen, L. N., Gard, J. M. C., Cleveland, H. H., Terris, S. T., et al. (1998). Dopamine DRD4 receptor polymorphism and attention deficit hyperactivity disorder. *Molecular Psychiatry, 3,* 419–426.

Rubia, K., Overmeyer, S., Taylor, E., Brammer, M., Williams, S. C. R., Simmons, A., & Bullmore, E. T. (1999). Hypofrontality in attention deficit hyperactivity disorder during higher-order motor control: A study with functional MRI. *American Journal of Psychiatry, 156,* 891–896.

Semrud-Clikeman, M., Steingard, R., Filipek, P. A., Biederman, J., Bekken, K., & Renshaw, P. F. (2000). Using MRI to examine brain–behavior relationships in males with attention deficit disorder with hyperactivity. *Journal of the American Academy of Child and Adolescent Psychiatry, 39,* 477–484.

Sherman, D. K., Iacono, W. G., & McGue, M. K. (1997). Attention-deficit hyperactivity disorder dimensions: A twin study of inattention and impulsivity-hyperactivity. *Journal of the American Academy of Child and Adolescent Psychiatry, 36,* 745–753.

Sherman, D. K., McGue, M. K., & Iacono, W. G. (1997). Twin concordance for attention deficit hyperactivity disorder: A comparison of teachers' and mothers' reports. *American Journal of Psychiatry, 154,* 532–535.

Smalley, S. L., Bailey, J. N., Palmer, C. G., Cantwell, D. P., McGough, J. J., Del'Homme, M. A., et al. (1998). Evidence that the dopamine D4 receptor is a susceptibility gene in attention deficit hyperactivity disorder. *Molecular Psychiatry, 3,* 427–430.

Solanto, M. V. (1984). Neuropharmacological basis of stimulant drug action in attention deficit disorder with hyperactivity: A review and synthesis. *Psychological Bulletin, 95,* 387–409.

Swanson, J. M., Flodman, P., Kennedy, J., Spence, M. A., Moyzis, R., Schuck, S., et al. (2000). Dopamine genes and ADHD. *Neuroscience and Biobehavioral Reviews, 24,* 21–25.

Swanson, J. M., Sunohara, G. A., Kennedy, J. L., Regino, R., Fineberg, E., Wigal, T., et al. (1998). Association of the dopamine transporter D4 (DRD4) gene with a refined phenotype of attention deficit hyperactivity disorder (ADHD). *Molecular Psychiatry, 3,* 38–41.

Tahir, E., Curran, S., Yazgan, Y., Ozbay, F., Cirakoglu, B., & Asherson, P. J. (2000). No association between low- and high-activity catecholamine-methyl-transferase (COMT) and attention deficit hyperactivity disorder (ADHD) in a sample of Turkish children. *American Journal of Medical Genetics, 96,* 285–288.

Tahir, E., Yazgan, Y., Cirakoglu, B., Ozbay, F., Waldman, I., & Asherson, P. J.

(2000). Association and linkage of DRD4 and DRD5 with attention deficit hyperactivity disorder (ADHD) in a sample of Turkish children. *Molecular Psychiatry, 5*, 404.

Todd, R. D., Neuman, R. J., Lobos, E. A., Reich, W., & Heath, A. C. (2001). Lack of association of dopamine D4 receptor gene polymorphisms with ADHD subtypes in a population sample of twins. *American Journal of Medical Genetics, 105*, 432–438.

Vaidya, C. J., Austin, G., Kirkorian, G., Ridlehuber, H. W., Desmond, J. E., Glover, G. H., & Gabrieli, D. E. (1998). Selective effects of methylphenidate in attention deficit hyperactivity disorder: A functional magnetic resonance study. *Neurobiology, 95*, 14494–14499.

Waldman, I. D., Rowe, D. C., Abramowitz, A., Kozel, S. T., Mohr, J. H., Sherman, S. L., et al. (1998). Association and linkage of the dopamine transporter gene and attention-deficit hyperactivity disorder in children: Heterogeneity owing to diagnostic subtype and severity. *American Journal of Human Genetics, 63*, 1767–1776.

Xu, C., Schachar, R., Tannock, R., Roberts, W., Malone, M., Kennedy, J. L., & Barr, C. L. (2001). Linkage study of the $x2A$ adrenergic receptor in attention-deficit hyperactivity disorder families. *American Journal of Medical Genetics, 105*, 159–162.

Zametkin, A. J., Nordahl, T. E., Gross, M., King, A. C., Semple, W. E., Rumsey, J., et al. (1990). Cerebral glucose metabolism in adults with hyperactivity of childhood onset. *New England Journal of Medicine, 323*, 1361–1366.

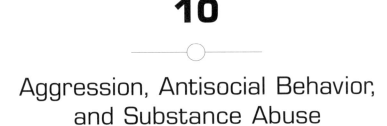

10

Aggression, Antisocial Behavior, and Substance Abuse

I must say first that there is not, nor is there ever likely to be found, a single gene or biological cause for antisocial behavior. The research on antisocial behavior and aggression does not suggest that there is a substantial group of people who are "born sociopaths." There is, however, a growing body of data showing that neurobiological factors play important roles in the development of aggressive and antisocial behavior. Not all of these factors are genetic. In this chapter I begin to show how early adverse environmental events might actually affect the brain and thus produce dysfunction. I also begin to examine the role of biological–environmental interaction in the etiology of maladaptive behavior. I examine aggression and antisocial behavior but narrow the focus in specific ways relevant to mental health clinicians.

Aggression (physical or verbal) may be a specific symptom of a mental disorder (such as conduct disorder [CD] or intermittent explosive disorder [IED]), or it may occur as a sequela of another disorder. The latter situation is not dealt with in this chapter. For instance, an autistic individual may hit or slap someone if his or her rituals are interrupted, or a schizophrenic may have command hallucinations to attack a member of his or her family. Treatment of the underlying condition is called for. This chapter concerns those individuals who engage in antisocial behavior or are aggressive as part of their primary mental disorder. Not all antisocial individuals are aggressive, nor do all individuals who show inappropriate aggression commit other antisocial acts, though the overlap is great. From a mental health perspective, I am concerned more with impulsive aggression and antisocial behavior than with well-planned, successful criminal activity. An insurance salesman may defraud his clients, but this individual may be quite normal in his interactions with family and friends. It is a moral question as to why he chose to betray the trust of his customers. Tragically, mentally healthy people may commit genocide, as was seen in the Holocaust and more recently in the Balkans. This chapter is concerned with aggressive and antisocial behavior that emerges in persons living in ordinary society and that often does not yield long-term gain for the individual him- or herself. For example:

> Mark is an 18-year-old young man who is currently in jail for burglary and heroin use. He was removed from his biological family at the age of 7 because of a history of extensive physical and sexual abuse. He was placed in a foster home but could not remain there because of frequent aggressive outbursts toward his foster siblings and destructiveness toward property. He was placed in a residential treatment facility. He was diagnosed with ADHD, and treatment with stimulant medication improved his hyperactivity and impulsivity. A family in the community became aware of his situation and adopted him. They made extensive efforts to deal with his behavior. Psychotherapy was attempted to help Mark deal with his abused past, but he would refuse to talk about it, saying he never thought about his abuse and that it had nothing to do with his current behavior.
>
> As he entered adolescence, he became more aggressive toward others and seemed to lack any feeling for his adoptive parents. At age 13 he began heavy use of alcohol, which was followed by use of marijuana. He was arrested several times for possession of marijuana and was placed in another residential facility. There, despite intensive psychotherapy, he made little progress. He regularly displayed an angry, irritable affect whenever frustrated. His lack of relatedness to others and his intense irritability led to the suspicion of a mood disorder, and he was treated extensively with antidepressants and mood stabilizers, with little result. He ran away from the treatment center; about 6 months after this he was arrested for burglary and was found in possession of heroin. He admitted that he had been snorting heroin since his elopement from the center.

Mark is most likely headed for a life of crime and frequent prison stays. Clearly, substance abuse is part of his problem, as it so often is in persons with severe behavior disorders, so I also consider the neurobiology of alcohol and substance abuse in this chapter.

IMPULSIVE AGGRESSION AND PERSONALITY DISORDER

Nationwide, crime statistics are stark and difficult to interpret. In 1976, 20 homicides were committed by persons ages 18–24 per 100,000 persons in that age group. By contrast, the homicide rate among teenagers ages 14–17 was only 10 per 100,000. By 1992, these rates had risen to 40 per 100,000 for young adults and 30 per 100,000 for 14- to 17-year-olds. By 1998, the homicide rate for both groups (as well as adults) had fallen significantly, and the reasons for both the rise and fall are not clear. It is quite likely that incarceration rates have removed many anti-social and aggressive persons from the community. The following statistics are astounding: In 1925 the United States imprisoned about 100 per 100,000 persons. This number remained constant until about 1975, when it began to rise. In the 1980s and 1990s the prison population exploded, rising to 450 per 100,000 by 1995! States are rapidly finding that maintaining such a massive prison system severely taxes their resources. Soon they will either have to raise taxes or sharply curtail other services. Thus is it critical for us to develop a better understanding of aggressive and antisocial behavior.

Patterns of Antisocial Behavior and Aggression

For some persons, such as Mark, antisocial behavior has a very early onset. For others, antisocial behavior does not begin until adolescence. People who show an early onset of antisocial behavior are far more likely to persist in that behavior into adult years than those who begin offending during the teen years. Other factors that predict persistence of antisocial behavior are, not surprisingly, severity and frequency of the antisocial acts. Children who show early onset of aggression and antisocial behavior are also more likely to have comorbid ADHD and learning disabilities.

A number of studies have shown that ADHD in early childhood, particularly when combined with family adversity and learning disability, is highly predictive of delinquent behavior during the teenage years. Rolf Loeber and colleagues examined the number of multiple criminal offenders in a sample of adolescents. Only 1.7% of adolescents without ADHD or CD were multiple offenders; among those with ADHD without CD, 3.4% were so classified. In contrast, 20.7% of adolescents with CD but no history of ADHD were multiple offenders. In the comorbid ADHD–CD group, nearly one-third (30.8%) had committed multiple crimes. Farrington and colleagues collected data on hyperactivity and conduct problems in a large nonreferred sample of schoolchildren and followed up on the number of juvenile convictions the participants acquired over time. Again, hyperactivity and conduct problems independently predicted delinquency: About 24% of children with ADHD had juvenile convictions (compared to 12.6% of controls), but 46% of the children with ADHD–CD had become delinquent. Thirty-five percent of children with CD in the absence of ADHD were later convicted of juvenile offenses. Thus it is not ADHD alone but ADHD in conjunction with the early onset of CD that particularly predisposes to later criminal behavior.

In 1993 Terri Moffitt reviewed the neuropsychology of conduct disorder and delinquency. She pointed out that delinquents showed an overall deficit of one-half standard deviation (about 8 IQ points) compared with nondelinquent peers. For delinquent samples as a whole, neuropsychological tests show statistically significant but clinically mild impairments in cognitive functioning. Few children with CD or delinquency are identified as brain damaged, as defined by the presence of severe signs such as aphasia or sensory loss. In the Dunedin (New Zealand) Multidisciplinary Health and Development study, Moffitt noted that IQ differences between offenders and controls varied greatly based on the seriousness of the offenses. Those adolescents who engaged in transient delinquency showed only a 1-point IQ difference relative to controls, whereas those aggressive delinquents who had been antisocial since early childhood showed a 17-point mean difference relative to controls. Many other studies have shown low IQs to predispose individuals to antisocial behavior; persons with above-average IQs are far less likely to engage in criminal activity, even when raised in high-risk environments.

As part of the Dunedin study, neuropsychological tests were administered to a large epidemiological sample of 13-year-olds. The sample was subdivided as follows: children with no history of ADHD or delinquency ($n = 558$), children with ADHD who had no history of delinquency ($n = 14$), delinquents with no history of ADHD ($n = 87$), and delinquents with ADHD ($n = 19$). The authors controlled for the effects of family adversity factors on test performance. Overall, the delinquents performed more poorly than the nondelinquents on the verbal, visual–motor integration, and visuospatial measures, but the two delinquent groups had very different neuropsychological profiles. Delinquents with ADHD scored significantly below the delinquents without ADHD on the verbal and visual–motor integration measures. Children with ADHD who did not become delinquent were not markedly different from controls on the neuropsychological measures. Similarly, delinquents without ADHD showed relatively good test performance. A similar effect of ADHD has been found in studies of executive function in CD and delinquency. In the New Zealand study, boys with ADHD and CD scored more poorly than those with either CD or ADHD alone on measures of executive function.

Moffitt then examined longitudinal data for 435 boys divided into the four groups mentioned previously. Delinquent boys without a history of ADHD did not begin their antisocial behavior until around age 13, whereas delinquent boys with ADHD showed antisocial behavior as early as age 5. Controls, delinquents without ADHD, and boys with ADHD but without delinquency were similar in verbal IQ and reading ability, whereas delinquents with ADHD showed deficits in both these areas. Delinquent boys with ADHD had experienced much greater family adversity than those in the other three groups. At follow-up at age 15, delinquents with ADHD had committed more aggressive acts of delinquency. Overall, there was a distinct pattern of symptoms in the ADHD boys who would become delinquent. Low verbal IQ was noted as early as age 3; ADHD was then diagnosed at age 7. These children also experienced greater family adversity. They then went on to commit more aggressive delinquent acts by age 15.

Neuropsychological deficits found in delinquent youths are of interest in the study of explosive rage, or intermittent explosive disorder (IED). Despite the long clinical use of the term, little is known about IED. The DSM-IV criteria are somewhat vague. IED consists of several "discrete episodes of failure to resist aggressive impulses that result in serious assaultive acts or destruction of property." Neither psychosis, a mood disorder, nor ADHD accounts for the aggressive acts, nor are they directly the result of a medical condition (i.e., Alzheimer's or other dementing disorders). Sometimes viewed as a possible variant of temporal lobe epilepsy, controlled studies have not in fact shown that explosively aggressive individuals have higher rates of epilepsy or abnormal EEGs (see Stevens and Hermann). The belief that aggressive outbursts could be triggered by a seizure led to the use of anticonvulsant medication as a treatment. Seizure medications such as carbamazepine and divalproex sodium (or valproic acid) can reduce aggressive outbursts even in the absence of a seizure disorder, as can treatment with lithium. One hypothesis that has emerged is that IED is related to mood disorder in some way, particularly as these individuals show such abnormal irritability. Moodiness, however, does not explain the relationship of the cognitive deficits to antisocial–aggressive behavior. Social information processing theory, developed by Kenneth Dodge and his colleagues, may provide a way of doing this.

There are various stages of social information processing. First, we must *encode* information about a social situation. This includes information about tone of voice, facial expression, and what type of setting we are in. Often a social cue is subtle, such as the raising of an eyebrow. Once encoded, social cues must be interpreted as either friendly, neutral, or hostile. Next we select a goal for our interaction (to obtain something or stop a hostile action) and generate possible responses (walk away, talk with the person, or be aggressive). Finally, we choose from among the responses. In choosing a response, we also have certain expectations about how successful those responses will be in getting us what we want.

In Dodge's studies, children view videotapes of social interactions in which possible conflict exists. Children are asked to interpret what went on in the tape and to discuss how they would respond and what they think the consequences of their actions would be. When looking at social situations, aggressive children encode fewer relevant cues and do not seek out additional information when the situation is ambiguous. They are more likely to interpret ambiguous cues as hostile. As for goal selection, aggressive children seek dominance and control and generate fewer potential responses to a problematic social situation. There is a negative correlation between the number of responses and the child's rate of aggression. In terms of response decision, aggressive children view aggression as producing more desirable outcomes—they are more likely to see aggression as leading to tangible rewards and peer-group approval and do not see their victims as suffering any real harm. The encoding and the response–decision phases are key, as these may differ in children with different subtypes of aggression.

Aggression has been subtyped in the research literature as proactive versus reactive. Although many aggressive children show aspects of both types of aggression, certain children can be reliability classified as having predominantly proactive (well planned, instrumental and affectless) or reactive (impulsive, hostile, and affective) aggression (see Vitiello and Stoff). In 1997, Dodge and colleagues classified both a large population of third graders and a group of adjudicated juvenile offenders as showing either proactive or reactive aggression. Participants viewed videotapes of social interactions. Each student was asked to imagine being the protagonist. In the community sample, encoding errors were found in the reactive aggressive children, whereas the proactive aggressive children were more likely to anticipate positive outcomes for aggression. Similar results were found for the offender sample. Reactively aggressive offenders made more encoding errors, whereas the proactively aggressive offenders expected aggression to reduce aversion. It is tempting to speculate that the reactive aggressive children have a neuropsychological deficit in encoding facial cues and other subtleties of social interaction and that the proactive aggressive children have learned (perhaps from the family environment) that aggression pays off.

These results necessitate a discussion of the possible role of physical abuse and family violence in children who become aggressive. Rates of family adversity are uniformly found to be higher among children with early-onset antisocial behavior. In the reactive aggressive groups described in the Dodge study, physical abuse and exposure to violence were higher relative to the proactive and control groups, both in the community and in offender samples. Dorothy Lewis and colleagues followed 95 incarcerated delinquents over many years. Her group found that 83% came from abusive families. The adolescent had either witnessed severe violence or had been physically abused him- or herself. Hans Steiner and colleagues examined 85 incarcerated boys in the California Youth Authority. Over 30% of the youths met full criteria for posttraumatic stress disorder (PTSD), and 20% met partial criteria. About 50% of the sample did not meet criteria for PTSD, even though half of these youths had in fact suffered a traumatic event. Intrafamilial violence (abuse, murder) was the most common stressor, followed by witnessing violent acts in the community.

Thus two different levels of family adversity could be involved in the development of aggression. Physical abuse can have deleterious effects on cognitive development, even if the abuse does not take the form of a brain injury (such as in an infant with a fractured skull). Physical abuse and neglect are usually associated with other types of dysfunction in the parent–child relationship: lack of bonding, eye contact, and language stimulation. These things, combined with the negative arousal that accompanies abuse, could interfere with the development of the brain mechanisms that underlie social cognition and affect regulation discussed in Chapter 7. If these things occur in an individual who is also at risk for ADHD, the combination results in the condition of IED. In contrast, those with proactive aggression may not have suffered the same level of abuse but saw aggressive behavior modeled by parents, siblings, or people in their neighborhoods. These individuals might be more neuropsychologically intact. Table 10.1 summarizes early- versus late-onset antisocial behavior in terms of the factors discussed thus far.

TABLE 10.1. Early- versus Late-Onset Antisocial Behavior

	Childhood onset	Adolescent onset
Comorbidity of ADHD	+++	++
Neuropsychological deficits	+++	++
Early abuse/neglect	+++	+
Genetic factors?	++	–
Persistence of antisocial behavior into adulthood	+++	+
Aggression subtype predominating	Reactive	Proactive

Genetics of Antisocial Behavior

The genetics of aggression per se has not been studied, but there has been substantial work on criminal behavior generally. Adoption studies show a modest genetic effect on antisocial behavior. In 1972 Schulsinger found, in studying adoptees with "psychopathy" (antisocial personality), a higher rate of psychopathy among the adoptees' biological relatives (14.4%) than among their adoptive relatives (7.6%). In the 1970s Raymond Crowe and Robert Cadoret both found that adopted-away offspring of antisocial parents showed higher rates of antisocial behavior than adopted-away offspring of noncriminal biological parents. Mednick and colleagues performed a major "cross-fostering" study. All Danish adoptions between 1924 and 1947 were reviewed. Cases fell into four groups, as shown in Table 10.2: children for whom neither the biological nor adoptive parent was antisocial (control group), children for whom *both* the biological and adoptive parent were antisocial (high-risk group), children of antisocial biological parents who were reared by nonantisocial parents, and children of nonantisocial biological parents who had antisocial adoptive parents. It was then determined whether the adoptees had criminal records of any kind. Examining the bottom row of Table 10.2, it can be seen that simply having an antisocial parent is not sufficient to increase the risk of having a criminal conviction; the two groups in the bottom row are not statistically different from each other. It is in the high-risk group, having both genetic and environmental risks for antisocial behavior, that a statistically significant increase of criminal convictions is found. This suggests that a gene-by-environment interaction is required to express antisocial behavior. It is important to note that even in the high-risk group, nearly 75% still did not have a criminal conviction.

Twin studies have also been informative on the genetics of antisocial behavior. In general, monozygotic (MZ) twins are more similar than dizygotic (DZ) twins in antisocial behavior, though heritability is lower

TABLE 10.2. Rate of Criminal Records of Adoptees in a Cross-Fostering Study (Mednick et al., 1984, 1987)

	Adoptive parents with antisocial history	Adoptive parents with no antisocial history
Biological parents with antisocial history	24.5%	20.0%
Biological parents with no antisocial history	14.7%	13.5%

than that found for ADHD. In a large study by Lyons and colleagues in 1995, the heritability for juvenile antisocial personality was quite low (0.07), whereas it was significant for adult antisocial personality (.43). DiLalla and Gottesman reviewed the literature on twin similarity for antisocial behavior. The concordance rate (how often the twins were both antisocial) differed in adult and juvenile studies. For juvenile studies, the concordance rates were .87 and .72 for MZ and DZ twins, respectively. For adult studies, the concordance rates were .51 for MZ twins and .22 for DZ twins. Again, the genetic effect was stronger for adult than juvenile antisocial behavior. At first this seems at variance with the earlier statement that early-onset CD is associated with persistence of antisocial behavior into adulthood. In these twin studies, juvenile delinquency was most often assessed. These studies would include many individuals with adolescent-onset CD in whom genetic factors were less likely to be prominent. These individuals often desist in their antisocial behavior by adulthood. The more "genetically loaded" individuals will have early onset in childhood, then persist in their antisocial acts through adolescence and into adulthood.

Joseph Biederman and colleagues at Harvard Medical School did a large family study that bears on the genetics of both ADHD and CD. They examined the rate of ADHD and CD among the relatives of two groups of patients: those with ADHD alone and those with a combination of ADHD and CD. Among the children with ADHD alone, a higher rate of ADHD, but not CD, was found among the relatives. The relatives of children with ADHD + CD showed a higher rate of both disorders, and the disorders cosegregated in the relatives. This means that the patient with ADHD + CD had relatives who also suffered from both ADHD and CD, rather than having one relative with CD and another with ADHD. This suggests that individuals with ADHD + CD are a distinct genetic subtype from those with ADHD without CD. How would genetic factors be involved in the development of antisocial or aggressive behavior? Genes mediating the development of the neuropsychological abilities might indirectly contribute to antisocial behavior by producing the impairments in cognition discussed earlier. Other genes might affect brain systems involved in regulating mood and impulse control (separate from those involved in ADHD). The serotonergic system has been most studied in this regard.

Serotonin in Impulsive and Aggressive Behavior

Chapter 4 discussed how extensively serotonin is distributed in the brain. After its release from neurons, serotonin is converted by a series of enzymes into 5-hydroxyindoleacetic acid (5-HIAA). It is instructive to look at some nonhuman primate data before examining the human data. In rhesus monkeys, 5-HIAA levels are under substantial genetic control (> 50% of the variance) and are highly consistent within individuals over time, although environmental factors can affect the development of the serotonin system. In adult rhesus monkeys, CSF 5-HIAA is highly associated with measures of both aggression and social competence. Low CSF 5-HIAA is associated with high rates of prolonged, inappropriate aggression in both males and females. In rhesus monkeys living in the wild, CSF 5-HIAA is positively correlated with prosocial behaviors such as grooming and physical proximity to other monkeys, whereas low CSF 5-HIAA is associated with increased intensity of aggression, more physical wounds, and greater risk taking. Monkeys low in CSF 5-HIAA were more likely to take long leaps from trees at dangerous heights. In 1996 Higley and colleagues collected CSF 5-HIAA from monkeys and followed them in the wild over a 3-year period; 46% of the monkeys in the low 5-HIAA group were dead at follow-up, most likely because of increased aggression.

Genetics are not the only factors influencing CSF 5-HIAA in monkeys. CSF 5-HIAA rises in monkeys who are introduced to a new social group, as well as when a new monkey is placed in an established group. Diet has an effect on both CSF 5-HIAA and aggression in nonhuman primates. A finding that human participants on cholesterol-lowering diets showed a slightly increased mortality from violence and suicide stimulated studies of the relationship of cholesterol and aggression. Kaplan and colleagues randomized cynomolgus monkeys to a high- or low-cholesterol diet for an 8-month period. The monkeys on a high-cholesterol diet had plasma cholesterol levels nearly three times higher than those on the low-cholesterol diet. The low-cholesterol group had significantly lower CSF 5-HIAA and higher ratings of aggression than the high-cholesterol group. These results are contrary to the stereotype of impulsive, aggressive children who consume too much fat or sugar. Equally important is the effect of season; in adult humans, CSF 5-HIAA is 40% lower in the late winter and early spring than in the summer and fall, although this seasonal pattern is not seen in children. Early rearing has an effect on the development of not only the serotonin but also other catecholamine systems. Kraemer and colleagues first studied the effects of social rearing on the development of biogenic amine systems in rhesus monkeys. Twelve infant male rhesus monkeys were reared by their mothers until the age of 10–14 months. This group was subdivided into those who continued to live with their mothers but were peer deprived and those who continued to live with their mothers and to have contact with peers. Another group of six infant monkeys was deprived of both mother and peer contact. These monkeys were finally introduced to peers at age 15–21 months. The mother-reared–peer-deprived monkeys were also introduced to peers at age 21–22 months. Serial measurements of CSF 5-HIAA, norepinephrine (NE) and homovanillic acid (HVA, the main metabolite of dopamine) were made throughout the monkeys' development.

5-HIAA declined steadily from birth to 24 months for all the infant monkeys, regardless of social-rearing group. The effects of social rearing were most pronounced on the correlations of serotonin indices with the measures of the DA and NE systems. By 22 months, monkeys reared with mothers showed strong, positive correlations of 5-HIAA with HVA, whereas no such correlation was noted in the other two groups of monkeys. These correlations suggest that social deprivation may disrupt the "entraining" of the DA and serotonin systems. I discussed in Chapter 4 how the NE, DA, and serotonin systems influence each other and are all involved in responding to stimuli; the Kraemer data strongly suggest that early experience influences how these systems interact with each other.

Studies of 5-HIAA in adult personality disorders show a striking consistency with those in nonhuman primates. A high negative correlation (–.78) between CSF 5-HIAA and ratings of aggression and suicide attempts has been found in men dishonorably discharged from the military. Marku Linnoila, Matti Virkkunen, and their colleagues have performed a large number of studies of 5-HIAA in aggressive individuals. Lower 5-HIAA levels were found in impulsive personality disorders relative to paranoid or passive–aggressive personality disorders. Men who had impulsively murdered a sex partner or their own children had lower CSF 5-HIAA levels than other violent criminals, and CSF 5-HIAA correlates negatively with ratings of hostility in normal volunteers. Criminals with high rates of recidivism and a history of suicide attempts had lower CSF 5-HIAA levels than less chronic offenders. Impulsive offenders with early-onset alcoholism and arsonists also show low levels of CSF 5-HIAA. In 1994 Virkkunen and colleagues compared four groups of individuals: 23 men with antisocial personality disorder (APD), 20 men with IED (both of these groups were highly impulsive), 15 nonimpulsive offenders, and 21 control participants. CSF 5-HIAA was significantly lower in the group with APD than in the control group, whereas the nonimpulsive offenders were significantly higher in CSF 5-HIAA than the controls. The offenders with IED also had a low glucose nadir during a glucose tolerance test, compared with the other groups. Both impulsive groups showed higher mean activity levels as measured by actometer counts, as well as a loss of the normal diurnal rhythm of activity. Testosterone was elevated in the group with APD relative to healthy volunteers.

Based on such studies, Linnoila and Virkkunen proposed a model of serotonin dysfunction in impulsive, alcoholic individuals. They hypothesized that there is decreased serotonin input into the nucleus suprachiasmaticus, a principal hypothalamic nucleus responsible for the maintenance of circadian rhythms that also plays a role in glucose metabolism. These authors suggested that deficient serotonin input to the suprachiasmaticus resulted in disturbed sleep, increased activity, and a tendency for glucose to fall to an abnormally low level during fasting periods. The dysphoria resulting from this disturbed state would then lower the threshold for impulsive, aggressive behavior. It might also result in an increased craving for alcohol to relieve the dysphoria.

Does low CSF 5-HIAA necessarily indicate a decreased release of serotonin in the brain? We cannot say for sure without measuring serotonin itself in the CSF, which is technically not possible. Neuroendocrine probe studies have been used to indirectly measure serotonin function in humans. Fenfluramine is an indirect central serotonin agonist. It enhances release of serotonin from neurons, blocks the reuptake of serotonin, and stimulates postsynaptic serotonin receptors. These actions in the hypothalamus ultimately cause the pituitary to release a large bolus of prolactin that can be measured in the plasma. CSF 5-HIAA correlates positively with the amount of prolactin released in response to fenfluramine. More prolactin would mean more serotonin had been released; thus more was metabolized to 5-HIAA. Thus one view would interpret a low prolactin response as suggestive of low serotonin release. On the other hand, if serotonin release is low, one would expect the serotonin receptors in the hypothalamus to upregulate (i.e., become more sensitive). Then administration of the serotonin agonist might cause an exaggerated release of prolactin. Thus caution is needed in interpreting clinical studies.

In 1989 Emil Coccaro and colleagues used this methodology in patients with personality disorders. Male patients with impulsive personality disorders and histories of suicide attempts showed a blunted prolactin response relative to controls and nonimpulsive depressed patients. A negative correlation was found between the peak prolactin level in plasma and ratings of aggression and hostility on several standardized ratings scales.

Molecular Genetic Studies of the Serotonin System

A family in the Netherlands has been identified who show an X-chromosome-linked behavior disorder and mild mental retardation. A mutation was identified in the gene that produces the enzyme MAO-A (monoamine oxidase). This enzyme is a key step in the breakdown of serotonin and dopamine. The mutation resulted in a severe deficiency of enzyme activity. Although the finding is intriguing, it is not known if the defective MAO-A gene directly influences aggression or whether it results in the mild retardation that in turn is associated with behavior disturbance. Because aggression and antisocial behavior in humans do not show an X-linked pattern of inheritance, it is unlikely that this particular genetic defect accounts for a great deal of antisocial behavior. The two members of the family with the mutation who were studied showed higher levels of serotonin and lower levels of 5-HIAA. Using advanced molecular techniques, the MAO-A gene can be knocked out of rodents; these rats show high levels of aggression, and their brains show low levels of 5-HIAA and very high levels of serotonin. Thus we should be careful not to interpret the low 5-HIAA studies as always indicating that serotonin is decreased in aggressive–impulsive disorders. Factors that interfere with the breakdown of serotonin could lead to decreased 5-HIAA while the serotonin amounts are in fact increased in the brain.

Recently the gene for tryptophan hydroxylase (TH), the critical enzyme in the production of serotonin, has been examined in impulse control disorders. The TH gene has U and L alleles, with the U allele the more rare of the two. Within the impulsive offender group the UU genotype had the highest CSF 5-HIAA concentration, and the LL groups had the lowest. (Recall that the impulsive offenders overall had lower CSF 5-HIAA levels). There was no relationship of TH genotype to CSF 5-HIAA in nonimpulsive offenders or controls. There was no relationship of TH genotype to psychiatric diagnosis (APD, IED, nonimpulsive offender, or controls), but among violent offenders (whether impulsive or nonimpulsive), having the L allele was associated with a greater number of suicide attempts. Although no definite findings have emerged, linkage studies are currently under way to determine whether mutations of the 5-HT_{2C} or 5-HT_{1D} receptors are linked to violent or antisocial behavior.

A polymorphism for the serotonin transporter (which governs the reuptake of serotonin into the neuron) has been much studied in anxiety and mood disorders. In the "short" (s) allele for this polymorphism, 44 base pairs are deleted from the DNA in the promoter region of the gene that activates its transcriptions. The s allele does not produce as much of the serotonin transporter as the long (l) allele. Theoretically, this would mean a person with the s allele would have more serotonin in the synaptic cleft after each neuronal impulse because of fewer transporters to remove it, but this has not been definitely established. As we shall see, alcoholics with the l allele may actually have fewer serotonin transporters. Two groups have found that persons with mood and alcohol abuse disorders who have an s allele are more likely to make violent suicide attempts.

Serotonin Studies in Aggressive Children

A number of studies have now examined serotonin function in children and adolescents. In 1990 Marcus Kruesi and colleagues first examined CSF monoamine metabolites in children with disruptive behavior disorders (DBD). The 29 children with DBD each had at least one comorbid diagnosis of ADHD, ODD, or CD, according to a structured interview. Twenty-one met criteria for ADHD at the time of the study; the other eight had past histories of ADHD. Twenty-two of the participants had either ODD or CD. All the participants were medication free for at least 3 weeks before the lumbar puncture. The contrast group was 43 children with obsessive–compulsive disorder (OCD), who were tapped under identical conditions as the DBD group. CSF 5-HIAA was significantly lower in the DBD group relative to the OCD group; all but one participant in the DBD group had levels of CSF 5-HIAA below the mean of the OCD group. Ratings of aggression against people correlated negatively with 5-HIAA in the DBD group but not in the OCD group. There were no correlations of 5-HIAA with either clinical or laboratory measures of impulsivity, but 5-HIAA did correlate positively with parent ratings of the child's social skills. The 29 children with DBDs were followed up 2 years later. All but one of the participants continued to meet criteria for a DBD at follow-up. 5-HIAA remained negatively correlated with overt physical aggression, and low 5-HIAA at baseline indicated a worse prognosis

The fenfluramine stimulation test has been done in children. In adult studies, nonaggressive individuals volunteer as controls and may participate in the study, even though there is no benefit to them. According to international ethical standards regarding research, however, children without psychopathology are not permitted to participate in studies that cannot benefit them if the study involves "more than minimal risk." The fenfluramine stimulation test involves placing an intravenous line to measure prolactin levels; thus studies with children do not involve normal controls but compare aggressive and nonaggressive children with ADHD or look for correlations of the aggressive behavior with the prolactin response. In some cases normal adolescents may volunteer for such studies. David Stoff and colleagues first did such studies. In teenagers, he found no difference between adolescents with conduct or oppositional disorders and controls. Jeffery Halperin and colleagues at Mount Sinai University in New York did the fenfluramine stimulation test in two groups of preadolescents with ADHD. In a younger group, the aggressive children showed an enhanced prolactin response compared with the nonaggressive group (the opposite of the adult finding), whereas in the older children there was no difference in prolactin response. Daniel

Pine (then at Columbia University) and colleagues did the fenfluramine stimulation test in 34 boys at risk for delinquency (based on the fact that their older brothers had been convicted of crimes). They found that the prolactin response correlated positively with ratings of aggression but also with ratings of family adversity.

Two conclusions can be reached from the preceding data. First, there may be a developmental aspect to serotonin's role in aggressive behavior. In young aggressive children, the prolactin response may be enhanced relative to nonaggressive participants, but by late childhood and adolescence it is no longer different. By young adulthood, the prolactin response becomes blunted in aggressive individuals relative to controls. Exactly how serotonin function itself is changing we cannot say, although we have some clues from neuroimaging studies, as I discuss shortly. The Pine study, like the Kraemer study of nonhuman primates, suggests a role for rearing in the development of the serotonergic system. This important latter point was lost in a controversy that enveloped the Mount Sinai and Columbia fenfluramine studies. Fenfluramine was one-half of the "fen-phen" combination in the weight reduction medication Redux that was later found to be associated with heart disease and withdrawn from the market. A single dose of fenfluramine given by mouth, as was done in these studies, did not present only undue risk. Nonetheless, the fact that fenfluramine was used and that aggressive behavior was being studied led to an uproar in New York, complete with street demonstrations and complaints to the National Institute of Mental Health. In Chapter 14, I return to the issue of the political and cultural aspects of studying antisocial and aggressive behaviors, because it is important that rumor and misconception not derail important work on the neurobiological contributors to antisocial behavior.

The Noradrenergic and Autonomic Nervous System in Antisocial Behavior

The autonomic nervous system (ANS), through its sympathetic and parasympathetic branches, both regulates critical life functions on a moment to moment basis and governs the "fight or flight" reaction. The ANS governs heart rate (HR) and skin conductance (SC); both of these measures have been found to be related to antisocial behavior. Fourteen studies, reviewed by Adrian Raine, have shown that the resting HR of children with CD is lower relative to controls. Raine and colleagues obtained psychophysiological variables on a community sample of 101 fifteen-year-old males in Great Britain. All socioeconomic classes were represented. Ten years later, police records were examined for criminal convictions. HR levels of those who would become criminals were significantly lower than those who were never convicted. Criminals-to-be also showed fewer nonspecific SC fluctuations during a rest period than noncriminals, but SC baseline level did not distinguish the groups. Criminals-to-be also showed more delta and theta power (i.e., slower, less arousal) on their EEGs. A discriminant function analysis using all four variables correctly classified 75% of the participants into criminal or noncriminal categories. A recent reanalysis of this data shows that the lowest HRs were found in those adolescents who would ultimately be convicted of violent crime. Increased autonomic activity proved to be a protective factor against developing antisocial behavior. A group of adolescents were identified who were already engaging in antisocial behavior at age 15 but who desisted and never obtained criminal convictions. They were compared with the criminals-to-be and with normals. The desistors showed even higher resting HRs and more nonspecific SCs than the normal controls.

Brennan and colleagues obtained HR and SC data in 50 men at risk for crime because they had criminal fathers. About half of these men became criminals themselves. They were compared with a group of criminals who had no family histories of crime and with a control group (neither fathers nor sons were criminals). Strikingly higher SCs and HRs were found in the men who did not commit crimes in spite of having criminal fathers. In contrast, the lowest HRs and SCs are found in adolescents who commit crimes despite coming from intact homes in higher social classes.

Decreased ANS arousal may translate to decreased fearfulness and a disinhibited temperament. Reviewing studies of SC in anxiety-provoking situations or in individuals with anxiety disorders, Fowles suggested that SC activity indexes inhibition. When there is no "social push" to crime (poverty, family dysfunction), ANS underarousal must be particularly marked to result in criminal behavior. In contrast, when a person is exposed to these social factors, high autonomic arousal may be a protective factor. High anxiety, better inhibitory control, or a tendency to withdraw from stimulation may lead a child in a high-risk environment away from antisocial behavior.

Neuroimaging Studies

A number of studies have shown decreased prefrontal glucose metabolism on positron emission tomography (PET) in persons with impulsive aggression relative to controls. Adrian Raine and colleagues reported on the brain metabolisms of a group of 41 murderers in 1997. Relative to controls, they found the murderers to have decreased activity in the prefrontal lobes and increased activation of the right amygdala. Those murderers who had committed impulsive, affectively driven crimes showed the greatest reduction in prefrontal metabolism, whereas the predatory murderers (proactive aggression) did not. Recently, Raine and his colleagues measured prefrontal cortex volume via MRI in 21 persons with APD, 26 substance abusers who were not antisocial, and 34 controls. The antisocials had significantly reduced white and gray prefrontal volumes relative to the other two groups. As in the preceding studies, the antisocials also had decreased HR and SC, and the decreased SC correlated with reduced gray matter prefrontal volume.

Recently PET studies have been completing the linking of cortical glucose metabolism to serotonin function. Larry Siever and colleagues administered fenfluramine to 6 impulsive–aggressive individuals and 5 controls and then measured brain glucose metabolism via PET. In normal volunteers, fenfluramine caused an increase in blood flow in the orbital frontal ventral medial cortex, as well as in the cingulate, whereas the impulsive–aggressive patients showed no change. Paul Soloff and his group at the University of Pittsburgh found similar results in 5 patients with borderline personality disorder (BPD) and 8 controls. This finding suggests that impulsive and aggressive individuals react differently to serotonin. The aggressive individuals do not activate the prefrontal cortex in response to serotonergic transmission. Finally, Sabine Herpertz and colleagues have examined the function of the amygdala in patients with BPD. They performed functional studies while both women with BPD and controls viewed photographs that were either neutral in emotional content or that were emotionally aversive (mutilated bodies, crying children, scenes of violence). The patients with BPD showed much greater activation of the amygdala than controls. Recall from Chapter 5 that the amygdala is particularly attuned to fearful stimuli and can override ongoing behavior to allow the initiation of an affectively charged response to threatening stimuli. Thus persons with impulsive–aggressive personality disorders may have either a constitutional or acquired overactivity of the amygdala that drives an emotionally charged response to events in the environment.

Putting It Together

Figure 10.1 conceptualizes how aggressive behavior might be mediated by neurobiological factors. It also continues the emphasis on how neurotransmitter systems interact in the governance of complex behaviors; focusing on impulsive, reactive aggression. Interpreting social situations and dealing with conflict with others is a complex process that is summarized in Box 1 in the figure. In dealing with others, we must use language and appreciate all the subtleties of the social interaction. Encoding

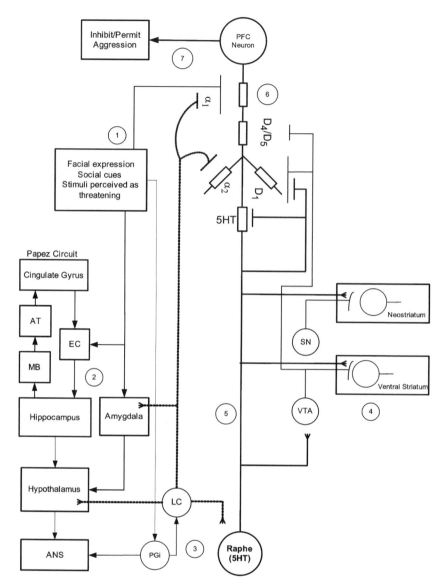

FIGURE 10.1. Interaction of brain systems in impulsive–aggressive behavior. See text for details

social cues, as in Dodge's model, also involves accurate interpretation of facial expression and reading people's intent. Cortical areas mediate these complex skills, as we saw in Chapter 7. Person with antisocial–aggressive behaviors are more likely to show neuropsychological deficits both in language and in visual–spatial areas. These deficits could be genetic in origin or be due to a lack of cognitive stimulation during early childhood. Information about the social situation is conveyed both to the hippocampus and amygdala (2), as well as to the paragigantocellularis (PGI) (3). The PGi activates both the locus coerulus (LC) and the sympathetic nervous system. The amygdala reacts to facial expression, particularly to faces deemed threatening. The hippocampus accesses long-term memory, asking what kind of outcome this social situation has yielded in the past. As is discussed in the next chapter, there are physical changes in the hippocampus of individuals who have experienced physical abuse. The ventral tegmental area (VTA) provides DA input to the prefrontal cortex, neostriatum, and nucleus accumbens (4). Recall from Chapter 5 that DA input to the NA will shift the balance of input to the prefrontal cortex toward the amygdala—that is, toward more immediate, affectively driven responses as opposed to more long-term, context-dependent behaviors.

In our model of ADHD, we emphasized the role of the NE and DA systems and the balance between them—NE being involved in alertness, orientation and working memory and the DA system being critical for both working memory and initiating action. Serotonergic mechanisms appear not to be heavily involved in ADHD, but they probably play a major role in aggressive–impulsive antisocial behavior. Follow the projections of the raphe serotonin neurons (5). Note that they synapse on the cell bodies of the VTA and substantia nigra (SN) but also provide input to ends of the axons of these neurons. Serotonin is released onto "heteroreceptors" located on the synaptic button of the DA neurons, and thus serotonin can regulate DA release at both the cell body and the axon terminal. As discussed in Chapter 4, the situation is not completely clear; under some circumstances serotonin may inhibit DA function. Given the multiplicity of serotonin receptors it is quite likely that serotonin both inhibits and facilitates DA, depending on the brain location and other neurotransmitter inputs.

In Chapter 4 I discussed how serotonin may maintain a balance between the NE and DA systems. In ADHD, a hyperdopaminergic status may lead to hyperactivity and impulsivity; but if the serotonin system is functional, it may serve to restrain the DA system when social stimuli are being processed. Because mood is being properly regulated, the individual does not experience intense, uncontrollable periods of irritability. Now suppose that there is a genetic malfunction in the serotonin system or that a history of abuse or neglect has resulted in a failure to program the NE, DA, and serotonin systems properly. Recall the neglected monkeys in Kraemer's study, as well as Pine's study showing that an adverse family environment was correlated with an enhanced prolactin response to fenfluramine. Serotonin input to the prefrontal cortex increases neuronal glucose utilization (6); along with input from NE and DA, the prefrontal neurons can act to inhibit aggressive behavior. The PFC connections to the amygdala directly inhibit activity in that structure, and PFC input to the hypothalamus will govern the output of the ANS. Thus the PFC can elect to turn off the "fight or flight" reaction.

Treatment Implications

One of the more obvious questions involves the roles of serotonergic drugs in the treatment of aggression. In 1989 Emil Coccaro and colleagues performed a double-blind placebo-controlled trial of fluoxetine (Prozac) in men with impulsive personality disorders. They found that the fluoxetine was helpful in reducing irritability and aggressive outbursts, even when the patient did not have a comorbid mood disorder. The drug was not a panacea for aggression. Psychiatrists have been routinely prescribing SSRIs for impulsive and irritable personality-disordered patients for the past decade. Although some are helped, many find no benefit. It is clear, however, that SSRIs do not induce violent behavior, though a number of patients experience restlessness or a sense of activation. We also cannot say that SSRIs achieve an antiaggressive effect by "increasing serotonin"; indeed, perhaps they down regulate the serotonin system, as they do in mood disorders. Chapter 11 tackles the mechanisms of action of antidepressants. Also of interest is that the newer, "atypical" neuroleptics also have a potent antiaggressive effect, even in nonpsychotic individuals, and that one of the mechanisms of action of these drugs is to *block* the serotonin 2_A receptor. Atypical neuroleptics have a variety of other neurochemical mechanisms, which I explore in Chapter 12. Haloperidal, an older neuroleptic with very little serotonin activity, has been shown to reduce aggression in conduct-disordered children. It is not used for this purpose now because of the risk these drugs have for tardive dyskinesia, but the finding suggests that blocking dopamine receptors may have an antiaggressive effect. Sedation is not a common side effect of haloperidal, suggesting that the effect is directly on aggression. Finally, mood stabilizers such as lithium and divalproex sodium (Depakote), drugs used in the treatment of bipolar disorder, also can reduce aggressive outbursts even when the patient does not have a mood disorder. Still, much more research is needed into the circuitry shown in Figure 10.1 before we have drugs that specifically target impulsive aggressive behavior. Eltoprazine, a compound that acts as an agonist at serotonin receptors, was tested in Europe and found to reduce aggressive behavior in mentally retarded people. The Food and Drug Administration (FDA) approves drugs only for disorders (except for things such as pain and fever), and when it became clear that the FDA would not consider approving the drug for the U.S. market, the company that had been researching it stopped further development of it. Again, I hash out these politically sensitive issues in Chapter 14.

The effects of early abuse on aggressive behavior and the association of biological changes in the individual with early adverse rearing should be sobering to us all. In Chapter 11 I discuss again how early stresses may write themselves into the brain. This way of thinking about environmental effects on behavior is different: In the past, when we have spoken of biological–environmental interactions, the biology has been assumed to be fixed and the environmental influence "psychological," somehow existing outside the brain. This led to the assumption that the effects of early abuse might not be permanent—after all, a "learned behavior" would go away when the environment changes, or an adult with an abusive past might erase the experience with a course of therapy. Many people with histories of abuse do overcome their tragic pasts and lead productive lives. The data presented thus far, however, should emphasize the need to stop early abuse and neglect as soon as possible and to do everything possible to prevent it. Many people like Mark may never recover if we do not.

ALCOHOL AND SUBSTANCE ABUSE

Alcohol and substance abuse are discussed in this chapter because, although these problems are associated with all mental disorders, they are particularly prevalent in persons with antisocial behavior and impulsive personality disorders. This is especially true of severe, early-onset alcohol and polysubstance abuse. Indeed, follow-up studies of children at risk have shown that severe substance abuse and dependence rarely occur in people without a history of early conduct problems. Many people experiment with substances and even engage in casual use, particularly in the young adult years, but they desist on their own. Only a small percentage of these experimenters go on to regular abuse and addiction. There seems to be something different about these individuals. Once addicted to a substance, they find it very difficult to stop their drug abuse, even when the consequences are grave. Witness the struggles of Darryl Strawberry, the baseball player, or the actor Robert Downey, Jr.: They destroyed careers that could have made them multimillionaires in order to pursue drugs. What is the biological substrate of such a destructive impulse? First, I look at how alcohol and illegal drugs might produce a "high," then examine some genetic mechanisms that might make some individuals more vulnerable to alcohol and substance abuse.

Mechanisms of Euphoria and Withdrawal

I have emphasized the role of dopaminergic projection from the VTA to the nucleus accumbens (NA) in the organism's experience of reward. Animals will press a button in their cages to activate an electrode that stimulates this pathway; they will also inject dopamine reuptake blockers such as cocaine and stimulants directly into the NA. This has led several scientists, including Roy Wise and George Koob, to hypothesize that drugs of abuse produce euphoria by having at least some of their action in that circuitry. Nora Volkow (discussed in Swanson & Volkow, 2001) and her colleagues have performed numerous PET studies in which adult volunteers are given intravenous (IV) stimulant or cocaine that contains positron-emitting atoms. This allows them to see where the drug binds in the brain. These potent dopamine reuptake blockers bind to the dopamine-rich area of the striatum. Interestingly, the high is experienced only during the period in which the drug is acutely blocking dopamine reuptake, that is, within a minute or so of administration. Although the drug remains bound to the reuptake site for several minutes, the high fades much more quickly. This suggests that it is the *rate of change* of dopamine in the NA that accounts for the high. When stimulants such as methylphenidate (Ritalin) are given by mouth rather than IV, the rate of binding to the DA receptor is much slower, and euphoria is not experienced, even though the methylphenidate ultimately reaches the same level of reuptake site binding as the IV-administered drug. This explains why treatment of ADHD with low-dose oral methylphenidate is not associated with a risk of abuse or addiction, whereas snorting or injecting the drug is. During these studies, Volkow and colleagues discovered a curious fact: Some of the volunteers experienced no euphoria at all to IV stimulant or cocaine, even though the PET study showed that the drug was clearly binding to their DA reuptake sites. This finding is consistent with the fact that many people will experiment with a drug of abuse but never go on to regular use because "it didn't do anything for me." Thus not all brains are the same when it comes to the experience produced by drugs of abuse.

Opiate drugs, such as heroin or morphine, exert their effects at the μ receptor, mimicking the effects of the endogenous opioid peptides. Small opioid peptide neurons are found around the VTA and the locus coeruleus (LC). Opiates appear to have different effects on these two neurotransmitter systems. As shown in Figure 10.2, opiate neurons inhibit the release of GABA from the small GABA interneurons around the

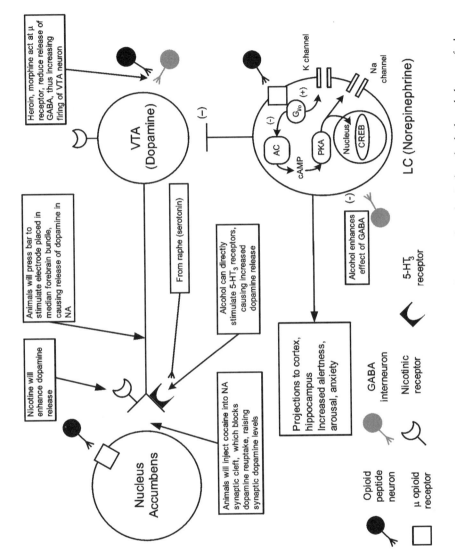

FIGURE 10.2. Brain systems mediating the production of euphoria by alcohol and drugs of abuse

VTA. With the VTA neuron released from GABA inhibition, its firing rate increases, and more dopamine is released into the NA. The opposite effect occurs in the LC. Opioid drugs directly stimulate the μ receptors on the LC, resulting in the stimulation of G proteins. The G_i protein will reduce the production of cAMP that will in turn lead to a reduction in protein kinase A (PKA). Among its many functions, PKA stimulates CREB, such that this protein, critical for controlling multiple genes, will be diminished. The G_o protein will activate a K channel; more K leaving the cell prolongs the after-hyperpolarization, leading to a more refractory, less active neuron. The opiates, in summary, reduce the activity of the LC. Because the LC normally promotes arousal and anticipatory anxiety, this action accounts for the opiates' antianxiety and sedating effects, whereas the increased activity of the VTA may account for some of the euphoria. Opiod peptide neurons occur throughout the brain, and part of the euphoria characteristic of the opiate drugs is produced through dopamine-independent mechanisms. The LC is also thought to be responsible for the mechanisms of withdrawal. The LC neuron somehow adapts to the chronic stimulation of the μ receptor: The activity of the cAMP-stimulated PKA pathway is up-regulated, in an attempt to counter the effects of the opiate. First, this leads to tolerance. Larger doses of opiates are needed to achieve the same effect. When opiates are discontinued, this up-regulated cAMP–PKA pathway now surges into action, massively increasing the firing of the LC and other sympathetic neurons. This increase causes the typical opiate withdrawal signs of excessive sympathetic nervous system activity: severe anxiety, sweating, dilated pupils, and a runny nose

Although they do not produce a "high" per se, cigarettes give much pleasure to chronic smokers and are highly addicting. Nicotine stimulates the VTA through nicotine receptors on the cell body, and it enhances the release of dopamine through similar receptors on the axon terminal. The active agent in marijuana (cannabis) is Δ^9-tetrahydrocannabinol (THC). It acts at specific cannabinoid receptors in the brain (not shown in the figure) to produce relaxation and mild euphoria.

After prolonged use, tolerance to THC results. Recently, it has been discovered that these cannabinoid receptors are stimulated by an endogenous neurotransmitter that has been named "anandamide" (from the Sanskrit word meaning "bliss"). Anandamide, however, is much less potent than THC. It is unclear why our brains produce this "natural marijuana," but anandamide does have analgesic effects. Interestingly, although one subtype of cannabinoid receptor is found primarily in the brain, another is found in the immune system; thus THC may have immunosuppressive effects.

The effects of alcohol are diffuse. It enhances the effects of GABA, and this, as shown in Figure 10.2, will decrease LC firing. Through direct stimulation of 5-HT$_3$ receptors on the dopamine nerve terminals, dopamine release is increased. Alcohol inhibits glutamate and NMDA receptors, leading to sedation. In toxic amounts, alcohol blocks sodium and calcium channels, which can lead to coma and death. In many alcoholics, acute withdrawal of alcohol leads to sudden rebound of neuronal excitability (due to reactivation of glutamate and NMDA receptors). This excess neuronal activity can lead to psychosis (delirium tremens, or "DTs") and seizures. If not treated with benzodiazepines, death may often ensue.

Withdrawal from opiates, marijuana, or cocaine is not life threatening but very uncomfortable. Cocaine users in particular will experience a craving for the drug, and recently a neuroimaging study of the craving process has been performed. Clinton Kilts and colleagues at Emory University performed PET studies in 8 men who were admitted to a hospital with cocaine addition. The men received three PET scans each. In the first, they imagined a neutral scene; in the second, they imagined scenes that conjured up use of cocaine; and in the third scan, they imagined an experience that made them angry. By subtracting the anger and drug-use scans from the neutral scans, the investigators could examine which brain regions were activated by drug craving. (All the participants reported that imagining drug use increased their desire to use cocaine.) Drug imagery resulted in strong activation of the amygdala and NA, highly consistent with the hypothesis that these areas are key in the actions of drugs of abuse, as well as in addiction.

Genetics of Alcohol and Substance Abuse

It is clear that alcohol and substance abuse problems run in families. The most substantial work has been done with alcoholism. In these studies, it became clear that alcohol abuse is a heterogenous disorder. Robert Cloninger and his colleagues have made distinctions between two major subtypes of alcoholism. Type 1 is characterized by a later age of onset, low levels of antisocial behavior and personality disorder, and high levels of guilt about alcohol abuse. These individuals often "lose control" of their drinking; they do not set out to get intoxicated, but one drink leads to another and another. In contrast, Type 2 alcoholics show very early age of onset (often in the teen years), high levels of antisocial behavior, and deliberate alcohol-seeking behavior. They show little guilt about their drinking behavior except in cases in which some consequence is harmful to them (i.e., being arrested for driving under the influence). Type 1 alcoholics tend to be anxious and to shy away from stimulation; they may drink to reduce their social anxiety, whereas Type 2 alcoholics are often risk takers, have low anxiety, and are easily bored. The similarity of Type 2 alcoholics to the impulsive, aggressive personality already discussed in this chapter should be apparent.

The two types of alcoholism show very different patterns of inheritance. M. Bohman, Sigvardsson, and Cloninger studied over 1,700 adoptees in Sweden. For Type 1 alcoholism, a gene-by-environment interaction was necessary for the adoptee to show the disorder. If a child with a Type 1 alcoholic parent was adopted by a Type 1 alcoholic, the child had about a 12% chance of developing Type 1 alcoholism (as opposed to the 4% rate in the general population). In contrast, children of Type 1 alcoholics did not show an increased risk if raised by nonalcoholic parents; and children with no genetic risk did not have an increased rate of alcoholism even if they were raised by a Type 1 alcoholic adoptive parent. The pattern for Type 2 alcoholism was quite different. Children of Type 2 alcoholics had a much greater rate of Type 2 alcoholism (17–18%) regardless of the alcoholism of the adoptive parent. Children of nonalcoholics did not have a higher rate of Type 2 alcoholism even when raised by a Type 2 alcoholic. That is, only genetics appeared to play a role in Type 2 alcoholism.

Genetic effects for the risk of abuse of other substances have been found as well. Tsuang and colleagues examined more than 1,800 MZ and DZ twins and calculated the heritability of substance abuse or dependence for various substances as follows: marijuana (.33), stimulants (.44), opiates (.43), and general drug abuse (.34). The effect of genetics on substance abuse and dependence is significant and may have some overlap with genetic risk for antisocial behavior. Many Type 2 alcoholics also abuse multiple substances. How could a genetic factor increase the risk of substance or alcohol abuse? If a person had high levels of genetically mediated anxiety or dysphoria as part of his or her baseline personality, he or she might be more prone to seek relief through drinking or drugs. This could be particularly the case in Type 1 alcoholism. Alternatively, individuals at risk might inherit some factor that causes their brains to react differently to alcohol or substances than do controls. This could predispose them to use excessively or to become addicted.

Over the past two decades, numerous studies of children of alcoholics have shown them to be more resistant to the effects of both alcohol and benzodiazepines than persons without strong family histories of alcoholism. In these studies, sons of alcoholics (SOAs) who do not yet abuse alcohol are compared with control participants. Both groups are given alcoholic beverages, and, even though the groups show similar blood levels of ethanol, the SOAs report feeling less intoxication and show less impairment on a measure of motor coordination. Normally, alcohol stimulates the release of cortisol and prolactin. These neurohormonal changes are diminished in SOAs, and in at least some studies SOAs show less EEG slowing in response to alcohol than controls do. Those SOAs who show the diminished response to alcohol are at the highest risk for future alcoholism. Thus one mechanism of alcoholism might be that those at genetic risk fail to get a "buzz" from a socially acceptable level of drinking. They increase their alcohol intake to enhance the effect, and these greater amounts place them at risk for addiction. In contrast, some people (particularly those of Asian descent) lack the liver enzyme alcohol dehydrogenase that breaks down alcohol. Such persons develop an intensely unpleasant flushing reaction to even small amounts of alcohol; they invariably give up drinking. Consequently, they are at very low risk for developing alcohol problems.

The Collaborative Study of Genetics of Alcoholism (COGA) examined more than 1,200 families to find polymorphisms linked to alcohol abuse and dependence. Markers on chromosome 4, near the gene for alcohol dehydrogenase, were associated with a lower than average risk of alcoholism. Markers on chromosomes 1 and 7 were related to a low risk of alcohol dependence, whereas a marker on chromosome 16 was associated with severe dependence. On event-related potentials (a form of EEG), alcoholics showed a reduced wave form (the P300), a wave that is normally produced in response to unexpected stimuli in the environment. (Reduced P300 is found in a number of mental disorders and is not unique to alcoholism.) Markers at chromosomes 2 and 6 appeared to be related to a reduced P300. Genes for the α, β, and γ subunits of the $GABA_A$ receptor are found on chromosome 5. Several studies have suggested that polymorphisms related to the genes for these subunits are associated with alcoholism. Because alcohol enhances the action of GABA, this is of definite interest. Recently Nakao Iwata and colleagues subdivided a group of 51 children of alcoholics according to their genotype for the $GABA_A$ receptor. Recall that the α subunit has six subtypes. The α_6 subtype has two forms: in one, a serine amino acid was substituted for proline in the amino acid structure of the protein. Adult children of alcoholics who had the serine substitution had less Valium-induced impairment of eye movement than controls, suggesting that they were more resistant to the effects of the benzodiazepine. Mark Schuckit and colleagues from the University of San Diego found that SOAs with a serine substitution were at a higher risk of developing alcohol problems than those with two proline alleles. Thus persons with a serine substitution might start drinking excessively because they are more resistant to the "normal" euphoric effects of usual doses of alcohol (step 1 in Figure 10.3).

Earlier I reviewed the data showing the likelihood of some sort of serotonergic dysfunction in individuals with impulsive aggression. Not surprisingly, serotonin has also been a focus of alcoholism research. SOAs from the Schuckit study who were homozygous for the long (l) allele of the serotonin transporter were also at high risk for alcoholism, particularly if they were also homozygous for the serine GABA α_6 subunit substitution. In controls, persons homozygous for the ll allele show increased serotonin transporter availability, whereas alcoholics homozygous for the long form show decreased serotonin transporter availability. Andreas Heinz and colleagues from the National Institute of Mental Health reported findings that suggest that individuals homozygous for the long form are more prone to damaging their transporters by chronic alcohol use (step 2 in Figure 10.3). With fewer transporters, more serotonin is available in the cleft to stimulate the autoreceptors, resulting in decreased serotonin neuron firing (step 3).

As was discussed in Chapter 4, the $5HT_3$ receptor is the only serotonin receptor subtype that is ionotropic in nature. As shown in Figure 10.2, serotonin neurons from the raphe may terminate on dopamine nerve terminals, and dopamine release is enhanced when $5HT_3$ receptors are stimulated. If baseline serotonin firing is reduced, as described previously, these $5HT_3$ receptors will up-regulate (step 4 in Figure 10.3). Interestingly, alcohol will directly activate the $5HT_3$ receptor, increasing dopamine release. Thus, when the alcoholic drinks, he or she may feel an enhanced euphoria because of alcohol's effect on the now oversensitive $5HT_3$ receptors. In a major clinical study, Bankole Johnson and his colleagues at the University of Texas Health Science Center at San Antonio performed a double-blind, placebo-controlled trial of the medication ondansetron (a $5HT_3$ blocker) in alcoholics. The medication was found to significantly cut the craving of alcoholics for drinking, especially in those with early-onset severe alcoholism. When on the active drug, the alcoholics had fewer drinks per day and were abstinent a greater number of days during the study than those on placebo. Here we see the benefit of biological research in this area—not to identify and stigmatize individuals but to develop treatments that have the potential to restore these individuals to health.

REFERENCES

Anthenelli, R. M., & Schuckit, M. A. (1997). Genetics. In J. H. Lowinson, P. Ruiz, R. B. Millman, & J. G. Langrod (Eds.), *Substance abuse: A comprehensive textbook* (3rd ed., pp. 41–51). Baltimore: Williams & Wilkins.

Bellivier, F., Szoke, A., Henry, C., Lacoste, J., Bottos, C., Nosten-Bertrand, M., et al. (2000). Possible association between serotonin transporter gene polymorphism and violent suicidal behavior in mood disorders. *Biological Psychiatry, 48*, 319–322.

Biederman, J., Faraone, S. V., Keenan, K., Benjamin, J., Krifcher, B., Moore, C.,

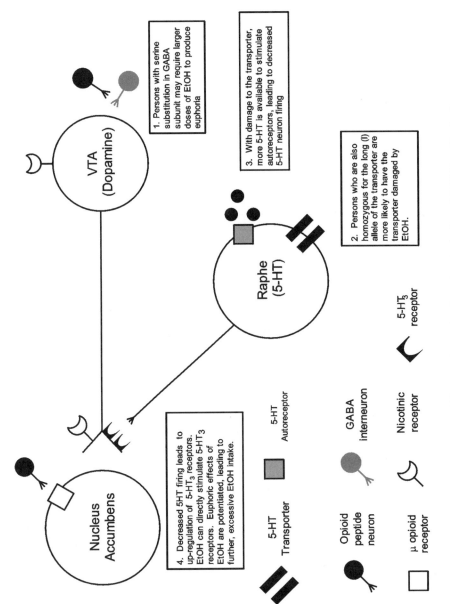

FIGURE 10.3. Possible genetic mechanisms in alcoholism (ETOH = Alcohol)

1. Persons with serine substitution in GABA subunit may require larger doses of EtOH to produce euphoria

3. With damage to the transporter, more 5-HT is available to stimulate autoreceptors, leading to decreased 5-HT neuron firing

2. Persons who are also homozygous for the long (l) allele of the transporter are more likely to have the transporter damaged by EtOH.

4. Decreased 5HT firing leads to up-regulation of 5-HT₃ receptors. EtOH can directly stimulate 5-HT₃ receptors. Euphoric effects of EtOH are potentiated, leading to further, excessive EtOH intake.

VTA (Dopamine)

Raphe (5-HT)

Nucleus Accumbens

5-HT Transporter

5-HT Autoreceptor

5-HT₃ receptor

Opioid peptide neuron

GABA interneuron

μ opioid receptor

Nicotinic receptor

et al. (1992). Further evidence for family–genetic risk factors in attention deficit hyperactivity disorder: Patterns of comorbidity in probands and relatives in psychiatrically and pediatrically referred samples. *Archives of General Psychiatry, 49,* 728–738.

Brennan, P., Raine, A., & Mednick, S. A. (1994). Psychophysiological protective factors for children at high risk for antisocial outcome. *Psychophysiology, 31,* S30.

Brown, G. L., Goodwin, F. K., Ballenger, J., Goyer, P., & Major, L. (1979). Aggression in humans correlates with cerebrospinal fluid metabolites. *Psychiatry Research, 1,* 131–135.

Bohman, M., Sigvardsson, S., & Cloninger, C. R. (1981). Maternal inheritance of alcohol abuse: Cross-fostering analysis of adopted women. *Archives of General Psychiatry, 38,* 965–969.

Brunner, H. G., Nelen, M., Breakfield, X. O., Ropers, H. H., & van Oost, B. A. (1993). Abnormal behavior associated with a point mutation in the structural gene for monoamine oxidase A. *Science, 262,* 578–580.

Brunner, H. G., Nelen, M. R., van Zandvoort, P., Abeling, N. G. G. M., van Gennip, A. H., Wolters, E. C., et al. (1993). X-linked borderline mental retardation with prominent behavioral disturbance: Phenotype, genetic localization, and evidence for disturbed monoamine metabolism. *American Journal of Human Genetics, 52,* 1032–1039.

Cadoret, R. J., Cunningham, L., Loftus, R., & Edwards, J. (1975). Studies of adoptees from psychiatrically disturbed biologic parents: 2. Temperament, hyperactive, antisocial, and developmental variables. *Journal of Pediatrics, 87,* 301–306.

Cloninger, C. R. (1989). Neurogenetic adaptive mechanisms in alcoholism. In K. L. Kelner & D. E. Koshland (Eds.), *Molecules to models* (pp. 375–387). Washington, DC: American Association for the Advancement of Science.

Cloninger, C. R. (1999). Genetics of substance abuse. In M. Galanter & H. D. Kleber (Eds.), *Textbook of substance abuse treatment* (2nd ed., pp. 59–66). Washington, DC: American Psychiatric Press.

Cloninger, C. R., Bohman, M., & Sigvardsson, S. (1981). Inheritance of alcohol abuse: Cross-fostering analysis of adopted men. *Archives of General Psychiatry, 38,* 861–868.

Coccaro, E. F., & Kavoussi, R. J. (1997). Fluoxetine and impulsive aggressive behavior in personality-disordered subjects. *Archives of General Psychiatry, 54,* 1081–1088.

Coccaro, E. F., Siever, L. J., Klar, H. M., Maurer, G., Cochrane, K., Cooper, T. B., et al. (1989). Serotonergic studies in patients with affective and personality disorders. *Archives of General Psychiatry, 46,* 587–599.

Crowe, R. R. (1978). Genetic studies of antisocial personalities and related disorders. In R. L. Spitzer & D. F. Klein (Eds.), *Critical issues in psychiatric diagnosis* (pp. 193–202). New York: Raven Press.

DiLalla, L. F., & Gottesman, I. I. (1991). Biological and genetic contributors to violence: Wisdom's untold tale. *Psychological Bulletin, 109,* 125–129.

Dodge, K. A. (1986). A social information processing model of social competence in children. In M. Perlmutter (Ed.), *Cognitive perspectives on chil-*

dren's social and behavioral development (pp. 77–125). Hillsdale, NJ: Erlbaum.

Dodge, K. A. (1993). Social–cognitive mechanisms in the development of conduct disorders and depression. *Annual Review of Psychology, 44,* 559–584.

Dodge, K. A., Harnish, J. D., Lochman, J. E., & Bates, J. E. (1997). Reactive and proactive aggression in school children and psychiatrically impaired chronically assaultive youth. *Journal of Abnormal Psychology, 106,* 37–51.

Farrington, D. P., Loeber, R., & Van Kammen, W. B. (1989). Long term criminal outcomes of hyperactivity–impulsivity–attention deficit and conduct problems in childhood. In L. N. Robins & M. R. Rutter (Eds.), *Straight and devious pathways to adulthood* (pp. 62–81). New York: Cambridge University Press.

Fowles, D. C. (1980). The three arousal model: Implications of Gray's two factor learning theory for heart rate, electrodermal activity and psychopathy. *Psychophysiology, 17,* 87–104.

Fowles, D. C. (1988). Psychophysiology and psychopathy: A motivational approach. *Psychophysiology, 25,* 373–391.

Gorwood, P., Batel, P., Ades, J., Hamon, M., & Boni, C. (2000). Serotonin transporter gene polymorphisms, alcoholism, and suicidal behavior. *Biological Psychiatry, 48,* 259–264.

Halperin, J. M., Newcorn, J. H., Kopstein, I., McKay, K. E., Schwartz, S. T., Siever, L. J., & Sharma, V. (1997). Serotonin, aggression, and parental psychopathology in children with attention deficit hyperactivity disorder. *Journal of the American Academy of Child and Adolescent Psychiatry, 36,* 1391–1398.

Halperin, J. M., Newcorn, J. H., Schwartz, S. T., Sharma, V., Siever, L. J., Koda, V. H., & Gabriel, S. (1997). Age-related changes in the association between serotonergic function and aggression in boys with ADHD. *Biological Psychiatry, 41,* 682–689.

Has America's tide of violence receded for good? (2000). *Science, 289,* 582–585.

Heinz, A., Jones, D. W., Mazzanti, C., Goldman, D., Ragan, P., Hommer, D., et al. (2000). A relationship between serotonin transporter genotype and in vivo protein expression and alcohol neurotoxicity. *Biological Psychiatry, 47,* 643–649.

Hermann, B. P., & Whitman, S. (1984). Behavioral and personality correlates of epilepsy: A review, methodogical critique, and conceptual model. *Psychological Bulletin, 95,* 451–497.

Herpertz, S. C., Dietrich, T. M., Wenning, B., Krings, T., Erberich, S. G., Willmes, K., et al. (2001). Evidence of abnormal amygdala functioning in borderline personality disorder: A functional MRI study. *Biological Psychiatry, 50,* 292–298.

Higley, J. D., King, S. T., Hasert, M. F., Champoux, M., Suomi, S. J., & Linnoila, M. (1996). Stability of interindividual differences in serotonin function and its relationship to severe aggression and competent social behavior in rhesus macaque females. *Neuropsychopharmacology, 14,* 67–76.

Higley, J. D., Mehlman, P. T., Higley, S. B., Fernald, B., Vickers, J., Lindell, S. G., et al. (1996). Excessive mortality in young free-ranging male nonhuman primates with low cerebrospinal fluid 5-hydroxyindoleacetic acid concentrations. *Archives of General Psychiatry, 53,* 537–543.

Iwata, N., Cowley, D. S., Radel, M., Roy-Byrne, P. P., & Goldman, D. (1999). Relationship between a GABAAα6 pro385Ser substitution and benzodiazepine sensitivity. *American Journal of Psychiatry, 156,* 1447–1449.

Johnson, B. A., Roache, J. D., Javors, M. A., DiClemente, C. C., Cloninger, C. R., Prihoda, T. J., et al. (2000). Ondanestron for reduction of drinking among biologically predisposed alcoholic patients. *Journal of the American Medical Association, 284,* 963–971.

Kaplan, J. R., Shively, C. A., Fontenot, M. B., Morgan, T. M., Howell, S. M., Manuck, S. B., et al. (1994). Demonstration of an association among dietary cholesterol, central serotonergic activity, and social behavior in monkeys. *Psychosomatic Medicine, 56,* 479–484.

Kilts, C. D., Schweiter, J. B., Quinn, C. K., Gross, R. E., Faber, T. L., Muhammad, F., et al. (2001). Neural activity related to drug craving in cocaine addiction. *Archives of General Psychiatry, 58,* 341.

Koob, G. F., & Nestler, E. J. (1997). The neurobiology of drug addiction. In S. Salloway, P. Malloy, & J. L. Cummings (Eds.), *The neuropsychiatry of limbic and subcortical disorders* (pp. 179–194). Washington, DC: American Psychiatric Press.

Kraemer, G. W., Ebert, M. H., Schmidt, D. E., & McKinney, W. T. (1989). A longitudinal study of the effect of different social rearing conditions on cerebrospinal fluid norepinephrine and biogenic amine metabolites in rhesus monkeys. *Neuropharmacology, 2,* 175–189.

Kruesi, M. J., Hibbs, E. D., Zahn, T. P., Keysor, C. S., Hamburger, S. D., Bartko, J. J., & Rapoport, J. L. (1992). A 2–year prospective follow-up study of children and adolescents with disruptive behavior disorders: Prediction by cerebrospinal fluid 5-hydroxyindoleacetic acid, homovanillic acid, and autonomic measures? *Archives of General Psychiatry, 49,* 429–435.

Kruesi, M. J., Rapoport, J. L., Hamburger, S., Hibbs, E. D., Potter, W. Z., Lenane, M., & Brown, G. L. (1990). Cerebrospinal fluid monoamine metabolites, aggression, and impulsivity in disruptive behavior of children and adolescents. *Archives of General Psychiatry, 47,* 419–426.

Lewis, D. O., Yeager, C. A., & Lovely, R. (1994). A clinical follow-up of delinquent males: Ignored vulnerabilities, unmet needs and the perpetuation of violence. *Journal of the American Academy of Child and Adolescent Psychiatry, 33,* 518–528.

Linnoila, M., & Charney, D. S. (1999). The neurobiology of aggression. In D. S. Charney, E. J. Nestler, & B. S. Bunney (Eds.), *Neurobiology of mental illness* (pp. 855–871). New York: Oxford University Press.

Linnoila, M., Delong, J., & Virkkunen, M. (1989). Monoamines, glucose metabolism, and impulse control. *Psychopharmacology Bulletin, 25,* 404–406.

Linnoila, M., & Virkkunen, M. (1992). Biologic correlates of suicidal risk and aggressive behavioral traits. *Journal of Clinical Psychopharmacology, 12,* 19S–20S.

Linnoila, M., Virkkunen, M., Scheinin, M., Nuutila, A., Rimon, R., & Goodwin, F. K. (1983). Low cerebrospinal fluid 5-hydroxyindoleacetic acid concentration differentiates impulsive from non-impulsive violent behavior. *Life Science, 33,* 2609–2614.

Loeber, R., Brinthaupt, V. P., & Green, S. M. (1988). Attention deficits, impulsivity, and hyperactivity with or without conduct problems: Relationships to delinquency and unique contextual factors. In R. J. McMahon & R. D. Peters (Eds.), *Behavior disorders of adolescence: Research, intervention, and policy in clinical and school settings* (pp. 39–61). New York: Plenum.

Lyons, M. J., True, W. R., Eisen, S. A., Goldberg, J., Meyer, J. M., Faraone, S. V., et al. (1995). Differential heritability of adult and juvenile antisocial traits. *Archives of General Psychiatry, 52,* 906–915.

McGee, R., Williams, S., Moffitt, T., & Anderson, J. (1989). A comparison of 13–year-old boys with attention deficit and/or reading disorder on neuropsychological measures. *Journal of Abnormal Child Psychology, 17,* 37–53.

Mednick, S. A., Gabrielli, W. F., & Hutchings, B. (1984). Genetic influences in criminal convictions: Evidence from an adoption cohort. *Science, 224,* 891–894.

Mednick, S. A., Gabrielli, W. F., & Hutchings, B. (1987). Genetic factors in the etiology of criminal behavior. In S. A. Mednick, T. E. Moffitt, & S. A. Stack (Eds.), *The causes of crime: New biological approaches* (pp. 74–91). New York: Cambridge University Press.

Mehlman, P. T., Higley, J. D., Faucher, I., Lilly, A., Taub, D. M., Vickers, J., et al. (1995). Correlation of CSF 5-HIAA concentration with sociality and the timing of emigration in free-ranging primates. *American Journal of Psychiatry, 152,* 907–913.

Mehlman, P. T., Higley, J. D., Faucher, I., Lilly, A. A., Taub, D. M., Vickers, J., et al. (1994). Low CSF 5-HIAA concentrations and severe aggression and impaired impulse control in nonhuman primates. *American Journal of Psychiatry, 151,* 1485–1491.

Moffitt, T. E. (1990a). Juvenile delinquency and attention deficit disorder: Boys' developmental trajectories from age 3 to age 15. *Child Development, 61,* 893–910.

Moffitt, T. E. (1990b). The neuropsychology of delinquency: A critical review of theory and research. In N. Morris & M. Tonry (Eds.), *Crime and justice* (pp. 99–169). Chicago: University of Chicago Press.

Moffitt, T. E. (1993). The neuropsychology of conduct disorder. *Development and Psychopathology, 5,* 135–151.

Moffitt, T. E., & Silva, P. A. (1988). Self-reported delinquency, neuropsychological deficit, and history of attention deficit disorder. *Journal of Abnormal Child Psychology, 16,* 553–569.

Nielsen, D. A., Goldman, D., Virkkunen, M., Tokola, R., Rawlings, R., & Linnoila, M. (1994). Suicidality and 5-hydroxyindoleacetic acid concentration associated with a tryptophan hydroxylase polymorphism. *Archives of General Psychiatry, 51,* 34–38.

Pine, D. S., Coplan, J. D., Wasserman, G. A., Miller, L. S., Fried, J. E., Davies, M., et al. (1997). Neuroendocrine response to fenfluramine challenge in boys. *Archives of General Psychiatry, 54,* 839–846.

Pine, D. S., Wasserman, G., Coplan, J., Fried, J., Sloan, R., Myers, M., et al.

(1996). Serotonergic and cardiac correlates of aggression in children. *Annals of the New York Academy of Sciences, 794,* 391–393.

Pine, D. S., Wasserman, G. A., Coplan, J., Fried, J. A., Huang, Y. Y., Kassir, S., et al. (1996). Platelet serotonin 2A (5-HT2A) receptor characteristics and parenting factors for boys at risk for delinquency: a preliminary report. *American Journal of Psychiatry, 153,* 538–544.

Raine, A. (1996). Autonomic nervous system factors underlying disinhibited, antisocial, and violent behavior. *Annals of the New York Academy of Sciences, 794,* 46–59.

Raine, A., Buchsbaum, M. S., Stanley, J., Lottenberg, S., Abel, L., & Stoddard, J. (1995). Selective reduction in prefrontal glucose metabolism in murderers. *Biological Psychiatry, 38,* 342–343.

Raine, A., & Jones, F. (1987). Attention, autonomic arousal and personality in behaviorally disordered children. *Journal of Abnormal Child Psychology, 15,* 583–599.

Raine, A., Lenz, T., Bihrle, S., LaCasse, L., & Colletti, P. (2000). Reduced prefrontal grey matter volume and reduced autonomic activity in antisocial personality disorder. *Archives of General Psychiatry, 57,* 119–127.

Raine, A., & Venables, P. H. (1984). Tonic heart rate level, social class and antisocial behaviour in adolescents. *Biological Psychology, 18,* 123–132.

Raine, A., Venables, P. H., & Williams, M. (1990a). Autonomic orienting responses in 15-year-old male subjects and criminal behavior at age 24. *American Journal of Psychiatry, 147,* 933–937.

Raine, A., Venables, P. H., & Williams, M. (1990b). Relationships between central and autonomic measures of arousal at age 15 years and criminality at age 24 years. *Archives of General Psychiatry, 47,* 1003–1007.

Raine, A., Venables, P. H., & Williams, M. (1995). High autonomic arousal and electrodermal orienting at age 15 years as protective factors against criminal behavior at age 29 years. *American Journal of Psychiatry, 152,* 1595–1600.

Schuckit, M. A., Mazzanti, C., Smith, T. L., Ahmed, U., Radel, M., Iwata, N., & Goldman, D. (1999). Selective genotyping for the role of 5-HT_{2A}, 5-HT_{2C} and $GABA_{\alpha 6}$ receptors and the serotonin transporter in the level of response to alcohol: A pilot study. *Biological Psychiatry, 45,* 647–651.

Schulsinger, F. (1972). Psychopathy: Heredity and enviroment. *International Journal of Mental Health, 1,* 190–206.

Siever, L. J., Buchsbaum, M. S., New, A. S., Spiegel-Cohen, J., Tsechung, W., Hazlett, E. A., et al. (1999). d,1–fenfluramine response in impulsive personality disorder assessed with (18F)fluorodeoxyglucose positron emission tomography. *Neuropsychopharmacology, 20,* 413–423.

Soloff, P. H., Meltzer, H. Y., Greer, P. J., Constantine, D., & Kelly, T. M. (2000). A fenfluramine-activated FDG–PET study of borderline personality disorder. *Biological Psychiatry, 47,* 540–547.

Steiner, H., Cauffman, E., & Duxbury, E. (1999). Personality traits in juvenile delinquents: Relation to criminal behavior and recidivism. *Journal of the American Academy of Child and Adolescent Psychiatry, 38,* 256–262.

Stevens, J. R., & Hermann, B. P. (1981). Temporal lobe epilepsy, psychopathology, and violence: The state of the evidence. *Neurology, 31,* 1127–1132.

Stoff, D. M., Pasatiempo, A. P., Yeung, J., Cooper, T. B., Bridger, W. H., & Rabinovich, H. (1992). Neuroendocrine responses to challenge with d1-fenfluramine and aggression in disruptive behavior disorders of children and adolescents. *Psychiatry Research, 43,* 263–276.

Swanson, J., & Volkow, N. (2001). Pharmacokinetic and pharmacodynamic properties of methylphenidate in humans. In M. V. Solanto, A. F. T. Arnsten, & F. X. Castellanos (Eds.), *Stimulant drugs and ADHD basic and clinical neuroscience* (pp. 259–282). New York: Oxford University Press.

Tsuang, M. T., Lyons, M. J., & Eisen, S. A. (1996). Genetic influences on DSM-III-R drug abuse and dependence: A study of 3.372 twin pairs. *American Journal of Medical Genetics, 67,* 473–477.

Virkkunen, M., Goldman, D., & Linnoila, M. (1996). Serotonin in alcoholic violent offenders. In G. R. Bock & J. A. Goode (Eds.), *Genetics of criminal and antisocial behaviour* (pp. 168–182). Chichester, UK: Wiley.

Virkkunen, M., & Linnoila, M. (1992). Psychobiology of violent behavior. *Clinical Neuropharmacology, 15*(Suppl. 1, Pt. A), 233A–234A.

Virkkunen, M., & Linnoila, M. (1993). Brain serotonin, type II alcoholism and impulsive violence. *Journal of Studies on Alcohol Supplement, 11,* 163–169.

Virkkunen, M., Nuutila, A., Goodwin, F. K., & Linnoila, M. (1987). Cerebrospinal fluid monoamine metabolite levels in male arsonists. *Archives of General Psychiatry, 44,* 241–247.

Virkkunen, M., Rawlings, R., Tokola, R., Poland, R. E., Guidotti, A., Nemeroff, C., Bissette, G., Kalogeras, K., Karonen, S. L., & Linnoila, M. (1994). CSF biochemistries, glucose metabolism, and diurnal activity rhythms in alcoholic, violent offenders, fire setters, and healthy volunteers. *Archives of General Psychiatry, 51,* 20–27.

Vitiello, B., & Stoff, D. M. (1997). Subtypes of aggression and their relevance to child psychiatry. *Journal of the American Academy of Child and Adolescent Psychiatry, 36,* 307–315.

Wise, R. A. (1987). The role of reward pathways in the development of drug dependence. *Pharmacotherapy, 35,* 227–263.

Wise, R. A. (1988). The neurobiology of craving: Implications for the understanding and treatment of addiction. *Journal of Abnormal Psychology, 97,* 118–132.

11

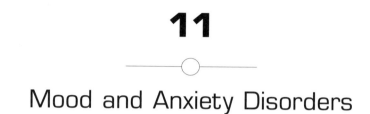

Mood and Anxiety Disorders

Mood and anxiety disorders are perhaps the most common disorders that present to mental health professionals. I focus on mood disorders first, as many of the proposed neurobiological systems involved in mood disorders are also implicated as factors in anxiety disorders. Consistent with this fact, antidepressant medications are increasingly being shown to be effective for the treatment of anxiety disorders such as panic disorder, posttraumatic stress disorder (PTSD) and obsessive–compulsive disorder (OCD).

MOOD DISORDERS

The lifetime prevalence of the mood disorders is striking: 10–25% of women and 5–12% of men will suffer an episode of major depressive disorder (MDD) at some point in their lives, and the lifetime prevalence of bipolar disorder is 1–2%. Mood disorders carry significant morbidity in terms of risk for substance abuse, suicide, psychiatric hospitalization, and lost productivity. The heterogeneity of the mood disorders complicates the study of their neurobiological factors. Over the years, Hagop Akiskal has written extensively on the classification of mood disorders. Figure 11.1 illustrates the spectrum of these conditions. Individual A normally experiences occasional brief episodes of sadness in response to stressors. Individual B has a "depressive temperament"—he or she is a person whose general outlook on life is pessimistic, brooding, introverted, and prone to guilt. Panel C shows a person who has clear-cut episodes of MDD but completely recovers between episodes, whereas individual D has dysthymic disorder, exhibiting a chronic pattern of de-

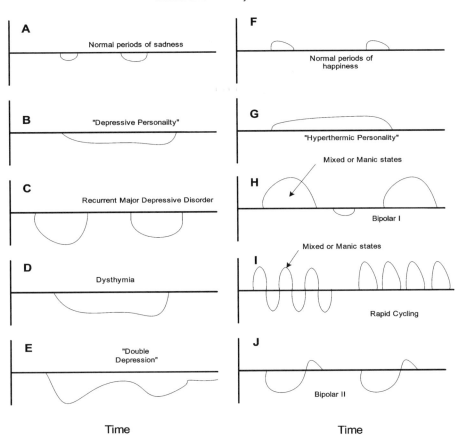

FIGURE 11.1. Patterns of mood disorder

pressed mood. Panel E illustrates "double depression": a person who first develops an episode of MDD but never completely recovers and continues to meet criteria for dysthymia until the next episode of MDD occurs.

The right side of the figure represents the bipolar spectrum. Panel F describes an individual who experiences appropriate periods of happiness when positive events occur in his or her life. Panel G illustrates a "hyperthermic" individual. This person is ordinarily very energetic, optimistic, and extroverted but does not meet full criteria for a mood disorder. Panel H is an example of bipolar I disorder; this individual has manic episodes that may or may not be interspersed with depressive episodes. Panel I shows a patient with rapid-cycling bipolar disorder who has at least four episodes of depression–mania in a year. Panel J shows a patient with bipolar II who has episodes of MDD but also has periods of hypomania. Mania and hypomania are distinguished by the degree of impairment the symptoms cause: The manic patient has become psychotic and required hospitalization, or the mania has caused marked impairment in social or occupational functioning (losing a job or a spouse, etc.). In hypomania the patient is never psychotic and does not require hospitalization, but impairment in social functioning is clearly observed by others. Hypomanic episodes in bipolar II generally last a shorter time than manic episodes in bipolar I. Mania itself can appear in a variety of mood states: elevated, expansive, and irritable. In the former two, the patient appears euphoric and cheerful (though abnormally so), whereas irritable patients can become severely angry and even paranoid. Complicating matters further is the concept of a "mixed" episode, informally referred to as "mixed mania" or "dysphoric mania." Technically, DSM-IV requires that patients with a mixed episode concurrently meet criteria for a manic episode and an MDD episode. In practice, "mixed mania" is more often used to categorize patients who are in an agitated state and show thought-process changes consistent with mania (flight of ideas, grandiosity) but who report depressed mood and suicidal ideation, along with their manic symptoms.

It should be clear that even experienced clinicians might struggle with diagnostic issues in patients with severe mood disorders. How does one distinguish a patient with rapid-cycling bipolar II (whose manic episodes are all mixed) from a patient with borderline personality disorder? A glance at the DSM-IV shows a considerable amount of overlap between the criteria for borderline personality disorder and those for mania and hypomania. Akiskal suggests, in fact, that borderline personality disorder is part of the bipolar spectrum. There is also debate regarding the age of onset of bipolar disorder. Once, both MDD and manic episodes were thought to be nonexistent in children; however, this is clearly not the case. Controversy does remain as to how common mania is in childhood. Furthermore the earlier the age of onset of a depressive episode, the greater the probability that the individual will develop a bipolar disorder, particularly a rapid cycling one. The fact that the field does not completely agree on the boundaries of the bipolar spectrum does present difficulties for neurobiological research, but progress has been steady.

Genetics of Mood Disorders

Family studies of mood disorders clearly implicate genetic factors. The relatives of persons with bipolar disorder have a risk of developing bipolar disorder that runs from 3–8%, whereas the relatives of patients with

MDD have an 8–17% chance of developing depression themselves. Twin studies of mood disorders show that monozygotic (MZ) twins are concordant for bipolar disorder about 58–70% of the time compared with a 16–24% concordance rate in dizygotic (DZ) twins. Heritability has been calculated to be about 0.8–0.9 for bipolar disorder and 0.45 for unipolar depression, suggesting a stronger genetic effect for the former.

Given the stronger genetic effect in bipolar disorder, it has been the focus of studies trying to link the disorder to a specific chromosome. In 1987 Egeland and colleagues found that a region in chromosome 11 was linked to bipolar disorder in the Old Amish, but this finding did not hold up. Currently, several locations on multiple chromosomes are of interest. Locations at chromosomes 4, 12, 13, 18 (two regions), 21, 22, and the X chromosome show at least some evidence for linkage to bipolar disorder, with the 18 and 22 regions showing the most robust evidence. At once, the polygenetic nature of mood disorders is evident. Some families with bipolar disorder show transmission through the maternal line, whereas in other families it appears to be maternally transmitted. Paternal transmission is found more often in families in which the 18-chromosome linkage is stronger, whereas maternal transmission could be the result of mutations in mitochondrial DNA or imprinting. Mitochondrial DNA is transmitted only via the ova (mitochondria being in the cytoplasm) and thus can come only from the maternal side. In imprinting, a gene is differentially expressed depending on which parent it is inherited from. For instance, a disease gene that has been inherited from one parent may not cause the disease because it has been inactivated by some process that is present only in that parent's genome. If the disease gene is inherited from the other parent, it is not inactivated, and thus it causes the condition.

The associations of the aforementioned chromosome regions to bipolar disorder require replication. Research also needs to focus on which genes are present at these sites and how they might be involved in mood disorders. Several genes of interest are found in the area of chromosome 18 linked to bipolar disorder. The gene for G_{olf} is located in that region; it codes for the alpha subunit of a G protein that was originally found in the olfactory area but is now known to be found throughout the brain. G_{olf} may interact with the D_1 receptor. This same area contains the gene for the enzyme inositol monophosphatase (IMP). Recall how phospholipase C, when activated by a G protein, cleaved phosphatidylinositol biphosphate (PIP_2) into IP_3 and DAG. IP_3 is then broken down (terminating its function) by a series of enzymes, one of which is IMP. Lithium inhibits IMP, and bipolar patients on lithium show decreased levels of inositol in their brains, as measured by magnetic resonance spectroscopy. Perhaps in some bipolar patients, the IMP gene is producing an unduly active form of the enzyme, which leads to an excessive amplification of the signal from neurotransmitters that use the PIP_2 second-messenger system.

The locus implicated in bipolar disorder at chromosome 22 is near to another locus that is involved in the disorder velocardiofacial syndrome (VCFS). VCFS has been associated with deletions of small parts of chromosome 22; people with this disorder suffer from facial deformities, mild mental retardation, and cardiac problems. About 30% suffer from psychosis, and there is debate as to whether patients with VCFS show a manic or a schizophreniform psychosis. Interestingly, both the 18 and 22 chromosome regions have been linked to schizophrenia, as well as bipolar disorder, suggesting that these disorders share some genetic factors. This may explain patients with schizoaffective disorder, who have symptoms of both illnesses (see Figure 11.2).

Also intriguing, the chromosome 22 region is close to the gene for the enzyme catechol-O-methyltransferase (COMT). (I discussed this enzyme in Chapter 9 in regard to ADHD.) Some studies suggested that the low-enzyme-activity allele for this enzyme that deactivates NE is associated with rapid-cycling bipolar disorder in adults. When bipolar disorder does occur in children, it tends to take a severe, rapid-cycling or "ultradian" pattern, in which several cycles may occur in a day. Recently, however, Barbara Geller and Edwin Cook did *not* find preferential transmission of the low-activity COMT allele to children with severe, ultradian bipolar disorder. We do not know for sure if the low-activity allele is in fact associated with rapid cycling, and not all researchers accept the validity of ultradian cycling in children with mood disorders. Thus further study of this issue is needed. COMT may play a role in schizophrenia, however, as will be shown in Chapter 12.

In Japanese patients bipolar disorder, with a polymorphism in mitochondrial DNA has been linked to the disorder, and patients with the

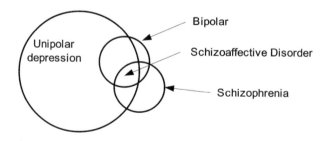

FIGURE 11.2. Overlap of bipolar disorder, unipolar depression, and schizophrenia

variant show differences in brain metabolism from those patients with the "wild type" allele. McMahon and colleagues did not find such an association with affective-disorder mitochondrial DNA polymorphisms in a European sample. Thus the Japanese work might not be confirmed in the long run. On the other hand, it is possible that genetic mechanisms of bipolar disorder are different (i.e., affective disorders evolved differently) in separate ethnic groups.

As I noted in Chapter 10, the gene for monoamine oxidase A (MAO-A) is located on the X chromosome, but studies linking polymorphisms at the MAO site to bipolar disorder have been mixed. For the other chromosome regions linked to bipolar disorder, no putative gene has yet been identified. There have been a number of negative studies looking at candidate genes that most investigators would have strongly suspected to be involved in the bipolar disorder. There do not appear to be any alterations in any of the five dopamine receptors in patients with bipolar disorder. Polymorphisms for corticotropin-releasing hormone (CRH), which is involved in the stress response, or for the CLOCK gene, which governs circadian rhythms, were not found to be different in patients with bipolar disorder. Genetics studies were negative for tyrosine hydroxylase, the enzyme involved in the synthesis of serotonin. Indeed, because so many antidepressants exert their effects through the serotonin system, one would expect genes for this system to be prime candidates to be altered in affective disorder, but studies have been mostly negative. In 1997 K. P. Lesch and colleagues found the short "s" allele of the serotonin transporter (introduced in Chapter 10) to have a modest relationship to anxiety traits in normal individuals, but it has not been found to be related to affective disorders per se. J. John Mann and colleagues examined the brains of 220 individuals; the sample consisted of persons with depression who had died of causes other than suicide, nondepressed controls, and 82 persons who had committed suicide. They genotyped the subjects for the s and l alleles of the serotonin transporter and also looked at the degree of serotonin transporter binding in the cortex of their brains. Individuals who had had major depression showed reductions in serotonin transporter binding throughout the brain; individuals who had committed suicide showed further reductions in serotonin transporter binding in the ventral prefrontal cortex. The s and l allele frequencies were not distributed differently in the individuals with or without major depression, and, curiously, the individual's genotype was not related to serotonin transporter binding in the brain. For the most part, other studies have not shown a relationship of the l or s alleles of the serotonin transporter to bipolar disorder. Bellivier and colleagues did show a modest relationship between possessing an s allele and a history of violent suicide attempts in depressed persons. This finding is consistent with the alterations in the serotonin system discussed in Chapter 10 in regard to impulsive personality disorders.

Patients with bipolar disorder often have other, comorbid psychiatric disorders, and this complicates genetic studies. For instance, patients with bipolar disorder have a higher than average risk of developing panic disorder. The research group of Alessandro Rotondo divided their sample of patients with bipolar disorder according to the presence or absence of panic disorder and examined mutations in the COMT and serotonin transporter genes. Only the patients *without* panic disorder showed a higher frequency of the s form of the transporter and the low-activity methionine-substituted COMT. This finding suggests the need to control for the comorbidity of various other disorders in these genetic studies, which is not always an easy task.

Studies of genes for the various serotonin receptors (5-HT_{2A}, 5-HT_{1A}, 5-HT_{2C}) have also been negative, though a recent study suggested that a polymorphism for the 5-HT_6 receptor might be associated with bipolar disorder. A gene for the ACTH receptor that lies on chromosome 18 and is thus of great interest also turned out not to be associated with affective disorder. None of the genes for the norepinephrine (NE) receptors have been implicated in affective disorders, nor have the genes for the NE transporter or dopamine β hydroxylase (the enzyme that converts dopamine into NE). To many clinicians, this may come as a surprise. We have known for years that most antidepressants block the reuptake of serotonin or NE in neurons; this fact has led to the hypothesis that derangements in these systems underlie the pathophysiology of mood disorders. Perhaps disturbances in these systems in affective disorder (which I review shortly) are downstream of the actual cause of the condition. First, a review of psychosocial factors in affective disorders is in order.

Life Events and Neurohormonal Response

It is clear that adverse life events contribute to the development of mood and anxiety disorders. Persons who were sexually or physically abused during childhood are up to four times more likely to develop major depression or commit suicide; child abuse is associated with an earlier age of onset of depression and greater chronicity of the depression. Other factors known to be related to affective disorders are early parental loss and nonspecific life stressors. As expected from heritability figures, these environmental stressors play a larger role in unipolar depression than in bipolar disorder. O. Agid and colleagues recently reviewed these data. Surprisingly, parental death is not as strongly associated with depression as parental separation is. Why should this be so? Parental separation (through divorce or abandonment) is more likely than parental death to be associated with impairment in the parent–child relationship. Consistent with this fact, depression within a group of adolescents who experienced separation from a parent was correlated with a lack of family support and weaker bonding with parents. A number of studies have shown that cold and distant parent–child relationships predispose not only to depression but also to heart disease and Type II diabetes.

People with depression clearly experience more general life stressors, but the role of these stressors in the etiology of depression is less clear. Many life stressors occur because of the depression (i.e., the individual suffers from low energy as a symptom of depression, performs poorly on the job as a result, is fired, and becomes more depressed as a result of the job loss). Twin studies have shown that the tendency to experience negative life events is itself influenced by genetics, separate from the genetic risk for the affective disorder itself.

We are now beginning to understand how such early stresses affect the neurobiology of the individual, leading to "scarring," that is, an abnormal neurohormonal response to future stressors. In Chapter 4, I discussed the work of the McGill University group on the role of maternal rat behavior on the development of the physiology of the offspring. Rats that are not handled or are not licked by the mother rat show increased corticotropin releasing factor (CRF) and enhanced LC activity (i.e., increased NE). They also express a form of the $GABA_A$ receptor that is less responsive to GABA and fails to inhibit LC activity. These "neglected" rats were more fearful and went on to repeat the "nonlicking" maternal style with their own pups. Interestingly, when the pups of "nonlicking" mother rats were adopted away to "licking" mother rats, the physiological changes in the pups were reversed, and they grew up to be less fearful. Similar findings have emerged in nonhuman primates. Mother monkeys and their infants can be placed in "variable foraging" demand situations. (See Heim and Nemeroff for a review of these data.) The amount of food that is available from day to day is unpredictable, and the mother must spend variable amounts of time foraging for food. On days when food is scarce, the mother has little time to interact with her infant, leading to a highly inconsistent rearing atmosphere for the infant. As a result, the infant monkeys show symptoms of depression and anxiety and have elevated levels of CRF in their cerebrospinal fluid. Of further interest, if CRF is injected directly into the cerebrospinal fluid of animals, they show clear signs of anxiety and fearfulness.

Recently, Christine Heim, Charles Nemeroff, and their colleagues performed an important study examining the effects of past abuse on a person's current neurohormonal functioning. They recruited 49 women as participants: 12 controls, 14 women with histories of abuse but no current depression, 13 women with histories of both depression and past abuse, and 10 depressed women with no histories of abuse. The investigators measured plasma ACTH and cortisol while the participants performed a stressful public speaking task. Women with histories of abuse, regardless of whether or not they were currently depressed, had much higher peaks of plasma ACTH during the stressor relative to the nonabused women. For cortisol, the abused depressed women had much higher levels than the other three groups. They suggested that the CRF system might be abnormally primed by the early abuse, leading to excessive cortisol secretion and activation of the NE system. Martin Teicher and his colleagues at McLean Hospital in Massachusetts have recently studied a large number of children admitted to the hospital, many of whom had histories of abuse. Four brain abnormalities were found in children with histories of abuse: (1) EEG abnormalities in the left hemispheres, (2) neuropsychological and neuroimaging evidence of deficit left-hemisphere functioning, (3) smaller corpus callosa, suggesting less communication between the hemispheres, and (4) increased cerebellar vermis activity. The left-hemisphere findings are most interesting in view of the data I reviewed in Chapter 7 regarding the left hemisphere being more involved in positive affect. As a result of left-hemisphere dysfunction, the right hemisphere may be more active, producing excessive negative affect.

Neurohormonal Status in Affective Disorder

The fact that many antidepressants block the reuptake of NE and serotonin led to extensive investigations of these systems in the 1970s and 1980s. These studies pursued the simple hypothesis that if antidepressants increased the amount of NE or serotonin in the synaptic cleft, then perhaps depressed patients suffered from deficiencies in one or both of these neurotransmitters. Similarly, because bipolar patients sometimes were "switched" into a manic state by antidepressants, it could be that manic patients suffered from the reverse: an excess of catecholamines that the antidepressant made worse.

The findings did not turn out to be that simple. James Maas and his colleagues in the National Institute of Mental Health (NIMH) Collaborative Program on the Psychobiology of Depression examined the amounts of NE and its many metabolites in the urine of depressed and manic patients, as well as in controls. These studies show that patients with affective disorders showed an increase in NE activity, consistent with *increased* sympathetic output in both depressives and manics. Subsequently, CRF, which increases activity of both the LC and the sympathetic nervous system (SNS), has been found to be elevated in patients with affective disorder. Depressed patients often have increased cortisol levels, and these levels are often not suppressed when patients are given dexamethasone, a drug that normally signals the pituitary to stop producing ACTH. If clonidine, which stimulates the α_2 postsynaptic NE receptor, is infused into the plasma, it normally causes a burst of growth hormone in normal persons; this response is blunted in people with major depression. This is consistent with the idea that high levels of circulating NE lead to down-regulation of the postsynaptic α_2 receptors.

It remains unclear whether the changes in the serotonin system found in affective disorders are related to depression or mania per se or to the risk of violent suicide or impulsive personality. As noted earlier, there appear to be fewer serotonin transporters in the cortex of persons with major depression, and several studies show the number of the 5-HT_{1A} and 5-HT_{2A} receptors to be decreased. Selective serotonin reuptake inhibitors (SSRIs) are clearly effective for depression, but it is not at all clear that there is a primary sertonergic dysfunction in affective disorders. Recently, tianeptine, a substance that enhances the uptake of serotonin (the opposite effects of the SSRIs), has been shown to have antidepressant properties. Clearly, our theories about how NE and serotonin are involved in affective disorder need some revision. Fortunately, some new ideas about how antidepressants exert their effects have emerged.

Antidepressant Response and Neuroprotective Factors

First, we must examine how antidepressants might affect neuron function over the long term. Figure 11.3 shows two neurons communicating with each other. In the upper panel, the neurons are synchronized, and when the presynaptic neuron fires, neurotransmitters are released and bind to postsynaptic receptors, triggering those neurons. Information flow is orderly. In the second panel, the neurons have become dysregulated. Note that the presynaptic neuron discharges excessively and that there is excessive noise after it has been stimulated. Excessive neurotransmitter is released, which causes postsynaptic receptors to become down-regulated. Note that the postsynaptic neuron does not receive information efficiently. In the third panel, a reuptake inhibitor has been administered acutely. Note that the synaptic level of the neurotransmitter increases dramatically, leading to the stimulation of both terminal and somatodendritic autoreceptors. This produces an acute attenuation in the presynaptic neuron firing rate. This is not the key therapeutic event, however. Antidepressants have a range of effects, which ultimately lead to the autoreceptors being down-regulated and the postsynaptic receptors (particularly in the case of the serotonin 5-HT_{1A} receptor) being up-regulated. As a result, "less is more"; the synchrony of the neuron

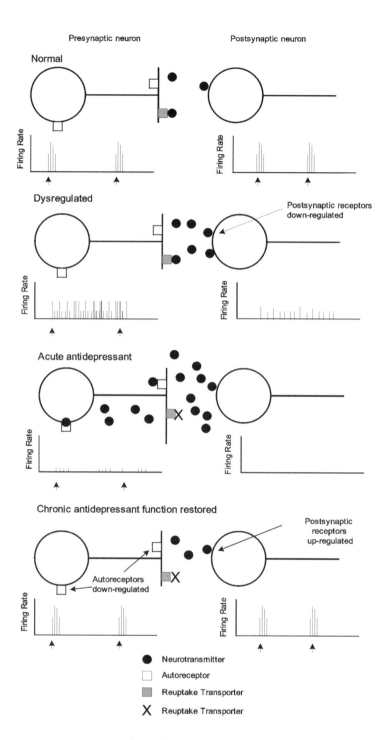

FIGURE 11.3. Hypothesized mechanisms of antidepressant action

pair is restored. Although less neurotransmitter is being released than in the dysregulated state, more neurotransmission occurs. Overall NE output drops after administration of antidepressants, as does level of 5-HIAA in cerebrospinal fluid (the main metabolite of serotonin). These changes occur in *both* systems, regardless of whether the patient is treated with an SSRI or an antidepressant that affects primarily NE.

Recent research has suggested that long-term, so-called neuroprotective effects may be critical in the actions of both antidepressants and mood stabilizers such as lithium and valproate. Table 11.1 shows the acute effects of common antidepressants on neurotransmitter reuptake and on various neurotransmitter receptors. Despite different mechanisms of action, the various antidepressants are of equal efficacy on average, though some patients will respond better to one than to another. Figure 11.4 shows these acute antidepressant effects, as well as longer term neuroprotective effects. The figure shows an NE neuron in the upper panel and a serotonergic neuron in the lower panel. The

TABLE 11.1. Acute Mechanisms of Action of Commonly
Used Antidepressants

Antidepressant class	5-HT reuptake inhibition relative to NE[a]	Other action
Tricyclic antidepressants		
amitriptyline (Elavil)	0.25	Block 5-HT$_{2A}$ receptors, block
imipramine (Tofranil)	0.5	α_1 receptors, antihistamine and
desipramine (Norpramin)	0.006	anticholingeric
SSRIs		
fluoxetine (Prozac)	13.3	
sertraline (Zoloft)	75	
paroxetine (Paxil)	70	
Bupropion (Wellbutrin)	0.16	Blocks reuptake of dopamine
Venlafaxine (Effexor)	6.0	5-HT effect predominates at low dose, NE effect at high dose
Nefazodone (Serzone)	4.0	Blocks 5-HT$_{2A}$ receptors
Trazodone (Desyrel)	26.6	Blocks 5-HT$_{2A}$ receptors and α_1 receptors
Mirtazapine (Remeron)	0.4	Blocks 5-HT$_{2A}$, α_2, and 5-HT$_3$ receptors; potentiates α_1 receptors

[a]That is, amitriptyline is only one-fourth as potent at blocking the reuptake of 5-HT than NE; paroxetine is 70 times more potent at blocking the reuptake of 5-HT than NE.

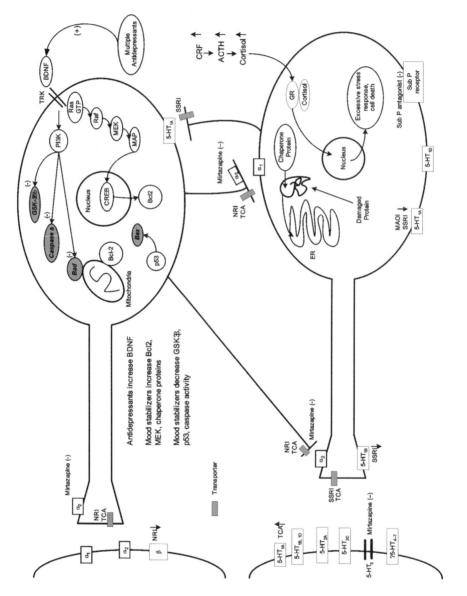

FIGURE 11.4. Neuroprotective and apoptotic factors in the genesis of mood disorders

serotonergic neuron has 5-HT_{1A} and 5-HT_{1D} receptors on its cell body and 5-HT_{1B} receptors on its axon terminal. As noted previously, SSRIs will down regulate these receptors. Tricyclic antidepressants (TCAs) block the reuptake of both norepinephrine and serotonin (though each TCA differs in its potency for effecting one or the other), and they all up-regulate the 5-HT_{1A} receptor. Antidepressants with NE reuptake block-ade properties (NRI) and some TCAs increase the amount of NE in the synaptic cleft. NE released onto α_1 receptors on the serotonin cell bodies will increase the serotonin neuron firing, whereas NE released onto α_2 receptors on the serotonin axon terminal will decrease serotonin release. The antidepressant mirtazapine blocks both α_2 autoreceptors on the NE neuron and the α_2 "heteroreceptors" on the serotonin axon terminal. Blocking the α_2 on the NE terminals (which normally inhibit NE release) causes an increase in NE neurotransmission. Extra stimulation of α_1 re-ceptors on the serotonin neuron increases serotonin cell firing. Blocking the α_2 receptors on the serotonin terminal (which normally inhibit sero-tonin release) further increases serotonin release. Thus, as with SSRIs, serotonin transmission is ultimately enhanced.

Antidepressants affect postsynaptic receptors differently. TCAs, mirtazapine, nefazodone, and trazodone all block 5HT_{2A} receptors, mirtazapine also blocks the 5-HT_3 receptors. It can be seen that NRIs will ultimately lead to postsynaptic NE β receptor down-regulation. Finally, a drug that inhibits the action of substance P and that has no ef-fect on serotonin or NE, has also recently been shown to have antide-pressant properties. For a deeper understanding of antidepressant mech-anisms, we must turn to the role of neuroprotective factors in the maintenance of brain health. As discussed, stress in a genetically vulner-able individual may lead to deleterious increases in CRF, ACTH, and cortisol. Cortisol binds to the glucocorticoid receptor (GR) and then en-ters the nucleus, where it influences the expression of genes. There, genes may produce proteins that are helpful acutely but that over the long term have negative effects on the neuron. In the upper neuron in Figure 11.4, various proteins are illustrated in the cytoplasm. Neuronal life and death are mediated by an exquisite balance of life-promoting (anti-apoptotic) and life-destructive (apoptotic) proteins ("apoptosis " means cell death). In the figure, apoptotic proteins are in grey. We again en-counter the tyrosine kinase system, which is stimulated by growth fac-tors, particularly by brain-derived neurotrophic factors (BDNF). Once BDNF activates the MAP kinase system (described in Chapters 3 and 4), the production of the protein Bcl-2 is increased. Bcl-2 has a variety of ef-fects, including prompting axon growth, turning off destructive en-zymes, and maintaining the integrity of mitochondrial membranes. The apoptotic proteins (Bad, caspase, GSK-3β, and Bax) encourage cell death. BDNF can activate the enzyme PI-3 kinase, which inhibits these apoptotic proteins. Overactivation of the antiapoptotic forces can lead to excessive cell growth (cancer), whereas excessive activation of apoptotic forces leads to neuronal degeneration.

In rats, severe stress decreases levels of BDNF in the hippocampus and leads to reductions in hippocampal volume. In patients with affective disorders and PTSD, a number of studies have shown enlargement of the cerebral ventricles and reduced gray matter. In particular, hippocampal volume has been found to be reduced in patients with a history of MDD, and the degree of reduction correlates with the lifetime duration of the depression. In a few cases, this reduction in the hippocampus may be visible to the untrained eye on the MRI scan. Recently, magnetic resonance spectroscopy (MRS) has been used in the study of affective disorder. In this technique, the signal is used to analyze aspects of the brain's chemical composition. The amount of N-acetyl-aspartate (NAA) is a good measure of neuronal integrity. Several studies have now shown decreased NAA in patients with bipolar disorder; other MRS studies have found evidence of abnormal energy regulation in the brain, mostly likely due to mitochondrial dysfunction.

Severe, unrelenting stress could lead to overactivation of apoptotic forces that destroy neurons, a process that leaves the patients vulnerable to another episode of affective disorder. It is well known that individuals with bipolar disorder, left untreated, will have more and more episodes of greater severity as they go through life. Others might have a genetic vulnerability to produce excessive apoptotic proteins or to fail to produce antiapototic substances in response to stress. These individuals might develop a affective disorders in response to the normal stressors of everyday life, even if they had not experienced abuse or neglect.

Growing evidence suggests that antidepressants enhance antiapoptotic forces. As shown in Figure 11.4, antidepressants, as well as electroconvulsive treatments, increase BDNF and enhance neurogenesis. Mood stabilizers such as lithium and valproic acid (Depakote) increase the production of Bcl2 and MEK (antiapototic) and inhibit proapoptotic proteins (Bad, caspase, and p53). Also of interest are the "chaperone proteins." As shown in the figure, chaperones lead a damaged protein to the endoplasmic reticulum (ER) to be broken down and thus act as the neuron's "garbageman." Chaperone proteins are activated during stress as yet another protective mechanism for the cell. Mood stabilizers increase the expression of the chaperone proteins. Thus we have a range of possible mechanisms for antidepressant and mood stabilizers, many of which may lead to a new generation of treatments for affective and anxiety disorders.

Neuroimaging in Mood Disorders

As noted, MRI and MRS studies have provided evidence of neuronal atrophy in affective disorders, particularly in those patients with multiple episodes of illness. Functional MRI and PET studies have focused primarily on patients with unipolar depression. This data has been succinctly reviewed by Helen Mayberg at the University of Toronto. Dr. Mayberg has produced a neuroimaging model of depression based on work with both patients and normal controls. Wayne Drevets of the University of Pittsburgh has also made important contributions in this area. Mayberg and her colleagues (Peter Fox, Mario Liotti, and Stephen Brannan, among others) had normal participants produce scripts of sad events in their lives. The participants then performed two PET studies. In the first, they listened to a neutral script; in the second, they listened to the sad script. By comparing the scans, the researchers could examine brain metabolism changes associated with transient sadness. The participants showed decreases in the dorsolateral prefrontal cortex, the dorsal and posterior cingulate gyrus, and inferior parietal lobe. In contrast, the normal participants showed increases in orbitomedial prefrontal cortex and hippocampus. Interestingly, a large number of PET studies have shown that, before treatment, depressed patients also show *decreased* dorsolateral prefrontal cortex metabolism and *increased* activity in the ventral limbic compartment (orbitomedial PFC, amygdala, hippocampus). Indeed, the decreased activity in the dorsolateral PFC may correlate with the cognitive impairments of depression, such as decreased concentration and poor memory. Mayberg and colleagues performed PET studies on patients with MDD before and after treatment with an SSRI. They then examined differences between responders and nonresponders: those who responded to drug treatment had higher rates of pretreatment activity in the anterior cingulate gyrus relative to controls, whereas the nonresponders had lower levels of activity in this area. I showed in Chapter 7 how the anterior cingulate plays a role in executive attention, recruiting "effort" for a task. Mayberg suggests that it also plays a role in modulating mood: When the anterior cingulate is intact, it helps to terminate sadness and depression by increasing activity in the dorsal compartment and decreasing activity in the ventral compartment. Increases in dorsal compartment activity correlate with improvements in cognition (more alertness, better concentration), whereas decreases in the ventral compartment activity correlate with improvement in vegetative symptoms of affective disorders (poor sleep, low energy, anxiety).

Using a ligand that binds to 5-HT_{1A} receptors, Wayne Drevets and colleagues have shown that the number of these receptors is decreased in depressed patients, particularly in those with past histories or family histories of mania. This is intriguing in view of the tendency of antidepressants to enhance serotonin neurotransmission. Very few functional imaging studies of manic patients have been done. In 1999, Hilary Blumberg and her colleagues at Cornell University compared 5 manic patients with 6 patients with bipolar disorder whose mania had resolved and 5 controls, using PET. The patients were on medication for bipolar disorder at the time of the scan. Compared with both the controls and euthymic patients, the manic patients showed decreased right dorsal lateral and orbitomedial PFC activity. Again, we see that the right hemisphere dysfunction is associated with mania, as left hemisphere dysfunction may be associated with depression.

ANXIETY DISORDERS

Anxiety disorders, such as PTSD, OCD, and panic disorders, are frequently comorbid with depressive disorders. As a result, much of the genetic research has focused on whether there is a separate genetic risk for anxiety and depressive disorders or whether these disorders share a common genetic vulnerability. Anxiety disorders, like affective disorders, run in families. Twin studies of panic disorders have shown a higher rate in MZ twins than in DZ twins. Similar results emerged for phobias, but clearly the genetic effect is less pronounced in anxiety than in affective disorders. As noted earlier, the short "s" allele for the promotor region of the serotonin transporter has shown a very modest relationship to anxiety levels in normal participants in one study. Until recently, genetic studies have not identified any specific chromosome region involved in anxiety disorders. In 2001, Monica Gratacos and her colleagues identified a region of chromosome 15 that appears to be associated with several anxiety disorders, including panic disorder, agoraphobia, social phobia, and simple phobia. One the investigators in this group, Antoni Bulbena, discovered a curious fact: Severely double-jointed persons have a rate of anxiety disorders four times that of the general population. This research group identified families with both joint hypermobility and anxiety disorders. They identified a region on chromosome 15 that was duplicated in 87% of the double-jointed people and 90% of the anxiety-disordered participants. When the group repeated the study in an independent sample, 97% of the patients with anxiety showed the duplication (called DUP25), as compared with only 7% of the controls. These are striking figures, so why hadn't these correlations been detected before? It seems that DUP25 is an unusual genetic mutation. What appears to be inherited is not a defective gene itself but a tendency for the genes in that area to be replicated. More interesting, the tendency to duplicate is not uniform in all cells of the body; that is, in some cells, the mutation leads to a doubling or tripling of the genes on chromosome 15 and in other cells of the body the mutation is silent. This effect is called "mosaicism," and it leads to a non-Mendelian pattern of inheritance, thus making it difficult to detect with traditional family studies. Why would this region be important in anxiety disorders? I return to that shortly.

The genetics of OCD is somewhat different from those of the other anxiety disorders because of its relationship to tic disorders. Persons with tic disorders have an elevated number of relatives in their families with OCD; conversely, people with OCD have more relatives than expected with tic disorders. It should be borne in mind, however, that not all studies have shown this relationship. I return to OCD shortly.

Panic Disorders

Patients with panic disorder can be induced to have a panic attack in the laboratory by a number of methods: breathing carbon dioxide, infusing lactic acid intravenously (lactic acid normally rises when a patient exercises vigorously), or injecting yohimbine, a drug that blocks α_2 receptors and increases the level of NE in the body. Patients with panic disorder produce much higher levels of plasma NE than do controls when administered yohimbine. In 1989 Jack Gorman and colleagues proposed abnormal brain stem regulation of the NE and serotonin systems, whereas in 1993 Donald Klein suggested that a panic attack represented the triggering of a "false suffocation alarm." That is, we naturally panic if our carbon dioxide levels rise; this is an instinctual response to get to fresh air. If this brain stem activity were too easily triggered by stimuli, the patient would not only panic at random but would come to associate whatever situation he or she was in at the time with the panic symptoms. This association in turn, would lead to phobic avoidance, which in some patients results in full agoraphobia. As research progressed in the 1990s, it became clear that this hypothesis would need revision. This hypothesis predicts that all panic attacks result in abnormal brain stem activation, but that is clearly not the case. Panic attacks do not always result in increases in plasma NE, heart rate, or other indices of brain stem activity, nor is there much evidence of brain stem abnormalities in patients with panic disorder at baseline. Thus, as with major depressive disorder, these peripheral changes in the NE system may be an effect rather than a cause of the disorder. Nonetheless, the recent work of Gratacos and colleagues implicating DUP25 in chromosome 15 does suggest a strong role for the NE system. A gene for the neurotrophin 3 receptor (NTrk3, part of the

Trk receptor system) resides in this area. The NTrk3 receptor is found on LC neurons. The duplicating process could give a patient a double dose of the NTrk3 neurons, leading to excessive proliferation of LC neurons. Conversely, if the abnormal duplicating process stopped in the middle of the NTrk3 gene, it might be broken and several dysfunctional copies produced. Without effective NTrk3 receptors, the antiapoptotic effects of the growth factors might not be realized.

Neuroimaging studies have addressed changes within the cortex. Reiman and colleagues published the first study utilizing PET in patients with panic disorder. They found increased cerebral blood flow in the hippocampus, and the increase was much greater on the right side. These studies were done with patients at baseline, that is, when they were not having panic attacks. Obviously, doing a neuroimaging scan in a patient who is having a full-blown attack is not easy. During a panic attack, patients begin to hyperventilate. The cerebral blood flow normally decreases during hyperventilation, but patients with panic disorder experience even greater decreases in blood flow. Gorman and his colleagues suggest that this may be due to overactivation of the NE system during the attack; NE restricts the volume of cerebral arterioles. They also point out that the parabrachial nucleus, a brain stem area that induces vasoconstriction, receives direct input from the amygdala and may be overactivated by the fear response generated by the amygdala. Interestingly, Gorman and colleagues showed that a patient with panic disorder who was successfully treated with antidepressants did not show as great a decrease in cerebral blood flow during hyperventilation as did acutely ill patients. In 2000, Gorman and colleagues revised their original hypotheses to emphasize the fear circuit that was discussed in Chapter 5 (Figure 5.2). They now suggest that panic disorder could represent a disturbance in the amygdala itself or in any of the other parts of this circuit, with the common pathway being an abnormal activation of the amygdala. Such a biological vulnerability would not be sufficient; early life stressors would also be required to trigger this excessive sensitivity. Finally, SSRIs might enhance serotonin neurotransmission in the amygdala (as described in Figure 11.3), dampening the abnormal amygdaloid activity.

Posttraumatic Stress Disorder

Structural MRI studies in patients with PTSD have shown hippocampal volume reductions similar to those found in affective disorder. PET studies have shown that left hippocampal blood flow is reduced (relative to the right hippocampus) in patients with panic disorder compared with controls. Patients with PTSD showed increased blood flow in the right amygdala and decreased flow in the left inferior frontal and middle temporal cortex. Again we see that decreased left-brain activity correlates with increased negative affect. Unlike depressed patients who showed an increase in metabolism of the ventral compartment, patients with PTSD (combat veterans) had decreased orbitofrontal metabolisms. These studies compared combat veterans with and without PTSD. Reviewing these studies, Dennis Charney and Douglas Bremner suggested that the orbitofrontal areas may suppress amygdala activity; dysfunction of the orbitomedial PFC might "disinhibit" the amygdala. Excessive amygdala activity could lead to an increase fear response when reminders of the trauma are present.

Patients with PTSD may also suffer from an overactive noradrenergic system. Antidepressants of all kinds also treat PTSD and panic disorders, but OCD responds only to SSRIs. We see that OCD is qualitatively different from the other anxiety disorders in a number of ways.

Obsessive–Compulsive Disorder

Both OCD and tic disorders run in families. Also, both of these disorders have a "motor" component. Persons with tics exhibit involuntary motor movements, whereas OCD patients engage in compulsions: doing the same movement (checking, hand washing) over and over. Obsessions, which are thoughts, also have a driven quality; the patient is "caught in a loop," ruminating on the same thing repeatedly. The term "caught in a loop" may also describe OCD at a neurological level. Review briefly the cortico-striatal-pallidal-thalamic loop involved in motor behavior discussed in Chapter 5. Recall how the striatal areas, when active in the direct pathway, inhibited the globus pallidus through GABA neurons. If the pallidal neurons are inhibited, they do not release GABA into the thalamus; thus the cortico-thalamic loop is indefinitely maintained. Lewis Baxter at the University of California at Los Angeles has reviewed the neuroimaging data in OCD. Like depressed patients, patients with OCD show increased activity in the orbitomedial PFC, but unlike depressed patients, they show higher activity in the head of the caudate nucleus. Baxter suggests that the orbitomedial PFC excessively "drives" the caudate, causing excessive GABA outflow to the pallidal areas. The cortico-thalamic loop is then difficult to interrupt, and the patient experiences an irresistible obsession or compulsion.

SSRIs are the only class of antidepressants that are helpful in OCD. This fact leads to the assumption that the serotonin system must be fundamentally disturbed in OCD. Probe studies have been performed in which drugs that increase serotonin activity have been given to patients with OCD and to controls. Although there are many inconsistencies, most of these studies show that these agents, administered acutely, *increase* OCD symptoms. In any case, SSRIs do not work acutely in OCD but, as in depression, take 4 to 8 weeks to reach their full effect. We saw that depressed patients taking SSRIs relapsed when they were given a serotonin-depleting drink. Patients with OCD treated with SSRIs *do not* relapse when given this drink. Genetic findings regarding serotonin system and OCD have been disappointing, as well. Neither the long nor the short allele of the serotonin transporter has been associated with OCD; recently, a polymorphism associated with the promotor region of the 5-HT_{2A} receptors was found to be associated with OCD, but only in women. Why, then, are SSRIs the only type of antidepressant found to be effective in OCD? Recall that the serotonin system, though not the NE system, has projections to the caudate nucleus. There may be no baseline deficit in the serotonin system in OCD, but by "tweaking" it with an SSRI we can "break" the abnormal striatal-pallidal-thalamic-cortical loop by improving serotonin transmission in the caudate.

Autoimmune phenomena may be involved in the pathophysiology of both tics and OCD. OCD has been observed among patients recovering from encephalitis. The immune systems of some people infected with the β-hemolytic streptococcal bacteria (such as "strep throat") sometimes turns against them. The body may produce antibodies that attack not only the bacteria but also the heart valves, leading to rheumatic fever. Rarely, the antibodies will attack the basal ganglia, producing Sydenham's chorea, a writhing-movement disorder. Interestingly, these individuals may develop OCD. Sue Swedo and her colleagues have described a number of cases in which children with strep infections acutely develop OCD. These cases have been referred to as "pediatric autoimmune neuropsychiatric disorders associated with strep" (PANDAS). Perhaps the genetic vulnerability to OCD in some individuals is not to the disorder itself but to a tendency to have an exaggerated autoimmune response to strep or other infectious agents. Strengthening this notion is the finding that patients with tic disorders (who often have a family history of OCD) have been found to have elevated concentrations of an antigen (D8/17) in white blood cells, which is linked to a risk for rheumatic fever.

REFERENCES

Agid, O., Kohn, Y., & Lerer, B. (2000). Environmental stress and psychiatric illness. *Biomedicine and Pharmacotherapy, 54,* 135–141.
Akiskal, H. S. (2000). Mood disorders: introduction and overview. In B. J.

Sadock & V. A. Sadock (Eds.), *Comprehensive textbook of psychiatry* (7th ed., pp. 1284–1297). Philadelphia: Lippincott Williams & Wilkins.

Akiskal, H. S., Bourgeosis, M. L., Angst, J., Post, R., Hans-Jurgen, M., & Hirschfield, R. (2000). Re-evaluating the prevalence of and diagnostic comparison within the broad clinical spectrum. *Journal of Affective Disorders*, 59, S5–S30.

Alda, M., Turecki, G., Grof, P., Cavazzoni, P., Duffy, A., Grof, E., et al. (2000). Association and linkage studies of CRH and PENK genes in bipolar disorder: A collaborative IGSLI study. *American Journal of Medical Genetics*, 96, 178–181.

Baxter, L. R. (1999). Functional imaging of brain systems mediating obsessive-compulsive disorder. In D. S. Charney, E. J. Nestler, & B. S. Bunney (Eds.), *Neurobiology of mental illness* (pp. 534–547). New York: Oxford University Press.

Bellivier, F., Szoke, A., Henry, C., Lacoste, J., Bottos, C., Nosten-Bertrand, M., et al. (2000). Possible association between serotonin transporter gene polymorphism and violent suicidal behavior in mood disorders. *Biological Psychiatry*, 48, 319–322.

Berrettini, W. H. (2000a). Genetics of psychiatric disease. *Annual Review of Medicine*, 51, 465–479.

Berrettini, W. H. (2000b). Susceptibility loci for bipolar disorder: Overlap with inherited vulnerability to schizophrenia. *Biological Psychiatry*, 47, 245–251.

Blier, P., & de Montigny, C. (1999). Serotonin and drug-induced therapeutic responses in major depression, obsessive-compulsive and panic disorders. *Neuropsychopharmacology*, 21, 91S–98S.

Blumberg, H. P., Stern, E., Ricketts, S., Martinez, D., de Asis, J., White, T., et al. (2000). Rostral and orbital prefrontal cortex dysfunction in the manic state of bipolar disorder. *American Journal of Psychiatry*, 156, 1986–1988.

Bowden, C. L., Koslow, S., Maas, J. W., Davis, J., Garver, D. L., & Hanin, I. (1987). Changes in urinary catecholamines and their metabolites in depressed patients treated with amitriptyline or imipramine. *Journal of Psychiatric Research*, 21, 111–128.

Charney, D. S., & Bremner, J. D. (1999). The neurobiology of anxiety disorders. In D. S. Charney, E. J. Nestler, & B. S. Bunney (Eds.), *Neurobiology of mental illness* (pp. 494–517). New York: Oxford University Press.

Crowe, R. R. (1999). Molecular genetics of anxiety disorders. In D. S. Charney, E. J. Nestler, & B. S. Bunney (Eds.), *Neurobiology of mental illness* (pp. 451–462). New York: Oxford University Press.

Desan, P. H., Oren, D. A., Malison, R., Price, L. H., Rosenbaum, J., Smoller, J., et al. (2000). Genetic polymorphisms at the CLOCK gene locus and major depression. *American Journal of Medical Genetics*, 96, 418–421.

Drevets, W. C., Gadde, K. M., & Krishnan, K. R. R. (1999). Neuroimaging studies of mood disorders. In D. S. Charney, E. J. Nestler, & B. S. Bunney (Eds.), *Neurobiology of mental illness* (pp. 394–418). New York: Oxford University Press.

Egeland, J. A., Gerhard, D. S., Pauls, D. L., Sussex, J. N., Kidd, K. K., Allen, C. R., et al. (1987). Bipolar affective disorders linked to DNA markers on chromosome 11. *Nature, 325,* 783–787.

Frazer, A. (1997). Pharmacology of antidepressants. *Journal of Clinical Psychopharmacology, 17,* 2S–18S.

Geller, B., & Cook, E. H., Jr. (2000). Ultradian rapid cycling in prepubertal and early adolescent bipolarity is not in transmission disequilibrium with Val/ Met COMT alleles. *Biological Psychiatry, 47,* 605–609.

Gorman, J. M., Kent, J. M., Sullivan, G. M., & Coplan, J. D. (2000). Neuroanatomical hypothesis of panic disorder, revised. *American Journal of Psychiatry, 157,* 493–505.

Gorman, J. M., Liebowitz, M. R., Fyer, A. J., & Stein, J. (1989). A neuroanatomical hypothesis for panic disorder. *American Journal of Psychiatry, 146,* 148–161.

Gratacos, M., Nadal, M., Martin-Santos, R., Pujena, M. A., Gago, J., Peral, B., et al. (2001). A polymorphic genomic duplication on human chromosome 15 is a susceptibility factor for panic and phobic disorders. *Cell, 106,* 367–379.

Heim, C., & Nemeroff, C. B. (1999). The impact of early adverse experiences on brain systems involved in the pathophysiology of anxiety and affective disorders. *Biological Psychiatry, 46,* 1509–1522.

Heim, C., Newport, D. J., Heit, S., Graham, Y. P., Wilcox, M., Bonsall, R., et al. (2000). Pituitary–adrenal and autonomic responses to stress in women after sexual and physical abuse in childhood. *Journal of the American Medical Association, 284,* 592–597.

Kato, T., Kunugi, H., Nanko, S., & Kato, N. (2000). Association of bipolar disorder with the 5178 polymorphism in mitochondrial DNA. *American Journal of Medical Genetics, 96,* 182–186.

Kendler, K. S., Makowsy, L. W., & Prescott, C. A. (1999). Causal relationship between stressful life events and the onset of major depression. *Archives of General Psychiatry, 156,* 837–841.

Klein, D. F. (1993). False suffocation alarms, spontaneous panics, and related conditions. *Archives of General Psychiatry, 50,* 306–317.

Koslow, S. H., Maas, J. W., Bowden, C. L., Davis, J. M., Hanin, I., & Javaid, J. (1983). CSF and urinary biogenic amines and metabolites in depression and mania. *Archives of General Psychiatry, 40,* 999–1010.

Lesch, K. P., Bengel, D., Heils, A., Sabol, S. Z., Greenberg, B. D., et al. (1997). Association of anxiety-related traits with a polymorphism in the serotonin transporter gene regulatory region. *Science, 274,* 1527–1531.

Liang, K., Johnson, E. I., Berrettini, W. H., & Overhauser, J. (2000). Identification of candidate genes for psychiatric disorders on 18p11. *Molecular Psychiatry, 5,* 389–395.

Maas, J. W., Koslow, S. H., Davis, J., Katz, M., Frazer, A., Bowden, C. L., et al. (1987). Catecholamine metabolism and disposition in healthy and depressed subjects. *Archives of General Psychiatry, 44,* 337–344.

Manji, H. K., Moore, G. J., Rajkowska, G., & Chen, G. (2000). Neuroplasticity and cellular resilience in mood disorders. *Molecular Psychiatry, 5,* 578–593.

Mann, J. J., & Arango, V. (1999). Abnormalities of brain structure and function in mood disorders. In D. S. Charney, E. J. Nestler, & B. S. Bunney (Eds.), *Neurobiology of mental illness* (pp. 385–393). New York: Oxford University Press.

Mann, J. J., Huang, Y. Y., Underwood, M. D., Kassir, S. A., Oppenheim, S., Kelly, T. M., et al. (2000). A serotonin transporter gene promoter polymorphism (5-HTTLPR) and prefrontal cortical binding in major depression. *Archives of General Psychiatry, 57,* 729–738.

Marek, G. J., & Aghajanian, G. K. (1998). The electrophysiology of prefrontal serotonin systems: Therapeutic implications for mood and psychosis. *Biological Psychiatry, 44,* 1118–1127.

Mayberg, H. S. (1997). Limbic-cortical dysregulation: A proposed model of depression. In S. Salloway, P. Malloy, & J. L. Cummings (Eds.), *The neuropsychiatry of limbic and subcortical disorders* (pp. 167–178). Washington, DC: American Psychiatric Press.

McMahon, F. J., Chen, Y. S., Patel, S., Brown, M. D., Torroni, A., DePaulo, J. R., & Wallace, D. C. (2000). Mitochondrial DNA sequence diversity in bipolar affective disorder. *American Journal of Psychiatry, 157,* 1058–1064.

Murphy, T. K., Goodman, W. K., Fudge, M. W., Williams, R. C., Ayoub, E. M., Lewis, M. H., et al. (1997). A peripheral marker for childhood-onset obsessive-compulsive disorder and Tourette's syndrome? *American Journal of Psychiatry, 154,* 402–407.

Reiman, E. M., Raichle, M. E., & Butler, F. K. (1984). A focal brain abnormality in panic disorder, a severe form of anxiety. *Nature, 310,* 683–685.

Reiman, E. M., Raichle, M. E., Robins, E., Butler, F. K., Herscovitch, P., Fox, P., & Perlmutter, J. (1986). The application of positron emission tomography to the study of panic disorder. *American Journal of Psychiatry, 143,* 469–477.

Reiman, E. M., Raichle, M. E., Robins, E., Mintun, M. A., Fusselman, M. J., Fox, P. T., et al. (1989). Neuroanatomical correlates of a lactate-induced anxiety attack. *Archives of General Psychiatry, 46,* 493–500.

Rotondo, A., Mazzanti, C., Dell'Osso, L., Rucci, P., Sullivan, P., Bouanani, S., et al. (2002). Catechol-O-methyltransferase, serotonin transporter, and tryptophan hydroxylase gene polymorphisms in bipolar disorder patients with and without comorbid panic disorder. *American Journal of Psychiatry, 159,* 23–29.

Sanders, A. R., Detera-Wadleigh, S. D., & Gershon, E. S. (1999). Molecular genetics of mood disorders. In D. S. Charney, E. J. Nestler, & B. S. Bunney (Eds.), *Neurobiology of mental illness* (pp. 299–316). New York: Oxford University Press.

Siever, L. J., Uhde, T. W., Jimerson, D. C., Lake, C. R., Silberman, E. R., Post, R. M., & Murphy, D. L. (1984). Differential inhibitory noradrenergic responses to clonidine in 25 depressed patients and 25 normal control subjects. *American Journal of Psychiatry, 141,* 733–741.

Sjoholt, G., Gulbrandsen, A. K., Lovlie, R., Berle, J. O., Molven, A., & Steen, V. M. (2000). A human myo-inositol monophosphatase gene (IMPA2) localized in a putative susceptibility region for bipolar disorder on chromosome 18p11.2: Genomic structure and polymorphism screening in manic–depressive patients. *Molecular Psychiatry, 5*, 172–180.

Swedo, S. E., Leonard, H. L., & Kiessling, L. S. (1994). Speculations on antineuronal antibody-mediated neuropsychiatric disorders of childhood. *Pediatrics, 93*, 323–326.

Teicher, M. H. (2000). Wounds that time won't heal. *Cerebrum, 2*, 50–67.

Vuoristo, J. T., Berrettini, W. H., Overhauser, J., Procktop, D. J., Ferraro, T. N., & Ala-Kokko, L. (2000). Sequence and genomic organization of the human g-protein golf gene (gnal) on chromosome 18p11, a susceptibility region for bipolar disorder and schizophrenia. *Molecular Psychiatry, 5*, 495–501.

Winsberg, M. E., Sachs, N., Tate, D. L., Adalsteinsson, E., Spielman, D., & Ketter, T. A. (2000). Decreased dorsolateral prefrontal N-acetyl aspartate in bipolar disorder. *Biological Psychiatry, 47*, 475–481.

12

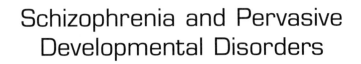

Schizophrenia and Pervasive Developmental Disorders

Schizophrenia and pervasive developmental disorders (PDDs) are among the most devastating of mental illnesses. Schizophrenia affects up to 1% of the population, and these individuals suffer severe impairment in their daily functioning. Two-thirds are totally disabled, a significant number are homeless, and 10% will eventually commit suicide. The prevalence of autism is debated, as the number of new diagnoses per year of autism is rising (although this may represent change in diagnostic practice rather a true increase in incidence). It may range between 1 in 500 to 1 in 2,500. Schizophrenia and autism–PDDs are qualitatively very different in terms of their life course and underlying pathophysiology, but they are discussed together here because of the similar severity of their impact on the patient's functioning.

SCHIZOPHRENIA

As was discussed in Chapter 1, Emil Kraepelin made the distinction between "dementia praecox" and manic–depressive illness. Kraepelin emphasized the early onset of disruption in thinking in dementia praecox with no return to healthy functioning. Eugen Bleuler later renamed the condition "schizophrenia," emphasizing as key features disturbance of relatedness and affect, loose associations (thought disorder), and difficulty determining reality and fantasy. These early investigators did not see hallucinations and delusions as primary to the disorder; indeed, these phenomena occur in other psychiatric disorders, as well. Yet the modern formulation of schizophrenia in DSM-IV emphasizes psychosis as the key feature. This change may have evolved because antipsychotic medications, particularly the older, "typical" antipsychotics were most successful in eliminating the positive symptoms, such as delusions and hallucinations, whereas the negative symptoms of flat affect, social withdrawal, impaired relatedness, and thought disorder often went unchanged. Yet these negative symptoms may be primary, as Kraepelin and Bleuler thought, whereas overt psychosis is secondary. Psychosis can occur in response to a wide variety of psychiatric disorders and brain insults (mood disorder, dementia, brain injury, or neurotoxins). Ming Tsuang and her colleagues discussed the need to reformulate the diagnosis of schizophrenia, returning to the emphasis on the negative symptoms, as well as neuropsychological deficits that occur before the psychosis. It has been known for many years that relatives of persons with schizophrenia often show mild signs of the disorder, such as odd thinking, dislike of social interaction, and problems with modulating affect. These individuals maintain adequate social functioning (i.e., holding jobs, completing school) and are never psychotic. Sometimes they meet criteria for schizoid disorder or schizotypal personality disorder, but often they do not fit into any current DSM-IV criteria. Tsuang and colleagues refer to this collection of symptoms as "schizotaxia." These individuals are predisposed to schizophrenia and may even respond to atypical antipsychotics (discussed later), which, unlike the typical antipsychotics, treat both positive and negative symptoms.

Any theory of schizophrenia must explain an important fact: Although persons with schizophrenia have a markedly reduced rate of producing offspring, the prevalence of schizophrenia has remained constant over many generations. Indeed, there are descriptions of schizophrenia back to antiquity. Thus something maintains the genetic predisposition to schizophrenia in the population. For instance, persons with schizotaxia may have adequate functioning to have children, but only some of the children may develop schizophrenia. The nonschizophrenic children pass the schizotaxic genes onto the next generation, maintaining them in the gene pool. Also, these schizotaxic genes many convey some other advantage. It is well known that higher levels of creativity and artistic accomplishment are found among people with bipolar disorder; less well known is that families of people with schizophrenia also contain individuals of considerable accomplishment. Bertrand Russell had both a son and a granddaughter with schizophrenia. Albert Einstein's son by his first marriage suffered from the disorder as did James Joyce's daughter Lucia. Thus schizotaxic genes, in certain situations, may lead to increased creativity or may, in combination with other events, produce schizophrenia. Finally, as noted in the preceding chapter, bipolar disorder and schizophrenia may not be as distinct as Kraepelin had first postulated. It is perhaps better to think of these two disorders as existing on a continuum. People with classic schizophrenia show poor premorbid functioning; then, in late adolescence or young adulthood, they begin to show flattening of affect, social withdrawal, and disordered thinking. Most then have a "first break" in which psychosis appears, consisting of hallucinations, paranoid or bizarre delusions, and disorganization of behavior. Good functioning is rarely, if ever attained. In contrast, people with classic mania have good premorbid functioning and an acute onset of mania at age 25–30 with good recovery after the first episode. The manic episode consists of euphoria, hypersexuality, flight of ideas, and pressured speech. Whereas people with schizophrenia are withdrawn and reclusive, the mania are expansive, intrusive, and inappropriately social. Between these two classic presentations, there are a significant number of patients who cannot be classified in either category—these patients are often referred to as "schizoaffective." The two disorders may share genetic vulnerabilities.

Genetics of Schizophrenia

Monozygotic (MZ) twins have a 48% concordance rate for schizophrenia compared with a 17% rate for dizygotic (DZ) twins. Nontwin siblings have only a 9% chance of both having schizophrenia, unless a parent is affected, wherein the risk jumps back to 17%. Heritability has been calculated to be .68. If both parents have schizophrenia, the risk of schizophrenia to the child is 46%. There is a clear genetic effect on schizophrenia but also an obvious role for environment, far more so than for ADHD or bipolar disorder. Of interest, too, is the difference in risk for the DZ twins and the nontwin siblings. Twins, of course, have a higher rate of complications during pregnancy and delivery, a factor that has turned out to play a role in schizophrenia.

Extensive work has been done searching for genetic markers linked to schizophrenia. A plethora of chromosome regions possibly related to the disorder have emerged, prompting skepticism among many in the field because a study that establishes one marker often fails to replicate the others. Brian Riley and Peter McGuffin at the Institute of Psychiatry in London have recently reviewed this work, emphasizing how difficult it has been to confirm findings of linkage. At the time of their review, no less than 14 markers had been implicated on chromosomes 1, 2, 4, 5, 6, 7, 8, 9, 10, 13, 15, 18, 22, and X. The regions on 18 and 22 may also be implicated in bipolar disorder, as discussed in the previous chapter. The COMT gene on chromosome 22 studied in ADHD and bipolar may also play a role in schizophrenia. Three widely separated areas of chromosome 1 have been linked to schizophrenia in different samples. This problem has been common in schizophrenia genetic studies: Even when studies agree that an area of a chromosome is linked to schizophrenia, the exact position of the locus has varied from study to study. This makes the search for a specific gene very difficult. Recently, J. K. Millar and colleagues found a disruption of a gene on chromosome 1 in a Scottish family with a 47% prevalence of the disorder. The function of the gene is not known, so it has been termed, "Disrupted in Schizophrenia Candidate-1" or DISC-1. The abnormality might be unique to this particular family, however. Further studies of the gene are underway. In 1988 Sherrington and colleagues found a marker on chromosome 5 linked to schizophrenia in one of the first molecular genetic psychiatry studies ever done, but the finding was not replicated and did not hold up after reanalysis. Recently, however, two new loci, one close to and the other distant from the Sherrington marker, have been found to be linked to schizophrenia. Chromosome 6 has been of interest because of the possibility that the area linked to schizophrenia might be close to the histocompatiblity complex allele (HLA), which helps govern the immune response. As is shown later, viral infections play a small role in schizophrenia, leading to speculation that the genetic vulnerability is related to the individual's immune response to infection. More data is needed, however. The q13–14 region of chromosome 15 has shown linkage to the p50 sensory gating deficit. Brain waves are measured in response to a sudden stimulus, such as a loud noise. The p50 is a positive EEG wave produced by the brain 50 msec after the stimulus. In normal participants, if a mild form of the stimulus is given before the main stimulus, the p50 is attenuated. People with schizophrenia fail to show this inhibition of their p50 to the main stimulus. The q13–14 region of chromosome 15 controls this trait, and within this region lies the gene for a subunit of the nicotinic cholinergic receptor. The cholinergic system is involved in arousal, as discussed in Chapter 4; furthermore, it is well known that people with schizophrenia smoke far more than average, and many patients report that smoking reduces their psychotic symptoms. If fully replicated, the chromosome 15 and nicotinic receptor linkages would imply a cholinergic deficit in schizophrenia.

The X chromosome is of interest because of the male predominance in schizophrenia and because the risk for schizophrenia in offspring is greater if the mother, rather than the father, has the disease. The region in which the X and Y chromosomes both have alleles is referred to as the pseudoautosomal region. T. J. Crow has suggested that an as yet unknown gene in the Xq21 region is responsible for lateralization in the human brain, that is, the segregation of functions into the left (primarily verbal) and the right (primarily nonverbal) hemispheres. Crow argues that the emergence of this gene made the development of language possible but also made individuals vulnerable to schizophrenia if the lateralization process did not complete itself. In neuroimaging studies, it has been found that people with schizophrenia often lack the brain asymmetries that normal individuals have: right frontal lobe larger than left, left temporal lobe larger than right. Linkage to the X chromosome remains weak, however. With the mapping of the human genome, there will be many more markers available to do a full genome scan in schizophrenia, resulting in more definitive work in this area.

Early Brain Insults in Schizophrenia

Consistent findings over three decades have linked adverse events during pregnancy and delivery to schizophrenia. Obstetrical complications appear to be particularly likely to increase the risk for schizophrenia; these include low birth weight, prematurity, the need for resuscitation after birth, or perinatal brain damage. People who develop schizophrenia are somewhat more likely to be born in the winter and early spring, when the mother is more likely to have been exposed to the influenza virus during pregnancy. During World War II, in the winter of 1944, the Netherlands was blockaded, producing a famine. Women who were in the second trimester of pregnancy during this period were more likely to bear children who later developed schizophrenia, suggesting that poor nutrition during critical phases of brain development is a risk factor in schizophrenia. Low maternal weight gain during pregnancy, small head circumference at birth, and low placenta weight also contribute to the risk of schizophrenia. During brain development, neurons migrate from the center of the brain to the periphery, where they establish networks with each other. In this period various molecules are produced that help guide neurons and axons to their locations. A molecule call "Reelin" is a key protein in brain development—it serves as a stop signal for neuronal migration. Two studies have shown that Reelin is reduced by 30–50% in the prefrontal cortex and hippocampi of schizophrenics. Obstetric complications often show correlations with MRI findings in schizophrenia, which are reviewed later. Finally, people with schizophrenia show a higher than expected rate of minor physical anomalies in various areas of their bodies. These include minor alterations in fingers, ears, mouth, and feet that do not affect function but that suggest a degree of fetal maldevelopment. These minor anomalies are not specific to schizophrenia, however; they are found in a number of psychiatric disorders, including fetal alcohol syndrome, autism, and learning disabilities.

It is important to note that the vast majority of people who have any of the early risk factors do not go on to develop schizophrenia. This fact has led to the "double hit" hypothesis, which suggests that a genetic risk is necessary but not sufficient for the development of schizophrenia. A genetic risk combined with one of the early insults just discussed would then lead to the expression of the disorder. Those who do not suffer an early brain insult might go on to develop schizotaxia or perhaps show no disorder at all. Genetics and perinatal insults operate early in life, but schizophrenia rarely has onset before adolescence. What accounts for this? First, children who will ultimately develop schizophrenia show subtle differences in a number of areas. They are thinner than average during childhood. Walker and colleagues studied home movies of people with schizophrenia as children and found that, compared with their normal siblings, children who were preschizophrenic showed more abnormal limb movements during the first 2 years of life. These abnormal movements tended to resolve after the age of 2, however. During the elementary school years, persons who will develop schizophrenia already show lower IQs and increased social withdrawal. These early signs are generally not noticeable to parents and teachers at the time. The development of schizophrenia may require a "triple hit"; that is, in addition to genetic risk and early brain insult, some factor triggered during adolescence may cause the final progression to schizophrenia.

Thomas McGlashan and Ralph Hoffman reviewed data that strongly suggest that people with schizophrenia show reduced synaptic connectivity. They have developed a computer model of hallucinations based on these data, which I discuss in the next section. Gray matter volume (i.e., neurons and their support cells) normally increases until age 5, when it begins to decline. During adolescence it begins a sharp decline, as synapses are "pruned"; this process is most marked in the frontal and parietal lobes. In a normal individual, this pruning eliminates unnecessary connections and optimizes brain flexibility to deal with new learning. McGlashan and Hoffman propose that in a vulnerable individual with too few synapses to begin with, the onset of the normal pruning process and can cause a severe impairment in information processing and the subsequent onset of schizophrenia. Alternatively, they propose that some individuals with schizophrenia have an overly aggressive pruning process (the "third hit"). Their model is consistent with the neuroimaging data.

Neuroimaging in Schizophrenia

Several decades of research examining brains—both postmortem and with structural MRI on live patients—have yielded consistent results. People with schizophrenia show decreased total brain volume and increased size of the cerebral ventricles. The frontal lobes and hippocampus appear to be particularly affected. A particularly useful strategy in studying brain structure in schizophrenia is to compare the brains of MZ twins discordant for schizophrenia. This allows the investigators to separate influences of genetic and other factors on brain structure. Recently, William Barre and colleagues studied 15 MZ and 14 DZ twins who were discordant for schizophrenia and compared them with 29 twin pairs, neither of whom had schizophrenia (the controls were matched for zygosity). In general, the correlation of the size of brain regions was higher for the MZ twins than for the DZ twins; that is, brain structure was more similar in the MZ twins. The investigators studied both intracranial volume (space inside the skull, which is set by early brain growth) and volume of the brain itself (whole brain volume). First, intracranial volume was reduced in the MZ twins discordant for schizophrenia. Second, frontal lobe size was decreased in ill MZ twins, relative to their healthy co-twins, in excess of the decrease in whole brain volume. This finding suggests that both the ill and healthy MZ twins had reduced early brain growth (particularly in the frontal lobe) but that only one of them developed the illness. Thus reduced early brain growth is a risk factor for schizophrenia, but it does not itself cause the disorder. In contrast, whole brain volume, as well as hippocampal volume, was reduced in the twins with schizophrenia regardless of zygosity. This additional decrease in brain size may be due to the schizophrenia disease process itself. The imaging data is consistent with the double-hit hypothesis: A genetic factor impairs early brain development, while some other factor triggers other events that lead to further decreases in brain volume.

Functional brain studies using both PET and MRI have shown decreased activity in the frontal lobes of people with schizophrenia relative to controls when they perform tasks such as the Wisconsin Card Sort Task, which tax working memory. Postmortem studies and magnetic resonance spectroscopy (MRS) studies in individuals with schizophrenia show reduced dendritic spines on neurons, decreased glutamate and GABA release, and decreased synaptic protein messenger RNA. Persons with schizophrenia are more likely to express a less functional version of the NMDA receptor. They have reduced N-acetyl aspartate (NAA) in the dorsolateral prefrontal cortex, implying decreased neuronal integrity. The amount of glutamic acid decarboxylase (the enzyme that is key to the synthesis of GABA) is reduced in the schizophrenic brain, and there are derangements in the GABA transporter that governs its reuptake. When reduced neuronal density is found in schizophrenic brains, there is no evidence of gliosis (i.e., signs of neuronal destruction by a toxic agent); rather, there are signs of maldevelopment. Clearly, a major malfunction has occurred in brain in people with schizophrenia. Recall that the valine-substituted form of the COMT enzyme has higher activity, and since COMT breaks down dopamine, this might lead to lower dopamine levels in the brain. Recently, Michael Egan and his colleagues showed that schizophrenics (as well as their unaffected siblings) who carried the valine-COMT variation showed poorer performance on neuropsychological testings; valine-COMT carriers also showed increased brain activation during cognitive tasks relative to methionine-COMT carriers. I will return to the possible implications of lower dopamine in the prefrontal cortex in the discussion of antipsychotic medications.

McGlashan and Hoffman describe a neural network computer simulation of speech perception and production that, under certain circumstances, will "hallucinate"; that is, it produces speech in the absence of input. The neural network has a verbal working memory that learns to recognize words from previous auditory input. The computer network has parallel processors that change the strength of their connections as they are exposed to stimuli. Thus, like the brain, the computer simulation has numerous synapses, and the experimenters can "prune" these synapses. Words are input, and the investigators look at how many words are correctly detected as a function of the degree of pruning. When less than 20% of the synapses are pruned, the neural network recognizes only about 60% of the words. When 20–40% of the synapses are pruned, the network recognizes over 80% of the words, suggesting that this is an optimal level of connectivity. When over 40% of the synapses are pruned, the recognition rate falls back again to only 60%, but the program begins behaving strangely. It begins to produce output, that is, produce words, even when there has been no input. The network has begun to hallucinate!

How does this relate to humans? Recall from Chapter 4 that the brain does not have separate areas for "thinking" and "perceiving." When we imagine something, the same areas of the brain are active as when we are actually seeing the object in front of us. This means that the brain must have a mechanism to tell what is real—that is, what is a signal from the outside world and what are our internal thoughts. The work of McGlashan and Hoffman suggest that without adequate connectivity, the brain may lose this crucial function.

Neurochemistry in Schizophrenia

Antipsychotic medications were discovered by accident. As with antidepressants, an attempt was made to reason backward from the mechanisms of actions of these drugs to a possible cause of schizophrenia. After a while, it became clear that the class of antipsychotics discovered in the period 1950–1980 all blocked dopamine (DA) receptors and that their effectiveness correlated with their ability to block the D_2 DA receptor. This led to the "DA theory of schizophrenia"—the simple idea that schizophrenia is caused by an excess of DA. This idea seemed bolstered by the fact that amphetamines, which increase the release of DA, can, when abused, cause psychosis, particularly in vulnerable individuals. There were, however, problems with this DA theory from the start. Antipsychotics eliminated all forms of psychosis besides those associated with schizophrenia, so it would have been more appropriate to speak of a DA theory of psychosis than one of schizophrenia. Antipsychotics blocked DA receptors immediately upon administration, but the psychosis took time to resolve. Finally, LSD, which has a serotonergic action, and PCP, which blocks the NMDA ion channel, both produce syndromes more akin to schizophrenia than the amphetamines do.

The DA theory of schizophrenia led to some obvious experiments. Did people with schizophrenia show evidence of increased DA activity in the brain? The principal way to explore this would be to assess the level of homovanillic acid (HVA, the prime metabolite of DA) in the cerebrospinal fluid of patients with schizophrenia versus controls. Rather than finding an excess of HVA, most studies showed either no difference or a decreased amount of CSF HVA relative to controls. Furthermore, it was found that low CSF HVA correlated with increased ventricle size, that is, people with schizophrenia might show decreased DA activity. Consistent with this, people with untreated schizophrenia show increased levels of D_2 DA receptors in their striata. This up-regulation of DA receptors may have occurred as a result of a DA deficit. This fact lead to a major revision of the DA theory of schizophrenia: that a DA deficit in the cortex might underlay negative symptoms, while excess DA in the mesolimbic system, particularly in the nucleus accumbens, might underlay positive symptoms such as hallucinations. When antipsychotics are administered, the DA neurons in the substantia nigra and ventral tegmental area actually increase their firing, possibly to compensate for the blockade of the DA receptor. After prolonged treatment, however, "depolarization block" sets in; that is, the DA neurons stop firing. Here there are critical differences between the older class of antipsychotics and newly developed atypical antipsychotics.

Differences between the typical and atypical antipsychotics are shown in Figure 12.1. The size of each slice of the pie represents how strongly the particular antipsychotic binds to that receptor subtype. Most of the time, this binding results in antagonism (blockade) of the receptor, though some receptor subtypes may be activated. Typical antipsychotics are divided into those of low and high potency. Haldol (haloperidol) is representative of the high-potency class; it is given in doses of 1–10 mg a day, strongly blocks DA receptors, and has minimal

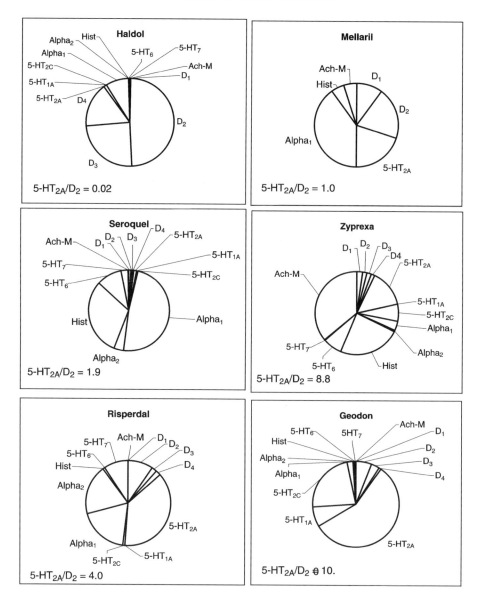

FIGURE 12.1. Receptor-blocking properties of antipsychotic medications

effects at serotonin or alpha norepinephrine receptors. Because it has such strong effects at DA receptors, it is far more likely to cause Parkinsonian-type symptoms (discussed later). Mellaril is the prototype for the low-potency neuroleptics. It is much less potent in blocking DA receptors and thus must be given in higher doses (200–800 mg/day) to achieve its effect. Because it so strongly blocks alpha norepinephrine, acetylcholine muscarine (Ach-M), and histamine (Hist) receptors, it is very sedating and causes dry mouth and increased appetite.

The four atypical antipsychotics presently in use are also shown in Figure 12.1. Note that Risperdal has less D_2 blocking activity than Haldol, yet it is effective against psychosis in the same dose range (1–6 mg). Note also the high degree of blockade of 5-HT_{2A} receptors, a feature shared by all the atypicals. Seroquel appears to have no D_2 or 5-HT_{2A} blocking capacity, but it simply has low potency to do so. Thus it is given at very high doses (200–600 mg/day) relative to the other atypicals. Geodon also blocks 5-HT_{2C} receptors, but it is not clear whether this has specific benefits in reducing psychotic symptoms. It also stimulates (has agonist effects) at the 5-HT_{1A} receptor. Like Mellaril, some of the atypicals have histamine and alpha noradrenergic blocking ability, which makes them sedating; when these effects are combined with serotonin receptor blockade, appetite increases dramatically. Thus the chief side effects for Seroquel, Zyprexa, and Risperdal is weight gain, though Geodon is less potent in this regard, perhaps due to its lower antihistaminic effects

Typical antipsychotics induce depolarization block in the terminal fields of both the ventral tegmental area and the substantia nigra. As discussed in Chapter 5, DA input to the neostriatum is critical for motor behavior. When DA input to this area deteriorates, Parkinson's disease results. Because typical antipsychotics block DA in this area, they cause Parkinson-like symptoms—tremor of the hands, bradykinesia (slow movements), and stiffness of the muscles (cogwheeling). The atypical antipsychotics, in contrast, do not induce depolarization block in the neostriatum and do not cause (except in rare cases) Parkinson-like symptoms. Atypical antipsychotics induce depolarization block only in the terminal field of the DA neurons whose cell bodies reside in the ventral tegmental area. These are the nucleus accumbens and prefrontal cortex, areas more likely to be involved in the thought disorder of schizophrenia than the neostriatum. Atypical antipsychotics also block 5-HT_{2A} receptors, though it is not known whether this is a critical mechanism of action in schizophrenia. Various antidepressants block 5-HT_{2A} receptors, but they are not effective in psychosis. The typical antipsychotic Mellaril also blocks the 5-HT_{2A} receptor. Finally, atypical antipsychotics are also effective for negative symptoms, whereas the older antipsychotic medications are not effective in this regard. Why this is so remains a mystery, but one theory focuses on the ratio of D_2 to $5\text{-}HT_{2A}$ blocking activity of the antipsychotics. As shown in Figure 12.1, the atypicals have relatively greater blocking at $5\text{-}HT_{2A}$ relative to D_2 (the larger the number, the greater the $5\text{-}HT_{2A}$ relative to D_2 antagonism). This combined antagonism has been thought to underlie their "atypicality" (i.e., more effective on negative symptoms, fewer motor-system side effects). It has been suggested that if $5\text{-}HT_{2A}$ receptors on DA terminals inhibit the release of DA, and that blocking these $5\text{-}HT_{2A}$ receptors with an atypical *enhances* the release of DA. This would be particularly important in the cortex, where there is thought to be a DA deficit. In the nigrostriatal and mesolimbic pathways, the atypical would block the D_2 receptors; in the accumbens this would be enough to eliminate positive symptoms since DA is thought to be elevated there. (In contrast, there are fewer D_2 receptors in the cortex, so the increased DA will bind to other DA receptors, perhaps enhancing cognition.) In the striatum, the binding of the atypical to the D_2 receptors is still lower than for the typical antipsychotics, resulting in fewer Parkinsonian effects relative to the these older agents. This theory is predicated on the concept that serotonin inhibits dopamine, but we saw in Chapter 4 that at least in humans, serotonin may facilitate the release of dopamine. More PET work in which DA release is measured in the presence of serotoninergic drugs is needed to resolve this issue. The antipsychotic amisulpride has been used in France for the treatment of schizophrenia for more than 20 years. It binds to D_2 and D_3 receptors in the limbic system, as opposed to the striatum. In a review, Stefan Leucht and colleagues found amisulpride to be as effective as other atypical antipsychotics. Thus the search for the neurochemical cause of "atypicality" must go on. A new class of drugs for schizophrenia, called DA system stabilizers, has recently been developed and is showing promise in clinical trials. While clearly acting as "atypicals", this class of drugs has minimal effects on the serotonin system. Aripiprazole is the prime example of this class. Aripiprazole is a "partial" DA agonist. A full agonist (like DA itself) binds to receptor and produces a full effect—say 100% activation of the enzyme. An antagonist (like haloperidol) blocks the receptor and the enzyme is not activated at all. A partial agonist may produce a 50% percent activation. This has very interesting properties. If no DA is around at baseline, the partial agonist produces an increase in DA action (50% better than nothing). In contrast, if the DA system is overactive (producing 150% enzyme activation), then when the partial agonist binds the receptor it produces a decline in DA action (50% rather than 150% activation of the enzyme). Stephen Stahl has referred to this as the "Goldilocks" effect—where DA action is "too hot" it reduces it, where is it "too cold" aripiprazole increases it, making things "just right." Thus the DA system stabilizers may increase DA in the cortex and reduce its action in the mesolimbic system.

Any theory of the neurochemistry of schizophrenia must go beyond DA: It must incorporate glutamate and serotonin and must explain how, if there is evidence of decreased DA functioning in schizophrenia, a DA blocker is helpful. Anthony Grace, whose work was reviewed in Chapter 9, has provided a model to do this. His model is incorporated into Figure 12.2. Grace distinguished between tonic and phasic DA release. Tonic release is the low level of DA that is chronically present in the synapse. The level of tonic release is governed by glutamergic input from other brain areas to the presynaptic terminals of the DA neurons. In panel A of Figure 12.2, it can be seen that the glutamate neurons from the PFC, amygdala, and hippocampus all have input to the DA neuron from the ventral tegmental area (1). This input raises tonic DA levels (2), which stimulate the DA autoreceptor (3); this autoreceptor stimulation in turn dampens phasic DA release (4). Phasic DA release is DA that is released in response to an action potential arriving at the nerve terminal, that is, in response to DA nerve stimulation. An appropriate amount of DA is released. Recall again from Chapter 9 that one of the roles of DA in the NA neuron is to gate stimuli from various sources; increased DA will lead to a greater amygdaloid input. Tonic release also influences the number of postsynaptic DA receptors (more tonic DA, fewer DA receptors; less tonic DA, more receptors). In panel A, the DA release is in balance with the number of postsynaptic receptors.

Panel B represents the possible situation in schizophrenia. The disease process has led to deterioration of glutamate input from the PFC and hippocampus. This deterioration is due to failures of neuronal migration in early development or to excessive pruning during adolescence. These primary cortical deficits underlie negative symptoms of schizophrenia. With less stimulation of the glutamate hetereoreceptors (1), less tonic DA is released (2), which leads both to autoreceptor understimulation (3) and an up-regulation of postsynaptic D_2 receptors.

Positive symptoms arise as shown in panel C of the figure. An axon potential reaches the DA nerve terminal, and, because DA autoreceptors remain understimulated (1 and 2), there is an excessive phasic release of DA (3). This excessive DA will stimulate the abnormal number of postsynaptic receptors, thus producing overstimulation of both the cortex and the NA by DA. The hippocampal process has already been weakened by the primary disease process; excessive DA input will further weaken it, resulting in an excessive gating of amygdaloid influences on behavior. The excessive DA disrupts the thought processes themselves to the point at which hallucinations and delusions emerge. A typical

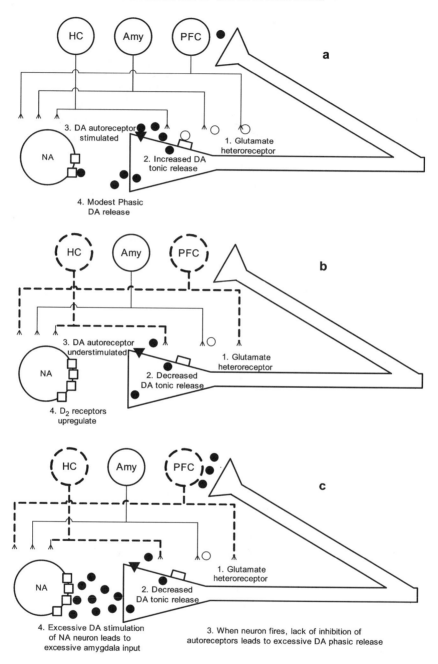

FIGURE 12.2. Hypothesized mechanism of antipsychotic action incorporating Grace's (1999) model of antipsychotic effects on dopamine neurotransmission

antipsychotic medication blocks the postsynaptic DA receptors, eliminating the positive symptoms, but often does not change the underlying disease process. Grace's model of antipsychotic action is similar to his theory of stimulant action in ADHD (both diseases showing decreased tonic and increased phasic DA release), but the symptoms are different because of the primary deterioration of frontal and hippocampal areas in schizophrenia, whereas ADHD might be related to a primary dysregulation of DA.

Serotonergic and GABA neurons have extensive input to cortical neurons. Perhaps as these cortical and hippocampal neurons deteriorate, the serotonergic input becomes more dysfunctional, simulating the effects of LSD on a normal brain. Blockading serotonin receptors seems to have an antischizophrenic effect only in combination with the DA blocking described previously, thus attention must be paid to the serotonin–DA antagonist ratio that differentiates the typical from the atypical neuroleptics.

Overview

Schizophrenia is a complex disease that may require a "triple hit." Polygenetic factors lead to a vulnerability to the disorder, but obstetric complications, infection, or malnutrition during pregnancy may be necessary to start the progression to the disorder. These same genes, in the absence of environmental stressors, may lead to schizotaxia or to some actual advantage (i.e., increased creativity). Children with preschizophrenic children may have subtle learning and motor problems as a result. The "third hit" may occur in adolescence with an overly aggressive pruning process. Frontal and hippocampal dysfunction results and underlies the negative symptoms, which are the primary features of the disorder. The deterioration in the glutamate frontal–hippocampal system dysregulates the DA system, producing positive symptoms of schizophrenia. Research to discover why atypical antipsychotics address negative symptoms is ongoing. New medications may be the result. Finally, the effects of early brain insults show the need to improve prenatal care to decrease the risk of schizophrenia.

AUTISM

Leo Kanner first described autism in the 1940s. Classically, children with autism appear to develop normally until 15–18 months of age, when a distinct and dramatic change takes place in their relatedness and language. They lose the ability to relate to others; in severe cases, they will cease to relate to their parents. Language stops developing or ceases to have a communicative function. The child stops saying "I" or "you" and may refer to himself in the third person. The child may say meaningless things repetitively or echo what others say. Eye contact is impaired. Odd, obsessive behaviors emerge: keeping the environment the same, collecting meaningless objects, or engaging in a certain action repetitively (turning lights on and off, running the water, etc.). There are stereotypical behaviors, such as toe walking and flapping; some children with autism become self-abusive or show irrational aggressive rages. Although some persons with autism have normal IQs (and a small minority may show savant behavior, such as Raymond in the movie *Rain Man*), most suffer from mental retardation. Autism was once a rare diagnosis. Clinicians tended to restrict it to the higher functioning group, who showed all the classic signs. In recent years, the diagnostic criteria have been broadened; clinicians and researchers refer to "autistic spectrum disorders" or PDD, as they are called in DSM. These are contrasted in Table 12.1.

Much media attention has been given to an alleged rise in the rate of autism over the past three decades, with some authorities claiming the rate of autism is closer to 1 out of every 250–500 persons rather than 1 out of 2,000. Because this "epidemic" occurred after the introduction of the measles, mumps, and rubella (MMR) vaccine, some individuals have focused on the MMR vaccine and immunological theories of autism. Eric Fombonne has criticized the data on which the claim of an increased incidence of autism was made. He pointed out that studies have not controlled for changing diagnostic processes: Children once diagnosed only as mentally retarded are now examined more closely and given an autism spectrum diagnosis. Furthermore, the diagnostic criteria have themselves been broadened to include children who would have been diagnosed with "childhood schizophrenia" or as "schizoid" according to earlier versions of DSM. Fombonne and colleagues examined rates of autism in successive birth cohorts from 1972 to 1985 and found no increase in incidence of the disorder. Thus the lower estimates of autism are more scientifically valid, and extensive research has *not* shown any association of autism or PDD with the MMR vaccine. Indeed, measles infection can lead to brain damage, which in turn could be a risk factor for a variety of mental disorders, especially mental retardation.

Genetics of Autism

Michael Rutter has recently reviewed the genetics of autism. Early theories of autism focused, tragically, on the parents as the cause of the disorder, but Rutter points out that, up to the 1970s, even geneticists were

TABLE 12.1. Contrasting Autism and the Pervasive Developmental Disorders

Disorder	Clinical features	Associated medical conditions	Prevalence and demographics	Prognosis
Autism	Early onset; impairments of language, relatedness; stereotypies present	Tuberous sclerosis; 15–30% with seizures	Male predominance; 1/2,000, claimed by some to be 1/500	Poor
Asperger's syndrome	Impairments of relatedness; stereotypies present; intact language; near normal or above-average IQ	None presently known	1/1,000	Variable
Rett's disorder	Early onset; head growth deceleration; loss of use of hands	X-linked mutation; MeCP2 gene, which regulates expression of multiple other genes, is defective	Females only; 1/15,000	Extremely poor
Heller's syndrome (childhood disintegrative disorder)	Sudden deterioration of language, social, and adaptive skills after age 2–4 years	Multiple medical conditions; 77% have seizures	Both genders	Extremely poor; early death by respiratory failure common
PDD	Autistic symptoms that do not meet full criteria	Variable	Depends on diagnostic criteria	Variable

241

dismissive of an inherited factor as a cause of autism. In the 1990s a number of twin studies were published that showed quite striking concordance rates in MZ twins (60%) versus DZ twins (5%). Heritability was calculated in excess of 90%. More interesting, it was noted that family members of the autistic patient who did not have autism nonetheless were more likely to have autistic features, such as mild social skill problems, aloofness, shyness, oversensitivity, and anxiety. For instance, a father of an autistic child had to drive the same exact route to work every day and insisted that he would never change his office. He was such a good employee, however, that the company abided by his request. As with schizophrenia, this broader phenotype helps explain how autistic genes maintain themselves in the population, as autistic individuals rarely reproduce. In his early work, Leo Kanner observed many high-functioning individuals among the parents of his patients with autism. Perhaps, as with schizophrenia, the genetic risk of autism also underlies other beneficial traits.

Molecular genetics has made some progress in autism and PDD. In 1998, the International Molecular Genetic Study of Autism (IMGSAC) found a linkage between autism and a region on chromosome 7. Between 3 and 15 genes may be involved in autism, however. There has been considerable study of the q11–13 region of chromosome 15. When the chromosomes of autistic individuals are examined for physical abnormalities (cytogenetic studies), the q arm of chromosome 15 is most likely to be abnormal. Abnormalities in this area are related to Prader–Willi and Angelman syndromes. The gene for the $GABA_A$ receptor is also near this region. Polymorphisms linked to the $GABA_A$ gene have been linked to autism. Edwin Cook and colleagues showed that, if the mother's chromosome 15 had a duplication of the q11–13 region and if this duplication were passed to the child, autism was more likely. In contrast, if the duplicated q11–13 region came from the father, the child would be normal, an excellent example of imprinting. Persons with autism who have the 15q11–13 duplication are more likely to show seizures or motor delays than are a typical sample of children with autism.

IMGSAC has recently published the results of whole-genome scans of autism in a large sample of families. This study confirmed the linkage of autism to chromosome 7, mentioned previously, as well as to a region on chromosome 16. Other sites on chromosome 2 and 17 were also implicated. Recently, Thomas Wassink and Joseph Piven and their colleagues reported a linkage of a gene on chromosome 7 to autism. The gene is called WNT2. Mice with WNT gene family mutations show disturbances of social interaction. Of particular interest, the polymorphism occurs in the gene itself (not in a marker nearby); thus the mutation is highly likely to lead to a malfunctioning protein. Patients with this mutation also tend to show more language impairment, suggesting that this gene is involved in language development.

The gene that causes Rett's disorder has been identified. It is on the X chromosome, and male infants who inherit it rarely survive past birth. It is dominant; a female needs only one X chromosome with the mutation to express the disorder. Females, however, always inactivate one of their X chromosomes. If the mutated X is inactivated, the individual may not develop the disorder but may still be able to pass it on to the next generation. Most patients with Rett's disorder, however, have had a spontaneous mutation and thus have no family history. The gene is called methyl-CpG-binding protein-2 (MECP2); mutations in this gene are found in 80% of Rett cases. The protein normally produced by the gene attaches methyl (-CH$_4$) groups to DNA; this actually turns off the transcriptions of genes. The mutant MECP2 fails to do this. MECP2 is highly expressed in the brain during development; perhaps it coordinates the activation of many genes in the proper sequence. In patients with Rett's disorder, the mutation fails to suppress transcription, genes are activated inappropriately, and, as they run amok, brain development is severely impaired. Research will examine whether similar genes alter brain development in autism or other PDDs.

Neuroimaging in Autism

A variety of findings from both MRI (structural and functional), MRS, and PET have given us a better sense of the nature of the brain dysfunction in autism. In 1987, Eric Courchesne and colleagues first reported a smaller cerebellar vermis in children with autism relative to controls. This area is distinct from the posterior vermis that was found to be decreased in children with ADHD. Decreased cerebellar size is found in a number of other neurodevelopmental disorders, and other groups have not confirmed the early finding. Even before the advent of neuroimaging, it was known that many autistic individuals have macroencephaly (larger than expected head relative to body size). Piven and Filipek both found that individuals with autism, relative to controls, have enlarged total brain volume (the opposite of what is found in schizophrenia). Piven found the temporal, parietal, and occipital (but not the frontal) lobes to be enlarged, whereas Filipek found that it was the white matter, rather the gray matter, that was increased. This is intriguing in view of the association of the disease tuberous sclerosis with autism. Tuberous sclerosis is an inherited illness characterized by seizures, mental retardation, and a red facial rash (*adenoma sebaceum*). Glial cells multiply abnormally and form "tubers," which then infiltrate and destroy the healthy brain tissue. Although only about 5% of chil-

dren with autism have tuberous sclerosis, up to 40% of patients with tuberous sclerosis have autism, and the autism is particularly likely if a tu-
ber infiltrates the temporal lobe.

MRS studies are suggestive of major abnormality of brain development. MRS can detect the amount of certain brain chemicals that vary in
quantity at different times of development. In particular, phospho-
monoesters (PME), which are the building blocks of neuronal membranes, are high during the 20 days of life when synapses are being
formed, whereas phosphodiesters (PDE), the breakdown products of
neuronal membranes, are at low levels in early life. Thus the PME:PDE
ratio is high in the first year of life, falling to around nearly 1 after the
first year. During old age, in which membrane breakdown begins to ex-
ceed synaptic growth, the PME:PDE ratio falls below 1. Another chemical, phosphocreatine (PCr), drops when the brain is in a hypermetabolic
state. Nancy Minshew and Jay Pettegrew of the University of Pittsburgh
measured these values in 11 high-functioning participants with autism
and 11 age- and IQ-matched controls. Individuals with autism had decreased PCr, suggesting an overall increase in brain metabolism. The
lower the patient's PCr, the worse his or hr performance on neuropsychological tasks. The PME:PDE ratio also correlated negatively with
cognitive functioning; as PDE levels rose and PME levels fell, the participants with autism did worse on the tasks. This suggests that autism is a
hypermetabolic state that leads to excessive breakdown of neuronal
membranes. Could these breakdown products be "piling up" in the
brain, leading to the increased brain volume? In tuberous sclerosis, abnormal brain matter also accumulates (though from a completely different cause than autism), and if the temporal lobe is affected, autism is
more likely.

Monica Zilbovicius and colleagues performed PET studies in children with autism and mentally retarded controls (groups matched for
IQ) while they slept. Blood flow was decreased to the temporal lobes bilaterally in those with autism relative to the controls, consistent with
earlier studies suggesting hypoperfusion of the temporal lobes. M.
Haznedar and Monte Buschsbaum at Mount Sinai School of Medicine in
New York compared high-functioning patients with autism and patients
with Asperger's syndrome on both PET and structural MRI. During the
PET study the patients performed a verbal learning task. The anterior
and posterior cingulate gyrus showed decreased metabolism, and the anterior cingulate showed decreased volume relative to controls. This is evidence of limbic system dysfunction in autism. When the amygdala is
damaged in monkeys, they develop Kluver–Bucy syndrome; they become
socially withdrawn and fail to distinguish animate from inanimate objects. Infant monkeys with amygdala lesions fail to develop normal at-

tachments, and they withdraw from other monkeys, showing, like children with autism, stereotypies and self-directed behavior. Recall the proximity of the amygdala to the medial temporal lobe. Baron-Cohen and colleagues recently discussed an "amygdala theory of autism," suggesting that damage to this area might lead to severe social deficits similar to those seen in the lesioned monkeys. They performed a functional MRI study with 6 high-functioning individuals with autism and 6 controls. Participants looked at pictures of the upper part of an individual's face that included the eyes, eyebrows, and lower forehead. They had to guess whether the eyes belonged to a male or a female and to describe the emotion of the individual. For normal individuals, detecting the emotion from the position of the eyes alone is quite easy, but the individuals with autism showed deficits on this task. More interesting, the individuals with autism failed to activate the amygdala as the control participants did.

Thus in autistic spectrum disorders it is possible that some process, most likely genetic, interferes with early brain development. At a point at which the brain should be producing synapses, it in fact begins to break down neuronal membrane, entering a hypermetabolic state. While the brain grows, its neurons fail to form synapses and achieve optimal connectivity. If connectivity fails in the amygdala–temporal areas, the "social brain" is adversely affected, and social attachments become impaired. The disease process is variable from one affected individual to the next, producing a range of severity from Asperger's syndrome to severe, classic autism.

CONCLUSION

It should be clear from this chapter that schizophrenia and autism–PDD are disorders of brain dysfunction on the same order as multiple sclerosis or Alzheimer's. Psychological treatments are still of great benefit. For instance, early and intensive language and social stimulation may attenuate the progression of autism; people with schizophrenia may benefit from highly intensive social rehabilitative efforts. In the 1960s a naive belief arose that schizophrenics, once freed from the "oppression" of the state hospitals, would flourish in the community with minimal assistance. It is clear that this view was as foolish as claiming that a paraplegic was a prisoner of his wheelchair who would be able to walk if he were thrown out of it. We must restore the mental health system that treated these individuals and give them the same intensity of treatment that would be given to any other patient with a devastating illness, such as cancer or Alzheimer's disease.

REFERENCES

Amir, R. E., Van den Veyver, I. B., Wan, M., Tran, C. Q., Francke, U., & Zoghbi, H. Y. (1999). Rett syndrome is caused by mutations in x-linked MECP2, encoding methyl-CpG-binding protein 2. *Nature Genetics, 23,* 185–188.

Andreasen, N. C. (2000). Schizophrenia: The fundamental questions. *Brain Research—Brain Research Reviews, 31,* 106–112.

Baron-Cohen, S., Ring, H. A., Bullmore, E. T., Wheelwright, S., Ashwin, C., & Williams, S. C. R. (2000). The amygdala theory of autism. *Neuroscience and Behavioral Reviews, 24,* 355–364.

Barre, W. F., van Oel, C. J., Hulshoff, H. E., Schnack, H. G., Durston, S., Sitskoorn, M. M., & Kahn, R. S. (2001). Volumes of brain structures in twins discordant for schizophrenia. *Archives of General Psychiatry, 58,* 33–40.

Bunney, W. E. Jr., & Bunney, B. G. (1999). Neurodevelopmental hypothesis of schizophrenia. In D. S. Charney, E. J. Nestler, & B. S. Bunney (Eds.), *Neurobiology of mental illness* (pp. 225–235). New York: Oxford University Press.

Byne, W., Kemether, E., Jones, L., Haroutunian, V., & Davis, K. L. (1999). Neurochemistry of schizophrenia. In D. S. Charney, E. J. Nestler, & B. S. Bunney (Eds.), *Neurobiology of mental illness* (pp. 236–245). New York: Oxford University Press.

Chakrabarti, S., & Fombonne, E. (2001). Pervasive developmental disorders in preschool children. *Journal of the American Medical Association, 285,* 3093–3099.

Cook, E. H., Courchesne, R. Y., Cox, N. J., Lord, C., Gonen, D., Guter, S. J., et al. (1998). Linkage-disequilibrium mapping of autistic disorder, with 15q11–13 markers. *American Journal of Human Genetics, 62,* 1037–1083.

Copolov, D., Velakoulis, D., McGorry, P., Carina, M., Yung, A., Rees, S., et al. (2000). Neurobiological findings in early phase schizophrenia. *Brain Research—Brain Research Reviews, 31,* 157–165.

Courchesne, E., Hesselink, J. R., Jernigan, T. L., & Yeung-Courchesne, R. (1987). Abnormal neuroanatomy in a nonretarded person with autism: Unusual findings with magnetic resonance imaging. *Archives of Neurology, 44,* 335–341.

Crow, T. J. (2000). Schizophrenia as the price that homo sapiens pays for language: A resolution of the central paradox in the origin of the species. *Brain Research—Brain Research Reviews, 31,* 118–129.

Egeland, J. A., Gerhard, D. S., Pauls, D. L., Sussex, J. N., Kidd, K. K., Allen, C. R., et al. (1987). Bipolar affective disorders linked to DNA markers on chromosome 11. *Nature, 325,* 783–787.

Fatemi, S. H., Earle, J. A., & McMenomy, T. (2000). Hippocampal CA4 Reelin-positive neurons. *Molecular Psychiatry, 5,* 571.

Filipek, P. A., Richelme, C., & Kennedy, D. N. (1992). Morphometric analysis of the brain in developmental language disorders and autism. *Annals of Neurology, 32,* 475.

Fombonne, E. (2001). Is there an epidemic of autism? *Pediatrics, 107,* 411–412.

Guidotti, A., Auta, J., Davis, J. M., Giorgi-Gerevini, V., Dwivedi, Y., Grayson, D. R., et al. (2000). Decrease in reelin and glutamic acid decarboxylase67 (GAD67) expression in schizophrenia and bipolar disorder: A postmortem brain study. *Archives of General Psychiatry, 57*, 1061–1069.

Grace, A. A. (2000). Gating of information flow within the limbic system and the pathophysiology of schizophrenia. *Brain Research—Brain Research Reviews, 31*, 330–341.

Haznedar, M. M., Buchsbaum, M. S., Wei, T. C., Hof, P. R., Cartwright, C., Bienstock, C. A., et al. (2000). Limbic circuitry in patients with autism spectrum disorders studied with positron emission tomography and magnetic resonance imaging. *American Journal of Psychiatry, 157*, 1994–2001.

International Molecular Genetic Study of Autism Consortium. (1998). A full genome screen for autism with evidence for linkage to a region on chromosome 7q. *Human Molecular Genetics, 7*, 571–578.

International Molecular Genetic Study of Autism Consortium. (2001). A genome wide screen for autism: Strong evidence for linkage to chromosomes 2q, 7q, and 16p. *American Journal of Human Genetics, 69*, 570–581.

Kanner, L. (1943). Autistic disturbances of affective contact. *Nervous Child, 2*, 217.

Kendler, K. S. (1999). Molecular genetics of schizophrenia. In D. S. Charney, E. J. Nestler, & B. S. Bunney (Eds.), *The neurobiology of mental illness* (pp. 203–213). New York: Oxford University Press.

Leucht, S., Pitschel-Walz, G., Engel, R. R., & Kissling, W. (2002). Amisulpride, an unusual "atypical" antipsychotic: A meta-analysis of randomized controlled trials. *American Journal of Psychiatry, 159*, 180–190.

McDonald, C., & Murray, R. M. (2000). Early and late environmental risk factors for schizophrenia. *Brain Research—Brain Research Reviews, 31*, 130–137.

McGlashen, T. H., & Hoffman, R. E. (2000). Schizophrenia as a disorder of developmentally reduced synaptic connectivity. *Archives of General Psychiatry, 57*, 637–648.

McNeil, T. F., Cantor-Graae, E., & Ismail, B. (2000). Obstetric complications and congenital malformation in schizophrenia. *Brain Research—Brain Research Reviews, 31*, 166–178.

Mehmet Haznedar, M., Buchsbaum, M. S., Wei, T. C., Hof, P. R., Cartwright, C., Bienstock, C. A., & Hollander, E. (2000). Limbic circuitry in patients with autism spectrum disorders studied with positron emission tomography and magnetic resonance imaging. *American Journal of Psychiatry, 157*, 1994–2001.

Millar, J. K., Wilson-Annan, J. C., Anderson, S., Christie, S., Taylor, M. S., Semple, C. A., et al. (2000). Disruption of two novel genes by a translocation co-segregating with schizophrenia. *Human Molecular Genetics, 9*, 1415–1423.

Minshew, N. J., & Pettegrew, J. W. (1996). Nuclear magnetic resonance spectroscopic studies of cortical development. In R. W. Thatcher, G. R. Lyon, J. Rumsey, & N. Krasnegor (Eds.), *Developmental neuroimaging* (pp. 107–126). San Diego, CA: Academic Press.

Piven, J., Arndt, S., Bailey, J., & Andreasen, N. (1996). Regional brain enlargement in autism: A magnetic resonance imaging study. *Journal of the American Academy of Child and Adolescent Psychiatry, 35,* 530–536.

Piven, J., Saliba, K., Bailey, J., & Arndt, S. (1995). An MRI study of brain size in autism. *American Journal of Psychiatry, 152,* 1145–1149.

Riley, B. P., & McGuffin, P. (2000). Linkage and associated studies of schizophrenia. *American Journal of Medical Genetics, 97,* 23–44.

Rutter, M. (2000). Genetic studies of autism: From the 1970s into the millennium. *Journal of Abnormal Child Psychology, 28,* 3–14.

Sanders, A. R., Detera-Wadleigh, S. D., & Gershon, E. S. (1999). Molecular genetics of mood disorders. In D. S. Charney, E. J. Nestler, & B. S. Bunney (Eds.), *Neurobiology of mental illness* (pp. 299–316). New York: Oxford University Press.

Sawa, A., & Snyder, S. H. (2002). Schizophrenia: diverse approaches to a complex disease. *Science, 296,* 692–695.

Sherrington, R., Brynjolfsson, J., Petursson, H., Potter, M., Dudleston, K., Barraclough, B., et al. (1988). Localization of a susceptibility locus for schizophrenia on chromosome 5. *Nature, 336,* 164–167.

Stahl, S. M. (2001a). Dopamine system stabilizers, aripiprazole, and the next generation of antipsychotics, part 1, "Goldilocks" actions at dopamine receptors. *Journal of Clinical Psychiatry, 62,* 841–842.

Stahl, S. M. (2001b). Dopamine system stabilizers, aripiprazole, and the next generation of antipsychotics, part 2: illustrating their mechanism of action. *Journal of Clinical Psychiatry, 62,* 923–924.

Tsuang, M. (2000). Schizophrenia: Genes and environment. *Biological Psychiatry, 47,* 210–220.

Tsuang, M. T., Stone, W. S., & Faraone, S. V. (2000, July). Toward reformulating the diagnosis of schizophrenia. *American Journal of Psychiatry, 157,* 1041–1050.

Wahlbeck, K., Forsen, T., Osmand, C., Barker, D. J. P., & Ericksson, J. G. (2001). Association of schizophrenia with low maternal body mass index, small size at birth, and thinness during childhood. *Archives of General Psychiatry, 58,* 48–52.

Walker, E., Lewine, R. J., & Neuman, C. (1996). Childhood behavioral characteristics and adult brain morphology in schizophrenia. *Schizophrenia Research, 22,* 93–101.

Wassink, T. H., Piven, J., Vieland, V. J., Huang, J., Swiderski, R. E., Pietila, J., et al. (2001). Evidence supporting WNT2 as an autism susceptibility gene. *American Journal of Medical Genetics, 105,* 406–413.

Zilbovicius, M., Boddaert, N., Belin, P., Poline, J. B., Remy, P., Mangin, J. F., et al. (2000). Temporal lobe dysfunction in childhood autism: A PET study. *American Journal of Psychiatry, 157,* 1988.

13

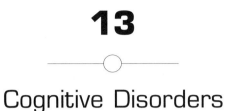

Cognitive Disorders

Disorders of language, learning, and memory can be divided into the developmental and acquired. Developmental cognitive disorders (the learning disabilities) are a failure to develop, during childhood, skills of language, speech, reading, or mathematics at a level commensurate with the individual's intelligence. Acquired cognitive disorders are a loss of the previously mastered skill, and this loss can be either acute (as in response to a stroke) or gradual, due to a degenerative disorder such as Alzheimer's disease. I focus here on the developmental disorders, as they are more likely to be found in the patients treated by mental health professionals. I touch on the degenerative disorders, but because they are of greater interest to clinicians working with an older population, a neuropsychiatry or geriatric psychiatry textbook should be consulted for more information on them.

Chapter 7 gave an overview of the cognitive functions of the cortex. Recall how cognitive functions were partitioned, with the left hemisphere handling verbal, conscious functions while the right hemisphere was dominant for nonverbal, visual–spatial functions. The right hemisphere also modulates emotion and is key to the recognition of facial expression. Table 13.1 shows the principal DSM-IV learning and communication disorders. Although I parse them by "right" and "left" brain, be aware that any complex function requires a smooth integration of the functioning of both hemispheres.

TABLE 13.1. Overview of Developmental Learning and Communication Disorders

	Developmental disorder				
Left brain	Stuttering	Phonological disorder	Reading disorder	Expressive language disorder	Mixed receptive–expressive language disorder
Features	Disturbance of speech characterized by sound and word repetitions and prolongations, broken words, excessive physical tension in word production. Receptive and expressive language skills adequate (person can write or sing without difficulty).	Speech sounds themselves are poorly articulated. Sound substitution is common (w for r), omission of consonants ("teve" for "Steve").	Oral language comprehension and speech are grossly normal, reading (and usually writing) are impaired. Cannot map sound to letters or decode (sound out) written words. Problems with processing rapidly changing visual stimuli?	Comprehends spoken language well, follows commands, but fails to express thoughts in words: limited vocabulary, making errors in tense, difficulty recalling words or producing sentences of age-appropriate length and complexity.	Combination of expressive language disorder with receptive language difficulties: inability to perceive differences in sounds, blending sounds to make words, recalling word meaning, and difficulty linking words to make comprehensible sentences.
Right brain	Mathematics disorder		Nonverbal learning disability (NVLD)		Asperger's syndrome?
Features	Mathematical ability below that expected for IQ. A heterogeneous set of problems may be present: difficulty with simple arithmetic operations (addition, subtraction), difficulty recognizing place, conceptualizing units of measure, problems with number sense (1,000 is much bigger than 10), inability to use symbols as in algebra. Blends into normal bell curve of mathematical ability.		Constellation of traits involving poor social skills, poor recognition of facial expression, poor modulation of affect, mathematics skills poor relative to verbal skills, poor motor coordination, impaired visual–spatial skills.		Extreme variant of NVLD? Severe deficits in communicative intent, language intact but cannot be used for normal social discourse.

Severity

LANGUAGE AND READING DISORDERS

Claudio Toppelberg and Theodore Shapiro described the major components of these disorders, including phonology, grammar, semantics, and pragmatics. Phonology is the ability to both perceive and make the sounds that compose words. Phonological processing is involved in both speech perception and reading. In the former, vibrations from the eardrum that characterize speech sounds are transduced into neural impulses that are in turn processed in the superior temporal cortex. A phoneme is a recognizable sound that could be part of a word ("ba" in ball). Infants as young as 1–4 months can discriminate these sounds. Wernicke's area then recognizes the combinations of the sounds as a word. In reading, the visual representations of the letter on the page are recognized as representing sounds, and a connection with Wernicke's area again must be made so that a word may be perceived. Grammar represents the rules of the language, consisting of morphology and syntax. A morpheme is the part of the word that conveys meaning or usage. The word "jumped" has two morphemes: "jump," which conveys meaning, and "ed", which conveys past tense. Syntax consists of the rules of the language, such as that an English sentence requires the order "subject–verb–object." Semantics is the understanding of words and sentences. Finally, pragmatics refers to the subtleties of the everyday use of language: taking turns when speaking and flexibility using language. When someone says, "He is a cool dude!" we immediately recognize that they are not talking about temperature. Pragmatics also involves the integration of purely verbal input with nonverbal cues: facial expression, tone of voice, and gestures. It comprises what has been called communicative intent, wherein much of what is communicated is inferred rather than directly stated. For instance, if I say to my wife, "Let's see a movie tonight," and she replies, "It's been a long day, I'm really tired," I infer that she does not want to go. She does not have to answer the question directly with a "yes" or "no." The basic rules of language—phonology, grammar, and word meaning—are handled predominantly by the left hemisphere, whereas the right hemisphere is more involved with pragmatics.

As shown in Table 13.1, stuttering and phonological disorder involve impairments of speech. Disturbances of phonology are found in reading and language disorders. Reading disorders (dyslexia) are the only developmental cognitive disorder that have been studied from a genetic perspective. Reading disorder affects about 9% of boys and 6.5% of girls of elementary school age. MZ twins were found to be 83% concordant for reading disorder compared with 23% concordance for DZ twins. When we read, we both break words down into their sounds and recognize whole words by sight. The former is critical for recognizing unfamiliar words and is the one young children strive to master during the early school years. Heritability has been found to differ for these two traits—it is much higher for phonological processing (.62) than for orthographic (sight) reading (.22). Elena Grigorenko and her colleagues searched for polymorphisms linked to reading problems. She found markers on chromosome 6 that were linked to problems with phonological processing, and problems with single-word identification were linked to a locus on chromosome 15. This genetic subtyping of reading problems is consistent with findings in acquired reading problems. Patients suffering injuries to the brain may develop either "surface dyslexia" (inability to read whole words while still being able to sound out words) or phonological ("deep") dyslexia in which phonological processing is impaired but whole-word reading is intact. Researchers have identified a family in England who have a specific language disorder; they are referred to as the "KEs" in the research literature. Affected members in this family cannot sequence their mouth movements to produce speech accurately, they cannot break words into phonemes, and they have a poor understanding of grammar. (For instance, if asked to complete the sentence, "Yesterday I wammed, today I will _____," they have difficulty making the correct future tense of "wam.") This language disorder has been linked to a gene on chromosome 7, FOXP2. In the mutation, a single guanine nucleotide is replaced by an adenosine. FOXP2 is a gene for transcription factors, which control the transcription of multiple genes; FOXP2 is particularly important in embryonic development of the brain. Recall from the previous chapter that regions on chromosome 7 have been linked to pervasive developmental disorders; these patients often suffer language disorders. Further study of this gene may help us understand the brain circuitry for language. Persons with language disorders other than the KE family need to be studied to see if mutations in this gene are a widespread cause of language problems generally.

For reading disorders, the problem with phonological processing is primarily in mapping the written letter to the appropriate sound, whereas in receptive language disorders the problem is at an auditory level. In severe cases, the child may not hear the difference between sounds. The blending of sounds into words is poor, or, if individual words are heard intact, they are not sequenced into sentences. Paula Tallal and her colleagues presented words to children with language impairments via headphones. When the words were presented at the normal rate of speed, the children had marked difficulty understanding them. The researchers then modified the speech sounds by means of a computer. In the first stage, the computer stretched out the speech sounds—"ball" would sound like "baa-ll." Next, they enhanced the transitional parts of the speech. For instance, in the word "captain," there is millisecond of silence between the "capt" and the "ain." The program would prolong this silence. To a normal person, the speech would end up sounding very odd indeed, yet this manipulation greatly enhanced the speech perception of these children. Furthermore, after practice with the computer, the children's general speech perception improved as well. Thus giving the children's brains more time to process the speech sounds was of benefit, and this is a clue to a possible global deficit in language and learning disorders.

Neuroimaging studies have focused primarily on reading disorders. Postmortem studies of people with dyslexia show evidence of neuronal disorganization in the temporal lobe. Control participants show an asymmetry of the temporal lobes, with the widest part of the temporal lobe (the planum temporale) being larger on the left side. People with dyslexia often, but not always, lack this asymmetry. Margaret Semrud-Clikeman and colleagues found that a lack of planum asymmetry was related to poor verbal comprehension and expressive language deficits. Functional imaging studies have also focused on left-hemisphere mechanisms. Before examining these studies, I should debunk a common myth: Dyslexia is not caused by any gross visual defects or "mirror writing." Reversing letters is quite common in young children up to the age of 8; a better predictor of reading problems is the child's inability to learn the relationship between letters and sounds or an unawareness of phonological phenomena such as rhymes. Two recent imaging studies illustrate brain pathology in dyslexia.

In 1998 Sally Shaywitz and colleagues performed functional MRI on 29 adults with dyslexia and 32 normal reader controls. They had the participants perform five tasks of increasing complexity while undergoing the scan. In the first task, participants had to say whether lines on a screen matched in their orientation or not (i.e., is //\ the same as \\\?). If people with dyslexia had gross visual deficits, the groups would be different on this task. Second, they were asked whether the pattern of cases of letters matched (Is bbBB the same as ccCC?). This task tapped into simple letter recognition. In the third task participants were asked whether two letters rhymed (i.e., T and V); this begins to tap into phonological processing. The fourth task required the participants to say whether nonsense words rhymed ("leat" vs. "jete"); this requires substantial phonological processing. Finally, the participants had to say whether two words (i.e., "car" and "truck") belonged to the same category; this stressed the semantic aspects of language. During the line-orientation tasks, the groups were not different in either performance or brain activation. As the tasks became more language oriented, the controls activated more of their left hemispheres, particularly the temporal lobe and angular gyrus. In contrast, those with dyslexia tended to activate the right hemisphere, and they showed significantly less activation of the temporal and angular gyrus areas than the controls. In contrast, the participants with dyslexia overactivated the inferior frontal lobe, perhaps reflecting the greater effort these individuals had put into the reading task.

English is a difficult language to learn because of its many irregular forms of spelling and verb usage. This has led to speculation that dyslexia is an English-language problem and that dyslexia is not seen in people who speak languages with more straightforward principles. Recently, Eraldo Paulesu and colleagues performed PET studies on people with dyslexia and controls who were of English, French, and Italian nationality. In all three nationalities, regardless of language, those with dyslexia showed significantly decreased left temporal lobe activity when engaging in reading. Thus the brain mechanism of reading and dyslexia appears to be universal. Dyslexia does affect an irregular language such as English or French more adversely, however.

I said earlier that people with dyslexia do not have any gross visual problems, and that was confirmed in the Shaywitz study. Recently, however, it has been shown that people with dyslexia may have some subtle visual deficits. There are two pathways from the retina to the lateral geniculate ganglion, which is a way station for visual information en route to the visual cortex. The parvocellular pathway appears to be important for processing visual stimuli that are stationary or highly contrasted by bright light. The other pathway, the magnocellular, processes visual information that is moving and is less concerned with the precise shape and location of the object. Individuals with dyslexia have difficulty detecting moving stimuli, even when they are nonverbal in nature. When they are performing tasks that require the detection of such stimuli, fMRI shows less activity in the magnocellular pathway relative to controls. Recall that Paula Tallal found that children with language impairments had trouble perceiving sounds when the nature of the sound was changing rapidly. In reading, the words do not appear to be moving, but, in fact, they are. As you read this, the book and your head are fixed, but your eyes are scanning back and forth across the page. The image of the letters and words on your retina is changing very rapidly. Perhaps a common defect in both reading and language disorders is that the left hemisphere cannot do its job of processing rapidly changing information. It would be intriguing if a gene related to dyslexia turned out to govern this central cognitive function.

At present, treatment of reading and language disorders focuses on direct remediation of the deficits in phonological processing. Techniques such as that developed by Tallal are promising, but most children with dyslexia receive intensive tutoring in phonics. No medication has been found that is helpful for dyslexia; stimulant medication is helpful only if a child has comorbid ADHD.

NONVERBAL LEARNING DISABILITIES

Of the right-hemisphere impairments, only mathematics disorder is currently in DSM-IV. The term "nonverbal learning disability" (NVLD) was developed by the Canadian neuropsychologist Byron Rourke to describe the set of deficits shown in Table 12.1. Mathematics disorder is a less well-researched category. It is thought to affect about 5% of the school-age population and, like reading disorder, it shows greater concordance in MZ twins relative to DZ twins. There is, however, a much greater variability in mathematical ability than in reading ability in the general population. In a typical middle-class suburban high school, almost all of the seniors will be reading at same level, but their math abilities will range from those who barely scraped through algebra to those who have already taken college calculus. Reading and mathematic problems often co-occur, but there are subtle differences between people with dyslexia who have problems with mathematics and those who have a pure mathematics disorder. People with dyslexia, obviously, cannot do word problems, and they also have difficulty memorizing and retrieving math facts (such as times tables). Persons with mathematics disorder, as shown in Table 13.1, fail to grasp basic mathematical concepts. Although they count well and learn their math facts, they have a poor sense of numbers and have difficulty understanding the concept of place. For instance, when we add 5 + 4, we automatically come up with an answer of 9. A young child may count sequentially on his fingers to get the answer. In contrast, if we must add 18 + 9, we shift to a more complex strategy. We recognize that the order of the numbers 1 and 8 is symbolic, the 1 representing 10s and the 8 representing units. In working memory, we add 9 + 8 to yield 17, place the 7 in the units column, and "carry" the one (i.e., 10) to the 10s column and add it to the 1 (10s) to yield the correct answer of 27. Watch a class of second graders trying to master this process, and you realize how complex it really is. A child with a mathematics disorder has trouble with the visual–spatial nature of multiple-digit numbers. He may, by counting, add 8 and 9 to get 17 and simply write 17 beneath the problem and then bring down the one to yield 117. When asked if 8 and 9 could add up to 117, he may reply "yes," showing his poor number sense. If an older child with mathematics disorder is given a problem such as, "Joe must travel 100 miles to New York. His car will travel 50 miles an hour. How long will it take to get there?" she simply cannot conceptualize the operations needed to solve it. Algebra and geometry are incomprehensible. What brain mechanisms have gone wrong?

Functional imaging studies have been performed showing that different areas of the brain are involved in rote arithmetic and complex mathematical processes. Examination of stroke patients over many years have shown that lesions to the left inferior parietal lobule may leave the patient without the ability to perform simple math calculations such as 2 + 2 = 4. Although such patients are unable to do simple math, they are often able to recognize as incorrect grossly inaccurate math results such as 2 + 1 = 18. Stanislas Dehanene and Laurent Cohen proposed that both the left and right interior parietal lobes are involved in processing numbers. If an arithmetic problem simply involves recalling a math fact or applying simple mathematical operations, the left parietal area is involved, and it interacts with the language areas. In contrast, bilateral inferior parietal activation occurs when mathematical reasoning is involved. When normal participants are asked to simply guess which answer is closest to being correct (Is 4 + 4 = 9 or 1?), bilateral activation of the inferior parietal is seen. Thus we see that number sense is dependent on the right hemisphere, which encodes numbers in a nonverbal format. Take the words "too" and "two," which sound identical. The left hemisphere takes the word "two" and matches to its verbal meaning, that is, the number 2. The left hemisphere also processes the rule that 2 + 1 = 3. But when it comes to the concept that the symbol 2 means two objects (#, #), the right hemisphere becomes involved.

As discussed in Chapter 7, the right parietal lobe is involved in a wide range of visual–spatial functions: geographical awareness, right–left discrimination, imaging objects in three dimensions, and time perception (understanding the relationship between the "big hand" and the "little hand" of the clock), among others. Interpretation of facial expression is a visual–spatial function. We instinctively observe the position of the eyes, eyebrows, and shape of the mouth; these images are instantly integrated to tell us that the person is sad, happy, irritated, or furious. We are capable of receiving and sending hundreds of emotional messages via our faces. If someone looks sad but tells us he is not, we are unconvinced; the nonverbal signs override the verbal ones. Byron Rourke studied a sample of children who performed well on tests of reading and spelling but did very poorly (relative to their full-scale IQs) on measures of arithmetic. Many of these children showed a range of deficits beyond math problems: poor motor coordination; social skills problems; flat, nonprosodic voices, and poor tactile discrimination, particularly on the left side of the body. They had problems with controlling their affect and mood, reporting a nonspecific depression not tied to any specific life event. Rourke followed up 8 of these children into adulthood; all showed poor employment and emotional adjustment, and some had developed schizophrenia. As Table 13.1 shows, at times nonverbal skills can be so impaired that social skills break down completely, possibly resulting in Asperger's syndrome.

At present there is no specific treatment for NVLD; remedial educational techniques are not so well developed as with dyslexia. Affective disorders that present with NVLD are treated with antidepressants in the usual fashion. Psychotherapists need to be aware of NVLD. Because these patients are verbal, they appear quite appropriate for psychotherapy at first, but they have trouble establishing a relationship with the therapist or dealing with abstract concepts. Insight is difficult to achieve. If there is a history of poor school performance despite good verbal skills, poor eye contact, or significant social awkwardness that does not respond to therapy, an NVLD should be considered and psychological testing done.

DEMENTIA

Decline of cognition in adulthood (dementia) may be either degenerative or nondegenerative. The nondegenerative dementias are caused by diverse medical etiologies: infection, chronic alcohol abuse, strokes, and autoimmune diseases (such as lupus). Degenerative dementia represents a process that causes the death of neurons that are intrinsic to the CNS. Alzheimer's disease (AD) is the most common and best known of these. As the population ages, the number of cases of AD will surely increase. Costs of nursing homes for people with AD are often a cause of personal bankruptcy and depletions of estates. Medicaid ends up paying these costs, and such end-of-life care represents a substantial portion of the health care budget. The hippocampus, one of the structures critical to memory, is most often the first structure to be affected. It undergoes marked atrophy. Mony De Leon and colleagues studied the hippocampus in a large number of elderly participants ages 65–90. They consisted of normal controls, persons with mild cognitive impairment, and two groups with mild and moderately severe AD. Data were analyzed by age group. At age 65, only 29% of normal controls showed hippocampal atrophy compared with 78% of those with mild cognitive impairment and 84% and 96% of those with mild and moderate AD, respectively. On microscopic examination of the brain, neurofibrillary tangles (found by Alzheimer himself) are the diagnostic feature of AD. These fibers are inside the neuron; they surround the nucleus and extend toward the dendrites. These are found first in the hippocampus, but they spread throughout the neocortex as the disease progresses. Once a neuron has died, the tangle may be left behind in the extracellular space. It is not clear where the neurofibrillary tangles come from. They appear to contain the same material as the microtubules, structures that normally transport substances throughout the neuron. The number of neurofibrillary tangles correlates with the severity of the dementia. Senile plaques, consisting of deposits of the protein amyloid-β peptide, are also seen in AD, although the correlation of these plaques with cognitive impairment is less strong than for the neurofibrillary tangles.

Substantial progress has been made in the molecular biology of AD. The gene for the amyloid precursor protein (APP) is found on chromosome 21. This is of interest because people with Down syndrome (who have an extra chromosome 21) are more vulnerable to AD. Ten different mutations in the APP gene have been linked to AD, although it accounts for only 2–3% of the cases of AD. Although the mutant gene is inherited as an autosomal dominant, how the mutation causes AD is unclear; indeed, the role of normal amyloid in the brain is also unknown. It has been suggested that, whereas the normal amyloid stimulates neuron proliferation and enhances the effects of nerve growth factors, the abnormally long amyloid produces the mutation that causes neuron death. Yury Verlinsky and colleagues reported on a woman who carried one of the APP mutations. She underwent preimplantation genetic diagnosis (PGD). In vitro fertilization was performed; the embryos were screened for the mutation, and healthy embryos were implanted. Thus the children born will not have a risk of early-onset Alzheimer's. This approach will work for single-gene mental disorders, as discussed in Chapter 14, but it will not be applicable to polygenetic disorders.

A small minority (5–10%) of AD cases have very early onset (age 28–60 years). Two genes, presenilin 1 (PS1) and 2 (PS2), found on chromosomes 14 and 1, respectively, have been linked to this early-onset form. Forty different mutations have been found in PS1 that cause early onset AD, whereas only two mutations in PS2 are related to this subtype. Both genes are found on chromosome 14. Interestingly, all the mutations of PS1 and PS2 also increase the production and deposit of amyloid; the mutated presenilins may cause an otherwise normal APP gene to produce the longer amyloid protein.

Apolipoprotein E (ApoE) is an important regulator of fat metabolism. The gene for it is found on chromosome 19. It appears to be linked to the majority of cases of AD. The ApoE gene has several alleles. $\epsilon 3$ is found in 75% of Caucasians, while $\epsilon 4$ and $\epsilon 2$ are found in 15% and 10% of Caucasians, respectively. The $\epsilon 4$ allele conveys a risk for AD; unlike the other genes, it is not an autosomal dominant. A person homozygous for $\epsilon 4$ has a much greater risk for AD (but will not inevitably develop it) than a heterozygote. The $\epsilon 4$ allele is also associated with poor recovery from head injury and poor outcome from elective cardiac bypass surgery. The ε4 allele also plays a role in amyloid deposits. The ApoE formed by the ε4 gene binds a protein called *tau*; this protein is part of the neurofibrillary tangles. This raises the possibility that the ApoE4 causes *tau* to produce the tangles and ultimate neuron death.

Research in AD has focused on neurotransmitter systems as well. The level of the enzyme choline acetyltransferase, which is responsible for the synthesis of acetylcholine, is markedly reduced in AD (38% of the level found in brains of controls). $5\text{-}HT_{2A}$, NMDA, and AMPA receptors are also decreased. Muscarinic receptors are increased in brains of people with AD, possibly representing an up-regulation due to decreased acetylcholine activity. A variety of medications that enhance acetylcholine function have been shown to be modestly effective in improving cognition in patients with AD, but they do not alter the long-term course. Research is focusing on developing drugs that would prevent the neurofibrillary tangles or amyloid deposits from forming. For this task, the discovery of the genetic mechanisms of AD will be invaluable.

REFERENCES

Dahaene, S., & Cohen, L. (1991). Two mental calculation systems: Case study of severe acalculia with preserved approximation. *Neuropsychologia, 29,* 1045–1054.

de Leon, M. J., Bobinski, M., Convit, A., & DeSanti, S. (1999). Neuropathological and neuroimaging studies of the hippocampus in normal aging and in Alzheimer's disease. In D. S. Charney, E. J. Nestler, & B. S. Bunney (Eds.), *Neurobiology of mental illness* (pp. 698–714). New York: Oxford University Press.

Demb, J. B., Boynton, G. M., Best, M., & Heeger, D. J. (1998). Psychophysical evidence for a magnocellular pathway deficit in dyslexia. *Vision Research, 38,* 1555–1559.

Demb, J. B., Boynton, G. M., & Heeger, D. J. (1998). Functional magnetic resonance imaging of early visual pathways in dyslexia. *Journal of Neuroscience, 18,* 6939–6951.

Francis, P. T., & Procter, A. W. (1999). Neurochemistry of dementia. In D. S. Charney, E. J. Nestler, & B. S. Bunney (Eds.), *Neurobiology of mental illness* (pp. 693–697). New York: Oxford University Press.

Gilger, J. W., Pennington, B. F., Harbeck, R. J., DeFries, J. C., Kotzin, B., Green, P., & Smith, S. (1998). A twin and family study of the association between immune system dysfunction and dyslexia using blood serum immunoassay and survey data. *Brain and Cognition, 36,* 310–333.

Grigorenko, E. L., Wood, F. B., Meyer, M. S., Hart, L. A., Speed, W. C., Shuster, A., & Pauls, D. L. (1997). Susceptibility loci for distinct components of developmental dyslexia on chromosomes 6 and 15. *American Journal of Human Genetics, 60,* 27–39.

Grigorenko, E. L., Wood, F. B., Meyer, M. S., & Pauls, D. L. (2000). Chromosome 6p influences on different dyslexia-related cognitive processes: Further confirmation. *American Journal of Human Genetics, 66,* 715–723.

Lai, C. S., Fisher, S. E., Hurst, J. A., Vargha-Khadem, F., & Monaco, A. P. (2001). A forkhead-domain gene is mutated in a severe speech and language disorder. *Nature, 413,* 519–523.

Paulesu, E., Demonet, J. F., Fazio, F., McCrory, E., Chanoine, V., Brunswick, N., et al. (2001). Dyslexia: Cultural diversity and biological unity. *Science, 291,* 2165–2167.

Rourke, B. P. (1989). *Nonverbal learning disabilities: The syndrome and the model.* New York: Guilford Press.

Semrud-Clikeman, M., Hynd, G. W., Novey, E. S., & Eliopulos, D. (1991). Relationship between neurolinguistic measures and brain morphometry in dyslexic, ADHD and normal children. *Learning and Individual Differences, 3,* 225–242.

Semrud-Clikeman, M., Steingard, R., Filipek, P. A., Biederman, J., Bekken, K., & Renshaw, P. F. (2000). Using MRI to examine brain–behavior relationships in males with attention deficit disorder with hyperactivity. *Journal of the American Academy of Child and Adolescent Psychiatry, 39,* 477–484.

Semrud-Clikeman, M., & Teeter, P. A. (1997). *Child neuropsychology: Assessment and interventions for neurodevelopmental disorders.* Boston: Allyn & Bacon.

Shaywitz, S. E., Shaywitz, B. A., Pugh, K. R., Fulbright, R. K., Constable, R. T., Mencl, W. E., et al. (1998). Functional disruption in the organization of the brain for reading in dyslexia. *Proceedings of the National Academy of Sciences USA, 95,* 2636–2641.

Sherrington, R., Hyslop, P. S., Hutton, M., Perez-Tur, J., & Hardy, J. (1999). The molecular biology of Alzheimer's disease. In D. S. Charney, E. J. Nestler, & B. S. Bunney (Eds.), *Neurobiology of mental illness* (pp. 650–658). New York: Oxford University Press.

Skottun, B. C. (1997). The magnocellular deficit theory of dyslexia. *Trends in Neuroscience, 20,* 397–398.

Stanescu-Cosson, R., Pinel, P., van de Moortele, P. F., Le Bihan, D., Cohen, L., & Dehaene, S. (2000). Understanding dissociations in dyscalculia: A brain imaging study of the impact of number size on the cerebral networks for exact and approximate calculation. *Brain, 123,* 2240–2255.

Stein, J., & Walsh, V. (1997). To see but not to read: The magnocellular theory of dyslexia. *Trends in Neuroscience, 20,* 147–152.

Tallal, P., Miller, S. L., Bedi, G., Wang, X., & Nagarajan, S. (1996). Language comprehension in language-learning impaired children improved with acoustically modified speech. *Science, 271,* 81–84.

Toppelberg, C. O., & Shapiro, T. (2000). Language disorders: A 10-year research update. *Journal of the American Academy of Child and Adolescent Psychiatry, 39,* 143–152.

Verlinsky, Y., Rechitsky, S., Verlinsky, O., Masciangelo, C., Lederer, K., & Kuliev, A. (2002). Preimplantation diagnosis for early-onset Alzheimer disease caused by V717L mutation. *Journal of the American Medical Association, 287,* 1018–1021.

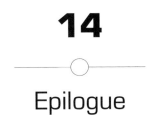

14

Epilogue

I conclude this study of neuroscience with a discussion of ethical and cultural issues that will surely attend its further advancement. Among these issues are the following:

1. What are the implications of the fact that genetics plays a major role in the development of mental disorders?
2. If environmental factors produce lasting changes in the brain and if these changes are linked to mental disorders, how will this affect public policy regarding the prevention of these illnesses?
3. How will advances in neuroscience change the way we treat patients?
4. What are the larger political dimensions of this clinical neuroscience? Does the changing view of mental disorders as diseases of the brain require changes in the way we deliver and fund mental health services? Will there be the "winners" and "losers" in such a realignment?
5. If certain maladaptive behaviors are brain based, how does this affect the principles of informed consent and the "right to refuse treatment"?

GENETICS AND THE FUTURE OF MENTAL HEALTH

Discussion of genetics in mental disorders, particularly in the lay media, conjures up images of Aldous Huxley's *Brave New World*, in which people are bred for their position in society. The great fear among many in

261

our society is that we are on the verge of a new eugenics movement. It is assumed that soon we will find "the gene" for this or that trait or disorder, and then we will move to prohibiting a person who carries "the gene" from having children. Such commentators seem to ignore the array of constitutional protections that would prohibit such actions even if the government would attempt such action. Why would anyone think that democratically elected Western governments, most of whom cannot force their citizens to recycle, could suddenly acquire the power to stop people from reproducing? Nonetheless, totalitarian governments might indeed pursue such a course. The People's Republic of China already enforces a one-child limit that has led to an imbalance in the sex ratio in that country; perhaps if a gene for compliance or acceptance of authority were found (an unlikely possibility), they might try to increase its allele frequency in the population. Others worry not about government coercion but about the effects of parental preference. Would parents find ways to screen embryos for an absence of ADHD, schizophrenic, or autistic genes and implant only the "healthy" embryos?

Such concerns, however, fail to recognize the three central facts about psychiatric genetics that I have emphasized in this book: mental disorders are polygenetic, genes and environment interact, and the genetic risk for mental disorder may also convey positive attributes. If a disorder has 10 to 30 genes that convey its risk, how is one to possibly "pick" an embryo that lacks all the risk genes? It is quite likely that such an embryo would not even be viable. Furthermore, no parent could control the gene-by-environment interactions that would invariably take place. Finally, having a child with no risk for ADHD, bipolar disorder, or schizophrenia might mean getting a child who has no capacity for spontaneity, intensity of feeling, or creativity. Thus widespread genetic engineering is unlikely ever to be pursued, and even if tried it would end because people would see it as ineffective. The greater issue is to protect people not from scientists but from scam artists: Individual practitioners outside the mainstream of science who would claim to be able to produce a genetically perfect child but in fact could do no such thing. We may have far more of a consumer protection issue than a true ethical dilemma.

The genetics of all diseases are studied not to breed a better society but to help the people who have the disease. By knowing what genes convey risk, we can discover which protein the gene ultimately produces. By learning how it is defective, we can develop new and more effective drugs. We will be entering the age of pharmacogenetics, that is, drugs designed for an individual's genotype. In short, we can have our genetic cake and eat it, too. There is no need to breed disease genes out of the population, as that would also remove the benefits they convey. Those unfortunate individuals for whom the genes did combine in an adverse way could be restored to health through our genetic knowledge. Of course, we may discover the genetic causes of a disorder long before we can effect a cure. During that time, people who suspect they are at risk (because of a family history of a disorder) would need to decide for themselves if they wished to be tested to determine if they carry the disease gene. This situation already confronts those with a family history of Huntington's disease, in which children of an affected parent have a 50% chance of developing the illness; genotyping can then tell them if they will or will not get the disease (and die from it) several decades later. Such dilemmas will become common as psychiatric genetics progresses. Naturally, people at genetic risk for any disease should be protected from discrimination, but this can be assured by appropriate legislation.

A great concern to many is that psychiatric genetics will bring a new eugenics, that findings will appear that suggest that ethnic and racial minorities are inferior to the majority group. So great is this concern that the Human Genome Project will not release any data about how persons of different ethnicity differ in terms of their genetic markers. But why do such critics assume that such findings are inevitable? Is not the reverse far more likely? Suppose a group of genes are clearly identified that predispose an individual to impulsive aggression. If these genes are found in all the world's racial and ethnic groups, is this not proof that no one group is more violent or dangerous than another? If the genetic predisposition to violence is proven to be the same for people of African and European ancestry, does this not clearly implicate the environment as the cause of differing crime rates between blacks and whites? Does this not create a moral imperative to correct the situation? One of the hidden benefits of genetic research is that it often ends up pointing the way to an environmental cause for the disorder.

Others worry about scientific fraud or unconscious bias. Could scientists, even without intending it, bias their experiments to "prove" that a disadvantaged minority was inferior? The demand of modern science for independent replication of findings means that bias or fraud cannot remain uncovered for long. Given the international nature of science, it is increasingly difficult to argue that all "white" scientists share the same bias. Today's scientists are not trying to prove racial inequality, so the motivation for fraud does not exist. The scientists of the early 20th century clearly were, and those who promoted the eugenics movement did so by *ignoring the science of their own time*. As early as 1925, Otto Klineberg showed that black children who moved to New York from the poverty of the Old South showed improvement in their IQ scores, and the psychologist Thomas Garth wrote in 1931 that "we have never, with all our searching . . . found indisputable evidence for belief in mental differences that are essentially racial." This should have been apparent to the eugenics advocates, but they proceeded in defiance of science, not because of it. It was a political and not a scientific movement.

ENVIRONMENTAL EFFECTS ON THE BRAIN

We have seen how perinatal complications and child abuse can cause permanent effects on brain functioning and how they can set the stage for schizophrenia, depression, and impulsive aggression. Obviously, our society must do more to ensure healthy pregnancies and deliveries. The brain grows in volume and increases its connectivity until age 5; both good nutrition and environmental stimulation are key to this process. Abuse and neglect can no longer be viewed as noxious psychological forces with limited effects once the abuse is stopped. They can be as deleterious to the brain as environmental toxins or head injury. Aggressive programs to stop child abuse and domestic violence will probably be key to preventing depression, suicide, and their fellow travelers, substance abuse and aggression. Given these effects, we must begin to question policies that delay intervention until the abuse is "severe," or that advocate leaving the child in an abusive home because it is less expensive than foster care. Prevention of child abuse must be aimed at parents when children are infants; abuse and neglect carried on during the critical early years of brain development may induce changes in the brain that will not be easily removed in later years.

THE DISEASE MODEL AND THE TREATMENT
OF MENTAL DISORDERS

For many clinicians, viewing mental disorders as brain diseases is a major paradigm shift. Psychiatry and clinical psychology are comfortable with a "disease model," whereas some other branches of the mental health profession may be less so. What do I mean by a disease model? Simply that mental disorders are no different from cancer or asthma. Asthma is caused by a combination of genetic (reactive airways) and environmental (allergens) factors; depression similarly has genetic and environmental etiological factors. In both diseases, the patient is in a state of poor health and comes to the health care professional (psychiatrist, psychologist, therapist) to get better. Isn't this obvious? For years, however, many in the mental health profession viewed mental illness as anything but a disease. In the 1960s, psychiatrists deemphasized their medical training, and later psychoanalytic writers tried to remove whatever biological leanings they found in Freud's original theory. Mental disorders were portrayed as a journey of self-discovery, a form of giftedness, or a revolutionary statement against an oppressive society. Novels such as *One Flew over the Cuckoo's Nest* and *Girl, Interrupted* portrayed the mentally ill as wiser than the mental health professionals caring for them—if only they could be "freed" from their oppression, they would be just fine.

As the mental health professions return to their scientific roots, it will take great effort to clear the detritus of this era. Mental health professionals have a duty to debunk and help our patients turn away from the "feel-good" nostrums of the "New Age," such as herbal supplements, "neurobiofeedback," or eye-movement training. Being a mental health professional means being a health care professional. We are not philosophers, spiritual guides, or magicians with a bag of tricks. Our goal is to relieve symptoms and to use techniques that have been validated by the scientific method. Many fear that the return to a disease model will mean an overreliance on psychopharmacology, but this need not be so. After all, in treating heart disease or arthritis, the health care field employs a variety of nonpharmacological techniques—diet changes, exercise, physical and occupational therapy. The disease model demands only that psychotherapy be grounded in science, and there is a wealth of data showing that behavior, cognitive, and specific interpersonal therapies are beneficial for a variety of mental disorders. We saw that cognitive behavior therapy for obsessive–compulsive disorder leads to changes in the brain as it reduces symptoms. Other forms of therapy may also alter disturbed brain processes, as well. Thus the neuroscience of mental disorders is likely to enhance rather than diminish psychosocial interventions, but only those which stand up to empirical validation.

NEUROSCIENCE OF MENTAL DISORDERS AND THE POLITICS OF HEALTH CARE

In no arena has straying from a disease model of mental disorders had a more deleterious effect than in the public mental health system. In the 1950s it was clear that the conditions in many state hospitals had deteriorated to an inhumane level, with little treatment being offered. With the introduction of antipsychotic medication and its great benefit, there was an opportunity to upgrade the state hospitals and provide intensive rehabilitative efforts. Sadly, this window of opportunity was lost. The community mental health movement held out the promise that effective treatment would be available locally, allowing patients to live and work at home. Services never materialized, due in large part to an unholy alliance of the left and right wings of American politics. Conservative state legislators saw the community mental health movement as a golden opportunity to shut down expensive state hospitals and off-load patients onto local communities or the federal government (through Medicaid and supplemental security income for the disabled). The left wing, caught up in the idea that mental illness was all psychological or a reaction to poverty, thought that getting patients out of the hospital was all that was needed. Once freed from the "incarceration" of the state hospital, the patient would only need some housing, a welfare check, and a friendly case worker to look after him or her. Thus did the problem of the homeless mentally ill arise in the 1970s and 1980s, and it is still with us today. Because mental disorders were not viewed as "real" diseases by either liberals or conservatives, community mental health systems were low on the public agenda and allowed to fall into the hands of political appointees. Although there are some fine community mental health centers around the country, all too many are run by lay persons far more concerned about who gets the contract for food services than about the quality of the care the patients receive.

Suppose that, over the past three decades, we had addressed the problem of cancer in the same manner in which we have approached mental health. Suppose we had listened to a faction of people who claimed, "Cancer doesn't really exist as a disease; it's the result of social conditions. Chemotherapy for cancer is drugging patients who don't know the side effects and can't make decisions for themselves. It's too expensive to keep cancer patients in hospitals or specialized treatment centers; let's just do all the treatment in a local doctor's office." Would we have made the kind of progress against cancer that we have? Not very likely. Recognizing the brain-based nature of mental disorders allows the mental health professionals to take the moral high ground in the debate about funding mental health treatment. Only when a congressman or state legislator feels as guilty about underfunding mental health treatment as he or she would about cutting funds for cancer research will progress be made. We must make the public understand that when they see a hallucinating homeless man on the street, they should react the same way as if they saw someone collapse and have a seizure. In the latter case, how many people would just walk away?

There are vested interests in the view that mental disorders do not exist or that they are not truly diseases. At one extreme, organizations such as the Church of Scientology attack the mental health profession. Hawkers of herbal products and other unproven treatments have a financial interest in increasing people's fears of psychopharmacology. The extreme left persists in the delusion that mental illness is simply a product of bad social conditions; their efforts to make the delivery of treatment more restrictive (i.e., making it more difficult to commit severely ill patients) places both the public and the patients at risk. The extreme right seeks to decrease both public and private spending on mental health services through budget cuts or managed care, spreading the view that the mentally ill really don't need such care. By explaining the brain-based nature of these disorders, we can begin to redress this situation.

INFORMED CONSENT AND FREE WILL

At what point are people no longer responsible for their behavior? When do they have the right to refuse treatment? The answers to these questions will surely change as we learn more about the neurobiology of mental disorders. The standard for "not guilty by reason of insanity" is quite difficult to meet; even when such a plea is entered, juries are loath to acquit. This is in large part due to the realistic fear that a patient will be released from a psychiatric hospital as soon as he or she is no longer deemed dangerous. Every adult has the right to refuse treatment unless declared incompetent by a court or unless he or she is engaging in behavior acutely dangerous to self or others. In the latter case, a person can be committed to a psychiatric hospital and, in most cases, required to accept treatment. As soon as the acute phase of the illness remits and dangerousness passes, the patient is released; if he or she stops taking medication, the illness may recur, and the cycle starts again.

Is this standard of acute dangerousness for commitment to a hospital outdated? Need we wait until a patient is demented to assign him or her a guardian? Compare the situation to tuberculosis (TB). In most states, persons who are infected with TB are required to receive treatment, even against their wills. Although almost all are treated as outpatients, some patients can be ordered to a sanatorium in order to be certain that they take their medication. This condition would include mildly ill patients who are not in acute danger, because TB's contagious nature puts the whole community at risk, even though many people can be exposed to TB and not develop the disease. We do not see an army of libertarians seeking to free "victims" of "forced antibiotic treatment." Why do we have a stricter standard for infectious disease than for mental disease?

Brain diseases often rob people of their insight. Yet we are as a society rightly reluctant to take away their right to decide for themselves. The time has come, however, to ask ourselves if by allowing people to go untreated we in fact take away their dignity, their productivity, and their attachments to others. With advances in genetics and neuroimaging, we should, in the future, be able to make diagnoses and prescribe treatment with much greater accuracy than we can today. For instance, if medications can stop a person from craving alcohol or illegal drugs, should he or she not be required to take them, just as the person with TB must take an antibiotic? Should we not stop the spread of both TB and drunk driving? We will, however, have to define a standard to govern when a person must be required to participate in treatment. A general theme might be that a treatment should be mandatory if it will prevent long-term deterioration (not just acute dangerousness) or if it will stop behaviors that adversely affect the health of an individual's family, particularly if the mental disorder impairs an individual's ability to be a parent.

What about personal responsibility? Suppose a violent patient is found to have dysfunctional frontal lobes and to carry genes that are linked to severe impulsivity. He or she is not psychotic, knows right from wrong, but finds it impossible to conform his or her behavior to the basic norms of society. Is the person responsible? There is no easy answer to this question, but we should begin to think about it, because such situations may soon be on us. Some might want to ban all such research because of the implications, but that would be a tragedy. We would lose our opportunity to understand and prevent violence, as well as to treat many violent patients. Still, if we decide that a person is biologically incapable of controlling his or her violent impulses, it would not be humane to jail that individual. Conversely, the individual could not be left to fend for him- or herself; some sort of long-term residential placement would be needed until a definitive treatment could be found. Conceptually, it would be no different from placing a person with Alzheimer's disease in an assisted living facility.

The immediate response of many is that government would use such power to confine dissidents or people who are just "different." Society could define, in legislation, the dysfunctional and harmful behaviors (violence, addiction) that would trigger the restrictions and mandatory treatment. It could be done with the supervision of a court and all required due process. Would there really be a danger of an oppressive society in such a state of affairs? If one studies the lives of great revolutionaries, those who truly confronted tyranny (Gandhi, Martin Luther King, Jr., Nelson Mandela), one does not find a history of impulsiveness or violence but an early life marked by reflection, deep attachments to others, and thoughtfulness. The violent, impulsive individual fills the ranks of the storm trooper, the suicide bomber, and those who perpetrate genocide. The tyrant depends on them. I am not suggesting that treatment of these impulsive violent people will end genocide or war, merely that changing their behavior will be a small step toward a better society, not a more intolerant one.

FINAL WORDS

In the 1850s a physician in a general practice must have felt very limited in what he could do for his patients. Infectious diseases raged, surgery was primitive and often unsuccessful—often his task was limited to comforting the dying. Yet within a number of decades great advances awaited. The germ theory, anesthesia, improved hygiene, all would soon revolutionize medical practice. At the beginning of the 21st century, we stand in the same place with regard to mental disorders. Our knowledge of the cause of these afflictions is growing, our medication and treatments are becoming more sophisticated, and with the proper resolve our generation of mental health professionals may see the greatest advances against mental illness since Pinel released the patients of Bicêtre from their chains. The chains we release will be those of the mind.

Index